ACCESS TO SURGER
500 SINGLE BEST ANSWER

C AND

TOMY

sTest

to your success

To my son, Roheen, who makes it all worthwhile.

ACCESS TO SURGERY: 500 SINGLE BEST ANSWER QUESTIONS IN BASIC AND APPLIED ANATOMY

Shahzad G. Raja

BSc, MBBS, MRCS

Specialist Registrar in Cardiothoracic Surgery

Department of Cardiothoracic Surgery

Western Infirmary

Glasgow

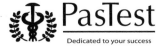

Dedicated to your success

© 2007 PASTEST LTD

Egerton Court
Parkgate Estate
Knutsford
Cheshire
WA16 8DX

Telephone: 01565 752000

First published 2007

ISBN: 1905635273

ISBN: 9781905635276

A catalogue record for this book is available from the British Library.

The information contained within this book was obtained by the author from reliable sources. However, while every effort has been made to ensure its accuracy, no responsibility for loss, damage or injury occasioned to any person acting or refraining from action as a result of information contained herein can be accepted by the publishers or author.

PasTest Revision Books and Intensive Courses

PasTest has been established in the field of postgraduate medical education since 1972, providing revision books and intensive study courses for doctors preparing for their professional examinations.

Books and courses are available for the following specialties:

MRCGP, MRCP Parts 1 and 2, MRCPCH Parts 1 and 2, MRCPsych, MRCS, MRCOG Parts 1 and 2, DRCOG, DCH, FRCA, PLAB Parts 1 and 2.

For further details contact:

PasTest, Freepost, Knutsford, Cheshire WA16 7BR

Tel: 01565 752000   Fax: 01565 650264

www.pastest.co.uk   enquiries@pastest.co.uk

Text prepared by Carnegie Book Production, Lancaster, UK

Printed and bound in the UK by Athenaeum Press, Gateshead

CONTENTS

ABOUT THE AUTHOR

Shahzad G. Raja BSc MBBS MRCS (Ed), passed the MRCS from the Royal College of Surgeons of Edinburgh in 2001. He is currently in the final year of specialist training in Cardiothoracic Surgery in Glasgow. He has been published in peer-reviewed medical journals. His interests lie in medical writing, undergraduate teaching and medical education.

PREFACE

Recent reforms in medical education in the United Kingdom have prompted replacement of multiple choice questions (MCQs) with single best answer questions: *Access to Surgery: 500 Single Best Answer Questions in Basic & Applied Anatomy* is the first book of its kind and provides 500 practice single best answer questions in basic and applied anatomy for candidates taking the surgical examinations. The book has primarily been written for surgical trainees with an emphasis mainly on surgical aspects of human anatomy. However, it can be used as a practice tool by undergraduate medical students as well as trainees in other medical disciplines (for whom anatomy can be a major examination hurdle).

Each question has been carefully formulated to cover a given topic in anatomy. All major aspects of anatomy are dealt with, being organised in a regional manner in nine sections under the headings: Upper Limb and Breast, Lower Limb, Thorax, Abdomen, Pelvis, Head and Neck, Brain and Cranial Nerves, Back and Spinal Cord, and Developmental Anatomy. The questions also cover the complete MRCS applied anatomy syllabus and are expected to be useful for the specialty FRCS candidates as well. This book contains a substantial number of patient-based questions or clinical vignettes that will enable prospective candidates to test their ability to integrate key basic anatomical concepts with relevant clinical problems. In addition, factual recall questions have also been included that probe for basic recall of facts. Detailed and comprehensive explanations, rather than just brief answers to questions have been provided so that candidates do not have to consult textbooks for clarification as is the case with most other MCQ books.

The questions in this book can be used in a number of ways: (i) as a diagnostic tool (pretest); (ii) as a guide and focus for further study; and (iii) for self-assessment. The least effective use of these questions is to 'study' them by reading them one at a time, and then looking at the correct response. These 500 practice questions are intended to be an integral part of a well-planned review as well as an isolated resource. If used appropriately, these questions can provide self-assessment information beyond a numeric score. Furthermore, the questions have been planned in such a way that this book can be used as companion to any textbook of anatomy.

I am hopeful that this book will prove a useful revision and self-assessment tool for all those involved in learning anatomy.

Shahzad G. Raja

2007

QUESTIONS

SECTION 1:
UPPER LIMB AND BREAST – QUESTIONS

For each question given below choose the ONE BEST option.

1.1 **While performing a radical mastectomy, the surgeon injured the long thoracic nerve. Which of the following muscles will be affected due to injury to the long thoracic nerve?**

- ○ A Anterior scalene
- ○ B Middle scalene
- ○ C Serratus anterior
- ○ D Subscapularis
- ○ E Teres major

1.2 **A motorcyclist involved in a hit-and-run accident was thrown from his motorcycle. He landed on the right side of his head and the tip of his shoulder, bending his head sharply to the left and stretching the right side of his neck. Subsequent neurological examination revealed that the roots of the fifth and sixth cervical nerves had been torn away from the spinal cord. What part of the upper limb will have diminished cutaneous sensations in this patient?**

- ○ A The back of the shoulder
- ○ B The top of the shoulder and the lateral side of the arm
- ○ C The pectoral region
- ○ D The medial side of the arm and forearm
- ○ E The tip of the little finger

3

1.3   A 75-year-old woman fell and fractured the olecranon process of her right ulna. The line of fracture passed through the superior surface and disrupted the attachment of a muscle. Which of the following muscles is most likely affected?

○   A   Brachialis
○   B   Flexor digitorum profundus
○   C   Flexor pollicis longus
○   D   Pronator teres
○   E   Triceps brachii

1.4   A motorcyclist fell from his bike. On arrival in A&E it was noticed that extension of his right humerus was severely limited. He has sustained injury to the:

○   A   Long thoracic nerve
○   B   Medial pectoral nerve
○   C   Suprascapular nerve
○   D   Thoracodorsal nerve
○   E   Upper subscapular nerve

1.5   A young boy fell from his skateboard, twisted his forearm and sprained his annular ligament. The annular ligament in the forearm:

○   A   Encircles the head of the radius
○   B   Encircles the head of the ulna
○   C   Encircles the styloid process of the radius
○   D   Goes from the olecranon fossa to the olecranon process
○   E   Spans the space between the ulna and radius

1.6 **Branches of the brachial artery contribute to the anastomotic circulation around the:**

○ A Acromioclavicular joint
○ B Elbow joint
○ C Glenohumeral joint
○ D Head of the humerus
○ E Scapula

1.7 **A rugby player sustained injury to his right supraspinatus muscle. Injury to the supraspinatus muscle will affect:**

○ A Adduction of the humerus
○ B Abduction of the humerus above the horizontal plane
○ C Lateral rotation of the humerus
○ D Initiation of abduction of the humerus
○ E Superior rotation of the scapula

1.8 **While performing mastectomy, the surgeon injured the lateral thoracic artery. The lateral thoracic artery:**

○ A Is a branch of the subclavian artery
○ B Is a branch of the brachial artery
○ C Accompanies the long thoracic nerve to the serratus anterior muscle
○ D Accompanies the thoracodorsal nerve to the serratus anterior muscle
○ E Emerges through the triangular space

upper limb

5

1.9 **A young gymnast sustained injury to a muscle that acts to depress the glenoid fossa directly. Which of the following is a muscle that acts to depress the glenoid fossa directly?**

○   A   Pectoralis minor

○   B   Serratus anterior

○   C   Pectoralis major

○   D   Latissimus dorsi

○   E   Supraspinatus

1.10 **The common flexor tendon of the forearm was avulsed from its attachment. Which of the following muscles originates from the common flexor tendon of the forearm?**

○   A   Flexor digitorum superficialis

○   B   Flexor digitorum profundus

○   C   Flexor pollicis longus

○   D   Pronator quadratus

○   E   Extensor carpi ulnaris

1.11 **Which of the following muscle combinations will work together to abduct the wrist?**

○   A   Pronator teres and brachioradialis

○   B   Palmaris longus and extensor digitorum

○   C   Extensor carpi radialis brevis and flexor carpi radialis

○   D   Extensor carpi radialis brevis and extensor carpi ulnaris

○   E   Supinator and extensor pollicis longus

1.12 Which of the following statements regarding adduction of the digits of the hand is CORRECT?

- A   The palmar interosseous muscles are the sole adductors of the digits
- B   The lumbrical muscles produce adduction of the digits
- C   There are two muscles that produce adduction of the thumb
- D   All of the adductors of the digits take at least part of their attachments from metacarpal bones
- E   Adduction of the digits will be affected by carpal tunnel syndrome

1.13 A victim of a road traffic accident has a severed nerve in her right upper limb resulting in loss of adduction of all the digits of the right hand. Which nerve controls adduction of all the digits of the hand?

- A   Ulnar nerve
- B   Median nerve
- C   Radial nerve
- D   Upper subscapular nerve
- E   Musculocutaneous nerve

1.14 During surgery to remove a lump from the axilla, a nerve originating from the lateral cord of the brachial plexus was injured. Which of the following nerves originates from the lateral cord of the brachial plexus?

- A   Ulnar
- B   Medial pectoral
- C   Suprascapular
- D   Lateral pectoral
- E   Thoracodorsal

upper limb

1.15 **A rugby player sustained spinal cord injury at spinal level C8. What is likely to be seen in this patient?**

○ A The brachialis muscle will be paralysed

○ B The muscles innervated by the radial nerve that would most likely be affected would be the most proximal ones

○ C The hypothenar muscles would be completely paralysed

○ D Innervation to the deltoid muscle would be affected

○ E The patient would be unable to flex their humerus

1.16 **The intertubercular groove of the humerus contains the:**

○ A Tendon of the pectoralis minor muscle

○ B Tendon of the long head of the triceps brachii muscle

○ C Tendon of the coracobrachialis muscle

○ D Tendon of the short head of the biceps brachii muscle

○ E Tendon of the long head of the biceps brachii muscle

1.17 **A young man presented in A&E following a street fight with profuse bleeding from the superior ulnar collateral artery. The superior ulnar collateral artery is a direct branch of which artery?**

○ A Ulnar

○ B Radial

○ C Brachial

○ D Profunda brachii

○ E Axillary

1.18 The primary ventral rami of the brachial plexus (rami = roots):

○ A Emerge from between the middle and posterior scalene muscles

○ B Are formed from spinal levels C7 to T3

○ C Do not give rise to any nerves directly

○ D Form the trunks of the brachial plexus

○ E Combine to form the cords of the brachial plexus

1.19 The muscle producing the main movement of the proximal radioulnar joint was paralysed following a stab wound to the cubital fossa. Which of the following muscles produces the main movement of the proximal radioulnar joint?

○ A Extensor carpi ulnaris

○ B Pronator teres

○ C Triceps brachii

○ D Brachioradialis

○ E Brachialis

1.20 Which of the following statements is CORRECT regarding the extensor retinaculum of the wrist?

○ A It is a direct extension of the axillary fascia

○ B The median nerve runs deep to it

○ C The tendon of the brachioradialis muscle runs through it

○ D It contains a compartment for the thenar muscles

○ E It prevents the tendons of the posterior compartment of the forearm from 'bowstringing' when the hand is extended at the wrist

upper limb

1.21 **To draw some blood from a patient's median cubital vein you will insert the needle in the:**

○ A Posterior aspect of the knee
○ B Femoral triangle
○ C Dorsal surface of the hand
○ D Anterior aspect of the elbow
○ E Deltopectoral triangle

1.22 **When you rest your elbows on a desk, what bony landmark of the upper limb are you resting on?**

○ A Styloid process of the radius
○ B Deltoid tuberosity of the humerus
○ C Olecranon process of the ulna
○ D Coronoid process of the ulna
○ E Radial tuberosity

1.23 **You examine a patient who has a rotator cuff injury. The rotator cuff comprises of a musculotendinous cuff surrounding the shoulder joint and consists of the supraspinatus, infraspinatus, subscapularis and one other muscle. Which muscle is that?**

○ A Deltoid
○ B Subclavius
○ C Long head of the biceps brachii
○ D Teres minor
○ E Coracobrachialis

1.24 **A patient has a fall on outstretched hand and fractures a bone at the wrist joint with which the distal end of the radius articulates primarily (when the wrist is in the anatomical position). Which bone is fractured?**

○ A Triquetrum
○ B Capitate
○ C Scaphoid
○ D Pisiform
○ E Trapezium

1.25 **What sort of a synovial joint is the elbow?**

○ A Ellipsoid
○ B Hinge
○ C Ball and socket
○ D Plane
○ E Bicondylar

1.26 **A road traffic accident victim injured a nerve, which resulted in loss of action of the muscle inserting on to the crest of the lesser tubercle of the humerus. Which nerve is damaged?**

○ A Radial
○ B Long thoracic
○ C Median
○ D Lower subscapular
○ E Axillary

upper limb

1.27 **A builder fell from a ladder and damaged the nerve that is posterior to the medial epicondyle of the humerus. This would most likely result in loss of:**

○ A Extension of the metacarpophalangeal joints of digits 4 and 5

○ B Flexion in the distal interphalangeal joint of digit 5

○ C Abduction of the thumb (digit 1)

○ D General cutaneous sensation from the skin overlying the thenar eminence

○ E Function of lumbricals 1 and 2

1.28 **A patient sustained damage to a muscle that forms the posterior wall of the axilla along with the scapula, subscapularis muscle and teres major muscle. Which muscle is damaged?**

○ A Latissimus dorsi

○ B Trapezius

○ C Pectoralis major

○ D Serratus anterior

○ E Supraspinatus

1.29 **A patient injured the posterior cord of the brachial plexus after being thrown off the back seat of a speeding motorcycle. The posterior cord of the brachial plexus generally contains nerve fibres from which level(s) of the spinal cord?**

○ A C5 only

○ B C5, C6 and C7

○ C C5, C6, C7, C8 and T1

○ D C7, C8 and T1

○ E C8 and T1

1.30 **A patient has spasm of the latissimus dorsi muscle. An analgesic is injected into the median cubital vein whence it goes into the heart, through the heart and is then distributed systemically. Imagine that the analgesic is flowing to the latissimus dorsi muscle. Identify a correct arterial sequence for the analgesic to reach that muscle, starting at the subclavian artery.**

○ A Subclavian – axillary – subscapular – thoracodorsal

○ B Subclavian – axillary – acromioclavicular – acromial

○ C Subclavian – axillary – supreme thoracic – intercostals

○ D Subclavian – axillary – thyrocervical trunk – suprascapular

○ E Subclavian – costocervical trunk – suprascapular

1.31 **Which of the following statements regarding the suprascapular nerve is CORRECT?**

○ A It courses superior to the suprascapular ligament en route to the supraspinatus muscle

○ B It contains nerve fibres from C5 and C6 spinal cord segments

○ C It innervates the teres minor muscle

○ D It provides cutaneous innervation to the posterolateral surface of the shoulder

○ E It branches from the middle trunk of the brachial plexus

1.32 **A typist complains of severe 'pins and needles' sensations on the dorsum of her left hand, over parts of the thumb and parts of digits 1 and 2. During physical examination, the patient has weakness of wrist dorsiflexion and finger extension. Which nerve is most likely to be injured?**

○ A Ulnar
○ B Radial
○ C Musculocutaneous
○ D Axillary
○ E Median

1.33 **A patient fractured the medial epicondyle of the humerus, resulting in laceration of an artery that courses posterior to the medial epicondyle of the humerus, with the ulnar nerve. Which artery is lacerated?**

○ A Superior ulnar collateral
○ B Anterior ulnar recurrent
○ C Radial collateral
○ D Middle collateral
○ E Interosseous recurrent

1.34 **The quadrangular space of the shoulder is an anatomical region bounded by the teres major and minor muscles, long head of the triceps brachii muscle and surgical neck of the humerus. The space contains the axillary nerve and the:**

○ A Circumflex scapular artery
○ B Radial nerve
○ C Posterior circumflex humeral artery
○ D Deep artery of the arm
○ E Thoracodorsal nerve

1.35 **A patient sustained a fracture of the humerus and injured the nerve that innervates the muscles of the anterior compartment of the arm. Which nerve is injured?**

- ○ A Median
- ○ B Musculocutaneous
- ○ C Radial
- ○ D Ulnar
- ○ E Axillary

1.36 **A patient injured the muscle that is an antagonist (has an opposing action) to the serratus anterior muscle, which is the primary protractor of the scapula. Which muscle is injured?**

- ○ A Levator scapula
- ○ B Rhomboid major
- ○ C Pectoralis minor
- ○ D Supraspinatus
- ○ E Deltoid

1.37 **A 52-year-old woman underwent a radical mastectomy to remove her left breast and all of the axillary lymph nodes on that side due to breast cancer. Postoperatively, the nurse giving her a bath noticed that she had a 'winged scapula' on the left side. This appearance is a result of damage to:**

- ○ A Axillary nerve
- ○ B Musculocutaneous nerve
- ○ C Lower subscapular nerve
- ○ D Medial pectoral nerve
- ○ E Long thoracic nerve

upper limb

1.38 **A young boy fell from his bike and dislocated the proximal radioulnar joint and stretched the annular ligament. This injury will make which movement very painful?**

○ A Elbow flexion

○ B Supination

○ C Elbow extension

○ D Shoulder abduction

○ E Radial deviation of the wrist

1.39 **During a triathlon biking accident, a rider fell and landed with the handlebar of her bike forced upward into her right axilla. Subsequently, while swimming in another triathlon event she found that her right arm tired so badly during the swimming portion that she could barely finish the event. During examination, it was found that movements involving adduction, medial rotation and extension of her arm were particularly weak and affected her swimming stroke. The nerve injured was the:**

○ A Accessory

○ B Dorsal scapular

○ C Lateral pectoral

○ D Medial pectoral

○ E Thoracodorsal

1.40 **After a penetrating wound in the area of the posterior axillary fold, a patient had weakness in extension and adduction of the arm. Which muscle is likely to be involved?**

○ A Latissimus dorsi
○ B Pectoralis major
○ C Levator scapula
○ D Rhomboideus major
○ E Trapezius

1.41 **A 28-year-old man suffered a Monteggia fracture of the elbow joint in a road traffic accident. Following this he is unable to extend the wrist and metacarpophalangeal joints, although the sensations are intact; the damage is most likely to be to the:**

○ A Radial nerve
○ B Median nerve
○ C Ulnar nerve
○ D Anterior interosseous nerve
○ E Posterior interosseous nerve

1.42 **A 42-year-old woman develops atrophy of the thenar eminence, but the sensation over it is intact; the damage is most likely to be to the:**

○ A Median nerve
○ B Ulnar nerve
○ C Radial nerve
○ D Musculocutaneus nerve
○ E Axillary nerve

upper limb

1.43 During a street fight a 25-year-old man suffered a blow over his right arm. Following that blow, he noticed some weakness in flexion of the elbow and supination of the arm. Which of the following nerves is most likely to be injured?

A Median

B Ulnar

C Radial

D Musculocutaneus

E Axillary

1.44 A rugby player sustained a right brachial plexus injury as a result of a rough tackle. Neurological assessment by the team doctor revealed that: (i) the diaphragm functions normally; (ii) there is no winging of the scapula; (iii) abduction cannot be initiated, but if the arm is helped through the first 45° of abduction, the patient can fully abduct the arm. From this amount of information and your knowledge of the formation of the brachial plexus, where would you expect the injury to be?

A Axillary nerve

B Posterior cord

C Roots of the plexus

D Superior trunk

E Suprascapular nerve

1.45 A young boy on a skateboard going downhill on a steep road at a high speed hit a large stone in the road, lost control and was thrown from his skateboard. He landed on the right side of his head and the tip of his shoulder, bending his head sharply to the left and stretching the right side of his neck. Subsequent neurological examination revealed that the roots of the fifth and sixth cervical nerves had been torn away from the spinal cord. Following the above injury, which of the movements of the arm at the shoulder would you expect to be totally lost?

◯　A　Adduction
◯　B　Abduction
◯　C　Flexion
◯　D　Extension
◯　E　Medial rotation

1.46 A 56-year-old man was found to have a squamous-cell carcinoma on the right forearm. He also had enlarged axillary lymph nodes on the same side. Following excision of the tumour from the forearm, all axillary lymph nodes lateral to the medial edge of the pectoralis minor muscle were removed. Which axillary lymph nodes would not be removed by this procedure?

◯　A　Apical
◯　B　Central
◯　C　Lateral
◯　D　Pectoral
◯　E　Subscapular

19

1.47 During a freak accident a medical student lacerates the anterior surface of his wrist at the junction of the wrist and hand with a piece of broken beer bottle. Examination reveals no loss of hand function, but the skin on the thumb side of his palm is numb. Branches of which of the following nerves must have been severed?

- A Lateral antebrachial cutaneous
- B Medial antebrachial cutaneous
- C Median
- D Radial
- E Ulnar

1.48 A front-seat passenger sustained a fracture of the surgical neck of humerus as a result of hitting the dashboard with his right shoulder during a high-speed head-on-collision. Which artery may be injured as result of this fracture?

- A Subscapular
- B Posterior humeral circumflex
- C Radial recurrent
- D Deep brachial
- E Circumflex scapular

1.49 Following a tough fight in the ring, a wrestler complained of pain in his shoulder when he brought his left forearm and hand behind his back while dressing. It was determined that the pain was caused by stretching of the lateral rotators of his arm during this motion. Which muscle was most likely to be involved?

- A Infraspinatus
- B Latissimus dorsi
- C Subscapularis
- D Supraspinatus
- E Teres major

1.50 An SHO punctures the skin on the medial side of her wrist with a contaminated needle. A few days later an infection is seen spreading up the medial side of her arm along the large cutaneous vein extending from the dorsum of her hand to the medial side of her arm. The vein involved is the:

- A Basilic
- B Brachial
- C Cephalic
- D Median cubital
- E Ulnar

1.51 During a bar fight a 26-year-old man suffered injury to his right axilla with profuse bleeding from an artery. He was rushed to A&E where on exploration it was discovered that a branch from the third part of axillary artery was transected. Which of the following arteries was most likely to be injured?

- A Anterior humeral circumflex
- B Lateral thoracic
- C Subscapular
- D Superior thoracic
- E Thoracoacromial

1.52 A glazier suffered a cut to his right thumb, which resulted in transection of the arteria princeps pollicis. The transected artery is a branch of the:

- A Brachial artery
- B Deep palmar arch
- C Radial artery
- D Superficial palmar arch
- E Ulnar artery

upper limb

1.53 A 25-year-old man sustained a cut just below the elbow in a street fight. The cut was muscle-deep and transected an artery which lies on the supinator muscle immediately below the elbow. Which of the following vessels was most likely to be injured?

- O A Anterior ulnar recurrent artery
- O B Common interosseous artery
- O C Dorsal carpal artery
- O D Posterior ulnar recurrent artery
- O E Radial recurrent artery

1.54 A 78-year-old woman had a fall and fractured a carpal bone in the distal row. Which of the following bones was most likely fractured?

- O A Lunate
- O B Pisiform
- O C Scaphoid
- O D Triquetral
- O E Trapezium

1.55 A 79-year-old woman fell and fractured a carpal bone that articulates with pisiform. Which of the following bones was most likely fractured?

- O A Capitate
- O B Lunate
- O C Triquetral
- O D Trapezium
- O E Trapezoid

SECTION 2:
LOWER LIMB – QUESTIONS

For each question given below choose the ONE BEST option.

2.1 **During a third-time redo mitral valve replacement, the surgeon decided to cannulate the femoral vessels in the groin before opening the chest. To expose the femoral vessels he divided the femoral sheath. Which of the following statements about the femoral sheath is true?**

○   A   The femoral sheath is formed by a prolongation downward of the pelvic fasciae

○   B   The femoral sheath invests the femoral vessels throughout their entire course

○   C   The femoral sheath has two compartments

○   D   The lateral compartment of the femoral sheath contains the femoral vein

○   E   The medial compartment is called the femoral canal

2.2 **A 45-year-old man was seen in surgical outpatients with varicosities in the territory of the left-sided small saphenous vein. The small saphenous vein:**

○   A   Begins anterior to the lateral malleolus as a continuation of the lateral marginal vein

○   B   Is accompanied by the saphenous nerve throughout its course

○   C   Ends in the great saphenous vein

○   D   Has nine to twelve valves

○   E   Is in close relation with the sural nerve in the upper two-thirds of the leg

2.3 **A 63-year-old man fractured his left fibula following a hit-and-run accident. On arrival in A&E he had significant bruising around the head of fibula. Clinical examination revealed loss of flexion of the foot at the ankle joint and weak extension of the phalanges. There was also impaired inversion and eversion of the foot. X-rays revealed a transverse fracture of the upper end of the fibula. Which of the following nerves is most likely to be injured in this patient?**

- A Tibial
- B Femoral
- C Deep peroneal
- D Superficial peroneal
- E Medial plantar

2.4 **A stab wound to the left thigh injured the superficial vein that terminates in the femoral vein within the femoral sheath. The injured superficial vein is the:**

- A Lesser saphenous
- B Sural
- C Obturator
- D Great saphenous
- E Tibial

2.5 **Injury at which spinal levels will affect the lateral femoral cutaneous nerve?**

- A L1, L2
- B L2, L3
- C L3, L4
- D L4, L5
- E L5, S1

2.6 **A patient has paralysis of the quadriceps femoris muscle. Which of the following movements will be affected in this patient?**

O   A   Extension of the leg
O   B   Flexion of the leg
O   C   Flexion of the thigh
O   D   Adduction of the thigh
O   E   Abduction of the thigh

2.7 **A young man was stabbed on the lateral aspect of the knee. Identify the correct superficial-to-deep sequence of structures traversed by the knife:**

O   A   Skin, tibial collateral ligament, lateral meniscus
O   B   Skin, fibular collateral ligament, popliteus muscle tendon, lateral meniscus
O   C   Skin, popliteus muscle tendon, tibial collateral ligament, lateral meniscus
O   D   Skin, popliteus tendon, fibular collateral ligament, lateral meniscus
O   E   Skin, anterior cruciate ligament, popliteus muscle tendon

2.8 **The nerve that passes through the obturator foramen:**

O   A   Is the nerve to the obturator internus muscle
O   B   Innervates the anterior compartment of the thigh
O   C   Arises from spinal levels L1 to L2
O   D   Innervates the medial compartment of the thigh
O   E   Contributes to the cutaneous innervation of the gluteal region

lower limb

2.9   **All of the muscles of the superficial posterior compartment of the leg insert onto the:**

○   A   Fibula
○   B   Talus
○   C   Calcaneus
○   D   First metatarsal
○   E   Cuboid

2.10   **The medial and lateral femoral circumflex arteries are usually direct branches of the:**

○   A   Obturator artery
○   B   Popliteal artery
○   C   Profunda femoris artery
○   D   External iliac artery
○   E   First perforating artery

2.11   **The short head of the biceps femoris muscle is innervated by:**

○   A   The common peroneal part of the sciatic nerve
○   B   The same nerve as the pectineus muscle
○   C   The same nerve as the piriformis muscle
○   D   The tibial part of the sciatic nerve
○   E   The same portion of the sciatic nerve as innervates the semitendinosus muscle

2.12   **Fracture of which of the following bones will affect the insertion of peroneus brevis muscle:**

○   A   Calcaneus
○   B   Navicular
○   C   Base of the first metatarsal
○   D   Proximal phalanx
○   E   Base of the fifth metatarsal

2.13 **What will be the result of a complete transection of the inferior gluteal nerve just as it emerges from the greater sciatic foramen?**

○ A The adductor part of the adductor magnus muscle would be affected

○ B Abduction of the thigh would be eliminated

○ C Muscles in the posterior compartment of the leg would be paralysed

○ D Extension of the thigh would be the action most affected

○ E Adduction of the thigh would be eliminated

2.14 **Which of the following statements regarding the obturator internus muscle is CORRECT?**

○ A It emerges from the pelvis through the obturator foramen

○ B It emerges from the pelvis through the lesser sciatic foramen

○ C It emerges from the pelvis through the greater sciatic foramen

○ D It shares innervation with the obturator externus

○ E It adducts the thigh

2.15 **Which of the following statements regarding the common peroneal nerve is CORRECT?**

○ A It gives rise to the nerve that supplies the anterior compartment leg muscles

○ B It branches to supply the intrinsic muscles of the foot

○ C It is closely approximated to the neck of the tibia

○ D It innervates the muscles that plantarflex the foot

○ E While part of the sciatic nerve, it innervates nothing in the posterior thigh

lower limb

2.16 Which of the following muscles acts on two joints?

○ A Vastus medialis
○ B Sartorius
○ C Adductor magnus
○ D Piriformis
○ E Adductor longus

2.17 The inferior gluteal nerve will be spared any deficit if a spinal cord injury occurs at or below the level of:

○ A L4
○ B L5
○ C S1
○ D S2
○ E S3

2.18 Which of the following arteries does not participate in the blood supply of the hip joint?

○ A Medial femoral circumflex
○ B Lateral femoral circumflex
○ C Femoral
○ D Obturator
○ E Pudendal

2.19 The femoral artery is found in which compartment of the femoral sheath?

- A Lateral compartment
- B Intermediate compartment
- C Medial compartment
- D Deep compartment
- E Superficial compartment

2.20 Which of the following structures is found in the anterior fascial compartment of the leg?

- A Superficial peroneal nerve
- B The fibular artery
- C Extensor hallucis muscle
- D Peroneus brevis muscle
- E Flexor digitorum longus muscle

2.21 The sartorius muscle:

- A Is a medial rotator of the thigh
- B Is innervated by the same nerve as the tensor fascia lata
- C Crosses only one joint
- D Lies deep to the adductor longus muscle
- E Will flex the leg at the knee joint

2.22 Which of the following statements is CORRECT regarding the long head of the biceps femoris muscle?

- A It arises from the same point as the gracilis muscle
- B It shares innervation with the gracilis muscle
- C It crosses two joints
- D It will plantarflex the foot at the ankle
- E It will extend the leg at the knee

lower limb

2.23 Which of the following statements regarding the muscles of the posterior compartment of the leg is CORRECT?

O   A   All pass deep to the extensor retinaculum

O   B   All pass deep to the flexor retinaculum

O   C   All of the posterior compartment leg muscles flex the leg

O   D   One of the posterior compartment leg muscles laterally rotates the femur

O   E   All are innervated by the femoral nerve

2.24 The gluteus medius muscle:

O   A   Flexes the thigh at the hip joint

O   B   Extends the thigh at the hip joint

O   C   Attaches to the linea aspera of the femur

O   D   Is supplied by the superior gluteal nerve

O   E   Is completely covered by the gluteus maximus muscle

2.25 A patient complains of deficit in the cutaneous field halfway down the anterior surface of the thigh. This:

O   A   Is due to damage to the sciatic nerve

O   B   Would result from compression of the ventral roots of L5 to S2

O   C   Would result from damage to a nerve accompanying the artery in the adductor canal

O   D   Could be the result of nerve damage during surgical procedures in the femoral sheath

O   E   Would result from damage to the nerve that innervates the pectineus muscle

lower limb

2.26 Innervation to the peroneus brevis muscle:

○ A Could be damaged by a fracture of the tibia

○ B Is by a nerve that is a direct branch of the femoral nerve

○ C Is by a nerve that is accompanied by an artery in the same compartment

○ D Is by the same distal nerve that innervates the peroneus tertius muscle

○ E Could be damaged by a fracture of the neck of the fibula

2.27 The linea aspera:

○ A Is a landmark on the tibia

○ B Is an attachment for the long head of the biceps femoris muscle

○ C Is inferior to the medial epicondyle of the femur

○ D Serves as an attachment for adductors of the thigh

○ E Is found on the inferior pubic ramus

2.28 Which of the following statements about the obturator artery is CORRECT?

○ A It enters the thigh immediately deep to the inguinal ligament

○ B It exits through the greater sciatic foramen

○ C It is a branch of the external iliac artery

○ D Its blood flow would be cut off by ligating the femoral artery

○ E It is found in the medial compartment of the thigh

lower limb

2.29 The first ligament to rupture with a plantar-flexion–inversion ankle sprain is the:

○ A Calcaneofibular ligament
○ B Posterior talofibular ligament
○ C Talotibial ligament
○ D Anterior talofibular ligament
○ E Tibiocalcaneal ligament

2.30 Posterior to the medial malleolus, the order of tendons from medial to lateral (anterior to posterior) is:

○ A Posterior tibial, flexor hallucis longus, flexor digitorum longus
○ B Posterior tibial, flexor digitorum longus, flexor hallucis longus
○ C Flexor hallucis longus, flexor digitorum longus, posterior tibial
○ D Flexor digitorum longus, flexor hallucis longus, posterior tibial
○ E Flexor hallucis longus, posterior tibial, flexor digitorum longus

2.31 What region of the os coxae are you sitting on right now?

○ A Ischial tuberosities
○ B Inferior pubic rami
○ C Ischial spines
○ D Posterior inferior iliac spines
○ E Pectineal line of the pubis

lower limb

2.32 **The semimembranosus muscle is responsible for what movement(s) in the lower extremity?**

○   A   Flexion of the hip and extension of the knee

○   B   Flexion of the hip and flexion of the knee

○   C   Extension of the hip and flexion of the knee

○   D   Extension of the hip and extension of the knee

○   E   Flexion of the hip only

2.33 **Which of the following is the CORRECT statement regarding the posterior compartment of the leg?**

○   A   The muscles plantarflex the foot and are innervated by the tibial nerve

○   B   The muscles dorsiflex the foot and are innervated by the common fibular nerve

○   C   The muscles plantarflex the foot and are innervated by the femoral nerve

○   D   The muscles dorsiflex the foot and are innervated by the tibial nerve

○   E   The muscles dorsiflex the foot and are innervated by the deep fibular nerve

2.34 **Which of the following muscles is attached to the tibial tuberosity?**

○   A   Pectineus

○   B   Vastus intermedius

○   C   Tensor fascia lata

○   D   Short head of the biceps femoris

○   E   Adductor brevis

lower limb

2.35 Following a stab injury a patient has his sciatic nerve cut as it exits the pelvis. Which of the following statements is CORRECT regarding this patient?

○ A Extension of the knee would be eliminated

○ B The long head of the biceps femoris muscle would be affected but not the short head

○ C There would still be cutaneous sensation over the anteromedial surface of the thigh

○ D The muscles in the anterior compartment of the leg would still be functional

○ E The sartorius and gracilis muscles would not be able to contract

2.36 Which artery branches from the deep femoral artery (deep artery of the thigh) and courses between the pectineus and iliopsoas muscles to supply the head and neck of the femur?

○ A Lateral descending femoral circumflex

○ B Medial femoral circumflex

○ C Superficial epigastric

○ D Lateral ascending femoral circumflex

○ E Obturator

2.37 Which of the following arteries predominantly supplies blood to the posterior compartment of the thigh?

○ A Superior gluteal

○ B Obturator

○ C Perforating

○ D Peroneal

○ E Genicular

2.38 **Which of the following arteries is the main source of blood supply to the muscles and tendons in the plantar region of the foot?**

○ A Anterior tibial artery

○ B Fibular artery

○ C Posterior tibial artery

○ D Superior genicular arteries

○ E Popliteal artery

2.39 **The presence of an 'anterior drawer sign' is indicative of damage to the:**

○ A Tibial collateral ligament

○ B Lateral meniscus

○ C Medial meniscus

○ D Posterior cruciate ligament

○ E Anterior cruciate ligament

2.40 **The artery of the round ligament of the head of the femur derives its blood supply via the:**

○ A Obturator artery

○ B Femoral artery

○ C Common iliac artery

○ D Superior gluteal artery

○ E Lateral femoral circumflex artery

2.41 **The popliteal fossa is bounded by the gastrocnemius, semimembranosus, semitendinosus and which other muscle?**

○ A Gracilis

○ B Sartorius

○ C Adductor magnus

○ D Biceps femoris

○ E Soleus

lower limb

2.42 **The lateral compartment of the leg containing the peroneus longus and brevis muscles is innervated by the:**

- O   A   Tibial nerve
- O   B   Common peroneal nerve
- O   C   Superficial peroneal nerve
- O   D   Deep peroneal nerve
- O   E   Sural nerve

2.43 **A footballer fell awkwardly as a result of a rash challenge. He sustained a blow to his left knee and was stretchered off the playing field. On examination of his injured knee the physiotherapist found excessive posterior movement of the tibia on the femur. The chief ligament preventing posterior sliding of the tibia on the femur is the:**

- O   A   Tibial collateral
- O   B   Fibular collateral
- O   C   Oblique popliteal
- O   D   Posterior cruciate
- O   E   Anterior cruciate

2.44 **Infection of which of the following structures will not lead to enlargement of superficial inguinal lymph nodes?**

- O   A   Ampulla of the rectum
- O   B   Lower part of the vagina
- O   C   Lower half of the anal canal
- O   D   Dorsum of the foot
- O   E   Penile urethra

2.45 **An athlete developed acute paronychia involving the big toe of his left foot. Which one of the following groups of lymph nodes is most likely to be inflamed due to this condition?**

O   A Vertical group of superficial inguinal lymph nodes

O   B Medial group of superficial inguinal lymph nodes

O   C Lateral group of superficial inguinal lymph nodes

O   D Deep inguinal lymph nodes

O   E External iliac lymph nodes

2.46 **A 25-year-old man attended A&E following a stab wound to the mid-thigh. On assessment, the wound was found to be involving the subsartorial (adductor) canal. Which of the following structures is most likely to be injured in this case?**

O   A Great saphenous vein

O   B Nerve to sartorius

O   C Nerve to vastus medialis

O   D Obturator nerve

O   E Popliteal artery

2.47 **A 60-year-old man arrived in A&E in cardiogenic shock following a massive anterolateral myocardial infarction. An intra-aortic balloon pump was inserted percutaneously through his left femoral artery. Which of the following statements regarding the femoral artery is CORRECT?**

O   A It is a continuation of the common iliac artery

O   B It lies outside the femoral sheath

O   C It has the femoral nerve lying lateral to it

O   D It can be surface-marked at the midpoint of inguinal ligament

O   E It pierces the adductor longus muscle

lower limb

2.48 A registrar exposes the right saphenofemoral junction for flush-ligation of the saphenofemoral junction to treat the varicosities involving the great saphenous vein. While exposing the saphenofemoral junction, which of the following structures is he most likely to see passing through the saphenous opening?

○ A Genitofemoral nerve

○ B Superficial circumflex iliac artery

○ C Saphenous nerve

○ D Superficial external pudendal artery

○ E Superficial external pudendal vein

2.49 A footballer received an injury to his left ankle in which the stud of the player from the opposite team pierced the skin, subcutaneous tissue and flexor retinaculum of the ankle. Which other structure passing under the retinaculum may be injured?

○ A Tibial nerve

○ B Tibialis anterior

○ C Quadratus plantae

○ D Anterior tibial artery

○ E Plantar arterial arch

2.50 **A patient has returned from the cardiac catheterisation laboratory following a coronary angiogram. The catheter was inserted through his right femoral artery. You advise the nurse looking after him to feel the pulsations of the dorsalis pedis artery in his right lower limb every half-hour for the next 4 hours. The most usual site for feeling the pulsations of the dorsalis pedis artery in the foot is:**

- A Just behind the medial malleolus
- B Just lateral to the tendon of extensor hallucis longus
- C Behind the tendon of fibularis tertius muscle
- D In the second dorsal metatarsal space
- E Just behind the lateral malleolus

2.51 **While walking barefoot on the beach, a 25-year-old woman sustained a deep laceration to the sole of her right foot from a broken beer bottle. There was profuse bleeding which was controlled with a pressure bandage and she was rushed to A&E where it was found that the deep plantar artery was severed. The deep plantar artery is a branch of the:**

- A Anterior tibial artery
- B Dorsalis pedis artery
- C Peroneal artery
- D Popliteal artery
- E Posterior tibial artery

lower limb

2.52 While walking barefoot on the beach, a 25-year-old woman sustained a deep laceration to the sole of her right foot from a broken beer bottle. There was profuse bleeding which was controlled with a pressure bandage and she was rushed to A&E where it was found that the belly of extensor digitorum muscle was lacerated and the lateral tarsal artery was severed. The lateral tarsal artery is a branch of the:

○ A Anterior tibial artery
○ B Dorsalis pedis artery
○ C Peroneal artery
○ D Popliteal artery
○ E Posterior tibial artery

2.53 A 26-year-old man sustained a firearm injury to the fibular side of his left leg, which fractured the fibula and lacerated an artery that is contained in a fibrous canal between the tibialis posterior and the flexor hallucis longus. Which of the following arteries was lacerated?

○ A Anterior tibial
○ B Dorsalis pedis
○ C Peroneal
○ D Popliteal
○ E Posterior tibial

2.54 **A 32-year-old man while cleaning windows fell off a ladder from a height of 2.4 m (8 ft) and landed on his feet. He fractured the tuberosity on the medial surface of his right navicular bone as result of this fall. Which of the following muscles may be affected by this injury?**

○　A　Extensor digitorum brevis

○　B　Flexor hallucis longus

○　C　Popliteus

○　D　Tibialis anterior

○　E　Tibialis posterior

2.55 **A 22-year-old football player fractured a bone in his right foot following a rough tackle. An X-ray of the foot showed the fractured bone to be situated at the medial side of the foot, between the navicular behind and the base of the first metatarsal in front. Which of the following bones was most likely fractured?**

○　A　Calcaneum

○　B　Cuboid

○　C　First cuneiform

○　D　Second cuneiform

○　E　Talus

lower limb

SECTION 3:
THORAX – QUESTIONS

For each question given below choose the ONE BEST option.

3.1 **A 44-year-old man developed chylothorax following trans-hiatal oesophagectomy. The chylothorax was attributed to iatrogenic injury to the thoracic duct. The thoracic duct:**

○ A Is the common trunk of all the lymphatic vessels on the right side of the head, neck and thorax

○ B Varies in length from 38 to 45 cm

○ C Extends from the first sacral vertebra to the root of the neck

○ D Enters the thorax through the vena caval hiatus of the thoracoabdominal diaphragm

○ E Have no valves to ensure free flow of chyle

3.2 **During a surface anatomy exam a second-year medical student was asked to identify the second costal cartilage on the chest of a fellow student. Which of the following structures will be palpated by the student to identify the second costal cartilage?**

○ A Costal margin

○ B Sternal notch

○ C Sternal angle

○ D Sternoclavicular joint

○ E Xiphoid process

3.3 **A 65-year-old man with a left-sided haemothorax following trauma had an X-ray to confirm the presence of blood in the left pleural space. In the erect posture the fluid would tend to accumulate in which part of the pleural space?**

○ A Costodiaphragmatic recess

○ B Costomediastinal recess

○ C Cupola

○ D Hilar reflection

○ E Middle mediastinum

3.4 **A patient with a pleural effusion is to undergo aspiration of fluid from the pleural space. From superficial to deep, identify the correct order of structures the needle must pass before it enters the pleural cavity:**

○ A External intercostals – innermost intercostals – internal intercostals – parietal pleura

○ B External intercostals – internal intercostals – parietal pleura – innermost intercostals

○ C Parietal pleura – innermost intercostals – internal intercostals – external intercostals

○ D External intercostals – internal intercostals – innermost intercostals – parietal pleura

○ E External intercostals – internal intercostals – innermost intercostals – visceral pleura

thorax

3.5 **While removing a mass from the back, the
thoracodorsal nerve (C6–C8) is accidentally
injured. Which muscle is most likely to be
affected?**

○ A Serratus posterior inferior

○ B Serratus anterior

○ C Levator scapulas

○ D Longissimus

○ E Latissimus dorsi

3.6 **A 65-year-old man underwent pulmonary
angiography following a suspected episode of
pulmonary embolism. The pulmonary angiogram
showed that the blood clot had occluded the
apical segmental pulmonary artery that supplies
the superior lobe of left lung. The blood clot
travelled to this segmental pulmonary artery
from a leg vein. Track the appropriate course of
the blood clot to the obstructed artery:**

○ A Inferior vena cava – right atrium – mitral valve – right
ventricle – pulmonary trunk – left pulmonary artery –
left superior lobar artery – left apical segmental artery

○ B Inferior vena cava – left atrium – mitral valve – left
ventricle – pulmonary trunk – left pulmonary artery –
left superior lobar artery – left apical segmental artery

○ C Inferior vena cava – right atrium – tricuspid valve
– right ventricle – pulmonary trunk – left pulmonary
artery – left bronchial artery – left apical segmental
artery

○ D Inferior vena cava – right atrium – tricuspid valve
– right ventricle – pulmonary trunk – left pulmonary
artery – left superior lobar artery – left apical
segmental artery

○ E Coronary sinus – right atrium – tricuspid valve – right
ventricle – pulmonary trunk – left pulmonary artery –
left superior lobar artery – left apical segmental artery

thorax

3.7 **Which of the following statements regarding the venous drainage of the heart is CORRECT?**

○ A The coronary sinus drains into the left atrium

○ B The anterior cardiac veins begin over the anterior surface of the left ventricle, cross over the atrioventricular groove (coronary groove) and directly drain into the left atrium

○ C The great cardiac vein is the largest tributary of the coronary sinus and this vein starts at the apex of the heart and ascends with the anterior ventricular branch of the left coronary artery

○ D The middle and small cardiac veins drain most of the areas supplied by the left coronary artery

○ E The coronary sinus drains into the great cardiac vein

3.8 **A patient presents with a clinically significant atrial septal defect (ASD). The ASD is most likely to be due to incomplete closure of which one of the following structures:**

○ A Foramen ovale

○ B Ligamentum arteriosum

○ C Ductus arteriosus

○ D Sinus venarum

○ E Coronary sinus

3.9 **A patient presents with a right bundle branch block due to blockage in the atrioventricular (AV) nodal artery. Part of the right bundle branch of the AV bundle is carried by which structure?**

○ A Pectinate muscles

○ B Anterior papillary muscle of the left ventricle

○ C Moderator band (septomarginal trabecula)

○ D Crista terminalis

○ E Chordae tendineae

3.10 You are asked to insert a chest drain anteriorly in the second intercostal space. To enter the right space you must correctly identify the second costal cartilage. The second costal cartilage can be located by palpating the:

○ A Costal margin
○ B Sternal angle
○ C Sternal notch
○ D Sternoclavicular joint
○ E Xiphoid process

3.11 After posterolateral thoracotomy surgeons like to infiltrate local anaesthetic both above and below the incision to block the nerves supplying the thoracic wall. The thoracic wall is innervated by the:

○ A Dorsal primary rami
○ B Intercostal nerves
○ C Lateral pectoral nerves
○ D Medial pectoral nerves
○ E Thoracodorsal nerves

3.12 An SHO has been asked to aspirate some pleural fluid for culture and sensitivity from the left pleural space of a 65-year-old man who has post-pneumonic effusion. If the SHO wants to aspirate the fluid with the patient sitting up in bed, where would the fluid tend to accumulate?

○ A Costodiaphragmatic recess
○ B Costomediastinal recess
○ C Cupola
○ D Hilar reflection
○ E Middle mediastinum

thorax

3.13 A corporal injured in a roadside explosion in Basra was found to have multiple small metal fragments in his thoracic cavity. He also had a pericardial effusion suggestive of a tear in the pericardium. He underwent emergency thoracotomy in the field hospital, which revealed that the pericardium was torn inferiorly. The surgeon began to explore for fragments in the pericardial sac. Slipping his hand under the heart apex, he slid his fingers upward and to the right within the sac until they were stopped by the cul-de-sac formed by the pericardial reflection near the base of the heart. His fingertips were then in the:

- A Coronary sinus
- B Coronary sulcus
- C Costomediastinal recess
- D Oblique pericardial sinus
- E Transverse sinus

3.14 A victim of anterior chest stabbing received a stab in a structure that is in close proximity to where the first rib articulates with the sternum. The structure most likely to be injured is the:

- A Nipple
- B Root of the lung
- C Sternal angle
- D Sternoclavicular joint
- E Xiphoid process

thorax

3.15 **A victim of anterior chest stabbing was brought to A&E with impending cardiac tamponade. There was a single puncture wound in the anterior chest 2 cm lateral to the left sternal border. An emergency thoracotomy revealed clots in the pericardium, with a puncture wound in the right ventricle. To evacuate clots from the pericardial cavity the surgeon slipped his hand behind the heart at its apex. A hand slipped behind the heart can be extended upwards until stopped by a line of pericardial reflection that forms the:**

- A   Cardiac notch
- B   Costomediastinal recess
- C   Hilar reflection
- D   Oblique pericardial sinus
- E   Transverse pericardial sinus

3.16 **A 25-year-old man was stabbed in the right supraclavicular fossa. The knife punctured the portion of the parietal pleura that extends above the first rib. This portion of the parietal pleura is called the:**

- A   Costodiaphragmatic recess
- B   Costomediastinal recess
- C   Costocervical recess
- D   Cupola
- E   Endothoracic fascia

thorax

3.17 **While performing thymectomy to remove a malignant thymoma, the surgeon is careful to avoid damaging an important nerve lying on and partly curving posteriorly around the arch of the aorta. Which of the following nerves is the surgeon trying to preserve?**

○ A Left phrenic
○ B Left sympathetic trunk
○ C Left vagus
○ D Right phrenic
○ E Right sympathetic trunk

3.18 **In a 6-week-old boy with a large subaortic ventricular septal defect, the cardiac surgeon decides to perform pulmonary artery banding through a left thoracotomy, as the child is not fit for surgical closure. To pass the tape around the pulmonary artery, the surgeon initially passes his index finger immediately behind the two great arteries in the pericardial sac to mobilise both the great arteries. The surgeon's index finger is inserted into which space?**

○ A Cardiac notch
○ B Coronary sinus
○ C Oblique pericardial sinus
○ D Coronary sulcus
○ E Transverse pericardial sinus

thorax

3.19 **During pericardiectomy, sudden bleeding was noticed due to accidental injury to a major vascular structure in the pericardium. The surgeon inserted his left index finger through the transverse pericardial sinus, pulled forward on the two large vessels lying ventral to his finger, and compressed these vessels with his thumb to control bleeding. Which vessels were these?**

    A Pulmonary trunk and brachiocephalic trunk

    B Pulmonary trunk and aorta

    C Pulmonary trunk and superior vena cava

    D Superior vena cava and aorta

    E Superior vena cava and right pulmonary artery

3.20 **A patient with a cystic swelling in his left chest underwent a computer tomography-guided biopsy. The radiologist inserted the biopsy needle into the ninth intercostal space along the midaxillary line to aspirate the swelling and obtain tissue for histological diagnosis. The swelling is most likely to be in which space?**

    A Cardiac notch

    B Costodiaphragmatic recess

    C Costomediastinal recess

    D Cupola

    E Oblique pericardial sinus

thorax

3.21 **A patient has loculated fluid in his right chest, which can be easily aspirated if the aspiration needle is inserted through the body wall just above the ninth rib in the midaxillary line. Where is this fluid located?**

- A Costodiaphragmatic recess
- B Costomediastinal recess
- C Cupola
- D Hilar reflection
- E Pulmonary ligament

3.22 **A 34-year-old woman with history of cough and weight loss for over a month is noticed to have a rounded opacity in the pleural cavity near the cardiac notch on her chest X-ray. The opacity is most likely to be present in the:**

- A Costodiaphragmatic recess
- B Costomediastinal recess
- C Cupola
- D Hilum
- E Pulmonary ligament

3.23 **A 25-year-old motorcyclist involved in a road traffic accident fractured a structure that articulates with the tubercle of the seventh rib. Which of the following structures is fractured?**

- A Body of vertebra T6
- B Body of vertebra T7
- C Body of vertebra T8
- D Transverse process of vertebra T6
- E Transverse process of vertebra T7

3.24 **A 28-year-old man suffered a gunshot wound, which entered immediately superior to the upper edge of the left clavicle near its head. He was in extreme pain, which was interpreted by the A&E physician as a likely indicator of a collapsed lung following disruption of the pleura. If that was true, what portion of the pleura was most likely to be punctured?**

- A Costal pleura
- B Cupola
- C Hilar reflection
- D Mediastinal pleura
- E Pulmonary ligament

3.25 **A specialist registrar is performing her first ductus arteriosus ligation. The consultant supervising her instructs her to be careful when placing a clamp on the ductus to avoid injury to an important structure immediately dorsal to it. To which of the following structures is the consultant referring?**

- A Accessory hemiazygos vein
- B Left internal thoracic artery
- C Left phrenic nerve
- D Left recurrent laryngeal nerve
- E Thoracic duct

thorax

3.26 **During a demonstration on anatomy of the lung the tutor asked one of the medical students to pass his index finger posteriorly inferior to the root of the left lung and identify the structure that is blocking the passage of the finger. Which structure would most likely be responsible for this?**

- A Costodiaphragmatic recess
- B Cupola
- C Inferior vena cava
- D Left pulmonary vein
- E Pulmonary ligament

3.27 **A patient with a malignant mesothelioma is to undergo pleuropneumonectomy, which involves removal of the entire pleura and lung on the affected side. Which of the following layers provides a natural cleavage plane for surgical separation of the costal pleura from the thoracic wall?**

- A Deep fascia
- B Endothoracic fascia
- C Parietal pleura
- D Visceral pleura
- E Transversus thoracis muscle fascia

3.28 **After cardiac surgery a patient is noticed to have a small effusion in the lowest extent of the pleural cavity, into which lung tissue does not extend. This part of the pleural cavity is known as the:**

- A Costodiaphragmatic recess
- B Costomediastinal recess
- C Cupola
- D Inferior mediastinum
- E Pulmonary ligament

thorax

3.29 **A medical student was asked by the supervising consultant to identify the sternal angle. The sternal angle is a landmark for locating the level of the:**

○ A Costal margin
○ B Jugular notch
○ C Second costal cartilage
○ D Sternoclavicular joint
○ E Xiphoid process

3.30 **A JHO is about to perform her first thoracentesis (remove fluid from the pleural cavity). If you were supervising her where would you ask her to insert the aspiration needle to avoid injuring the lung or neurovascular elements?**

○ A The top of interspace 8 in the midclavicular line
○ B The bottom of interspace 8 in the midclavicular line
○ C The top of interspace 9 in the midaxillary line
○ D The bottom of interspace 9 in the midaxillary line
○ E The top of interspace 11 in the scapular line

3.31 **A 28-year-old man was stabbed in the left chest. The tip of the knife entered the pleural space just above the cardiac notch. The lung was spared as it would only occupy this space during deep inspiration. Which of the following structures was pierced by the knife?**

○ A Anterior mediastinum
○ B Costodiaphragmatic recess
○ C Costomediastinal recess
○ D Cupola
○ E Pulmonary ligament

thorax

3.32 **During a gross anatomy exam a medical student was asked to identify the left lung. Which of the following features found only in the left lung will this student use to identify the left lung?**

○ A Cardiac notch

○ B Horizontal fissure

○ C Oblique fissure

○ D Superior lobar bronchus

○ E Three lobes

3.33 **A 40-year-old patient with sarcoidosis has enlarged tracheobronchial lymph nodes. Which of the following nerves would be most vulnerable to irritation in this patient?**

○ A Right phrenic

○ B Left phrenic

○ C Right recurrent laryngeal

○ D Left recurrent laryngeal

○ E Right vagus

3.34 **A 26-year-old man involved in a bar brawl was stabbed in a part of the left lung that might partially fill the costomediastinal recess in full inspiration. Where was the knife stuck in this man?**

○ A Apex

○ B Cupola

○ C Hilum

○ D Lingula

○ E Middle lobe

3.35 **A 50-year-old man underwent exploratory thoracotomy for resection of a right lung tumour. On entering the chest the surgeon decided that the tumour was not resectable as it was crossing the oblique fissure. The oblique fissure of the right lung separates what structures?**

- A Lower lobe from lingula
- B Lower lobe from upper lobe only
- C Lower lobe from both upper and middle lobes
- D Lower lobe from middle lobe only
- E Upper lobe from middle lobe

3.36 **A 32-year-old man was stabbed in the back during a bar fight with a knife that just nicked his left lung halfway between its apex and the diaphragmatic surface. Which part of the lung was most likely to be injured?**

- A Hilum
- B Inferior lobe
- C Lingula
- D Middle lobe
- E Superior lobe

3.37 **A 3-year-old boy is brought in with coughing, and his mother tells you that he had been playing with some beads and had apparently aspirated one. Where would you expect it most likely to be?**

- A Apicoposterior segmental bronchus of the left lung
- B Left main bronchus
- C Lingular segment of the left lung
- D Right main bronchus
- E Terminal bronchiole of the right lung, lower lobe

thorax

3.38 **An anatomy demonstrator is teaching medical students about the right lung. Which of the following statements regarding the right lung made by the demonstrator is CORRECT?**

○ A It is slightly smaller than the left lung

○ B It has a lingular segmental bronchus

○ C It occupies the rightmost portion of the mediastinum

○ D Its upper lobar bronchus lies behind and above the right pulmonary artery

○ E It has the right phrenic nerve passing posterior to its lung root

3.39 **While mobilising the descending aorta to repair an aortic coarctation in a 3-week-old baby, a surgeon accidentally cuts the first aortic intercostal arteries. Which of the following structures might be deprived of its main source of blood supply as a result of this iatrogenic injury?**

○ A First posterior intercostal space

○ B First anterior intercostal space

○ C Left bronchus

○ D Right bronchus

○ E Fibrous pericardium

3.40 **A 78-year-old man with pseudobulbar palsy, lying supine in bed, aspirates one of his tablets into his lungs while swallowing. It would be most likely to end up in which of the following bronchopulmonary segments?**

○ A Anterior segmental bronchus of the right superior lobe

○ B Medial segmental bronchus of the right middle lobe

○ C Superior segmental bronchus of the right inferior lobe

○ D Medial basal segmental bronchus of the left inferior lobe

○ E Inferior segmental bronchus of the lingular lobe

3.41 A medical student is observing a respiratory physician perform a flexible bronchoscopy. As she passes the bronchoscope down the trachea, she asks the medical student to identify a cartilaginous structure that resembles a ship's keel and separates the right and left main stem bronchi. This structure is the:

○ A Carina
○ B Cricoid cartilage
○ C Costal cartilage
○ D Pulmonary ligament
○ E Tracheal ring

3.42 A patient has a tumour crossing the minor (horizontal) fissure. This fissure separates:

○ A The lower lobe from the lingula
○ B The upper lobe from the lingula
○ C The lower lobe from both the middle and upper lobes
○ D The lower lobe from the middle lobe
○ E The middle lobe from the upper lobe

3.43 An 82-year-old man who has been bedridden and lying supine for many weeks in a nursing home has developed a right lung abscess that is draining by gravity into one particular region of the lung. Where is the most likely site of fluid accumulation?

○ A Apical segment of the upper lobe
○ B Lingula
○ C Lower lobe
○ D Middle lobe
○ E Superior segment of the lower lobe

thorax

3.44 A 32-year-old man was shot in the chest. The bullet punctured a vessel that courses across the mediastinum in an almost horizontal fashion. Which of the following vessels was injured?

○ A Left subclavian artery

○ B Left subclavian vein

○ C Left brachiocephalic vein

○ D Left internal jugular vein

○ E Left common carotid artery

3.45 A 76-year-old man presented in a surgical outpatient clinic with oedema of the left upper limb due to poor venous return. Examination revealed an aneurysm of the ascending aorta that was impinging on a large vein lying immediately anterosuperior to it. Which of the following veins was most likely to be obstructed?

○ A Azygos

○ B Internal thoracic

○ C Left brachiocephalic

○ D Left superior intercostal

○ E Right brachiocephalic

thorax

3.46 **While performing oesophagectomy through a right thoracotomy the surgeon suddenly noticed a gush of blood. After controlling the haemorrhage he realised that there was tear in a large venous structure located in the posterior mediastinum that empties into the superior vena cava. Which of the following venous structures was most likely to be injured?**

  A Azygos vein

  B Basilic vein

  C Brachiocephalic vein

  D Cephalic vein

  E External jugular vein

3.47 **While excising a tumour of the thymus gland the surgeon accidentally injured a vein lying immediately posterior to the thymus. Which of the following vessels is most likely to be injured?**

  A Left brachiocephalic vein

  B Left pulmonary vein

  C Left bronchial vein

  D Right pulmonary artery

  E Right superior intercostal vein

thorax

3.48 While performing a surgical procedure in the mid-region of the thorax the surgeon accidentally injured an important structure that lies immediately anterior to the thoracic duct. Which of the following structures was most likely to be injured?

- A Aorta
- B Azygos vein
- C Oesophagus
- D Superior vena cava
- E Trachea

3.49 A 42-year-old man was diagnosed with a tumour of the posterior mediastinum. Such a tumour is most likely to compress which of the following structures?

- A Arch of the aorta
- B Oesophagus
- C Inferior vena cava
- D Pulmonary trunk
- E Trachea

3.50 While performing extended mediastinal lymph node dissection for a squamous-cell carcinoma of the right upper lobe bronchus, a patient's right sympathetic trunk was accidentally severed just cranial to the level of spinal nerve T1. Which function would be left intact in the affected region?

- A Arrector pili muscle activity
- B Dilation/constriction of blood vessels
- C Sweat production
- D Visceral reflex activity
- E Voluntary muscle activity

3.51 A 76-year-old man with a complaint of dull chest pain of 3 months' duration, with a normal electrocardiogram and cardiac enzymes, underwent a computed tomographic scan, which showed a mass lesion involving a structure in the middle mediastinum. Which of the following structures could be involved?

○ A Aortic arch
○ B Ascending aorta
○ C Descending aorta
○ D Oesophagus
○ E Thoracic duct

3.52 During investigations for chest pain in a 32-year-old man computed tomography showed a large mass in the posterior mediastinum. Which of the following structures could be involved?

○ A Aortic arch
○ B Ascending aorta
○ C Innominate artery
○ D Lymph glands
○ E Superior vena cava

3.53 Which of the following vertebrae is the lowest limit of the superior mediastinum?

○ A First lumbar
○ B Fourth thoracic
○ C Second thoracic
○ D Seventh cervical
○ E Third thoracic

thorax

3.54 **A 42-year-old man is to undergo oesophagectomy. While mobilising the oesophagus in the neck, for anastomosis with the stomach tube on the left side, the operating surgeon must be careful about avoiding injury to which of the following vital structures?**

O   A   Innominate artery

O   B   Innominate vein

O   C   Internal carotid artery

O   D   Sympathetic chain

O   E   Thoracic duct

3.55 **While performing left pneumonectomy the surgeon must avoid injury to which of the following vital structures that leaves an impression on the mediastinal surface of the left lung?**

O   A   Aortic arch

O   B   Azygos vein

O   C   Innominate artery

O   D   Inferior vena cava

O   E   Superior vena cava

SECTION 4:
ABDOMEN – QUESTIONS

For each question given below choose the ONE BEST option.

4.1 A 35-year-old man was received in A&E following blunt abdominal trauma. On arrival he was in shock. He was resuscitated and rushed to the operating theatre for emergency laparotomy. On entering the peritoneal cavity the operating surgeon noticed a torn gastrosplenic ligament with a large clot around the spleen. Which of the following arteries is most likely to be injured in this case?

○ A Splenic
○ B Left gastric
○ C Short gastric
○ D Middle colic
○ E Left gastroepiploic

4.2 A 22-year-old Asian girl with a tuberculous perforation of the ileum underwent exploratory laparotomy. The small bowel was matted due to adhesions and it was difficult for the specialist registrar to differentiate ileum from jejunum. Which of the following features is typical of the jejunum?

○ A It is narrow
○ B It has thinner and fewer vascular coats
○ C The circular folds of its mucous membrane are small
○ D It occupies the right iliac region
○ E It has sparse aggregated lymph nodules

4.3   **The lumbar plexus is related to the psoas major muscle. It is situated in the posterior part of the psoas major, in front of the transverse processes of the lumbar vertebrae. Its branches emerge on either the lateral or the medial sides of this muscle. Which of these nerves lies immediately medial to the psoas major muscle?**

- A   Iliohypogastric
- B   Ilioinguinal
- C   Lateral femoral cutaneous
- D   Obturator
- E   Femoral

4.4   **Which of the following statements regarding gonadal venous drainage is CORRECT?**

- A   The right ovarian vein drains into the right renal vein
- B   The left testicular vein drains into the inferior vena cava
- C   The left ovarian vein drains into the left renal vein
- D   The right testicular vein drains into the right renal vein
- E   The right and left ovarian or testicular veins drain into the same vessel

4.5   **What is the normal location of the major duodenal papilla?**

- A   Superior part of the duodenum
- B   Ascending part of the duodenum
- C   Descending part of the duodenum
- D   Horizontal part of the duodenum
- E   Duodenal bulb

abdomen

4.6   **While performing laparoscopy the surgeon identified the medial umbilical folds on the deep surface of the anterior abdominal wall. The medial umbilical folds are caused by the:**

○   A   Urachus
○   B   Inferior epigastric vessels
○   C   Obliterated umbilical veins
○   D   Obliterated umbilical arteries
○   E   Round ligaments of the uterus

4.7   **A patient with a history of duodenal ulcer presents in A&E with symptoms of acute haemorrhagic shock. Emergency endoscopy revealed that the duodenal ulcer has perforated the posterior wall of the first part of the duodenum. The haemorrhage is most likely to be from which of the following arteries?**

○   A   Splenic
○   B   Superior mesenteric
○   C   Gastroduodenal
○   D   Left gastric
○   E   Left hepatic

4.8   **Which of the following branches of the abdominal aorta is unpaired?**

○   A   Coeliac artery
○   B   Inferior phrenic artery
○   C   Renal artery
○   D   Middle adrenal artery
○   E   Gonadal artery

abdomen

4.9 **In a patient with gastric carcinoma, the radiologist reported that the lymph nodes around the coeliac trunk are enlarged. The coeliac trunk:**

○ A Is the arterial supply to the embryonic midgut

○ B Is accompanied by the coeliac vein

○ C Arises from the lateral surface of the abdominal aorta, at about the level of the first lumbar vertebra

○ D Gives rise to the splenic, left gastric and common hepatic arteries

○ E Is surrounded by the aorticorenal ganglion

4.10 **The duodenojejunal flexure is held in place by which of the following structures?**

○ A Greater omentum

○ B Suspensory ligament (of Treitz)

○ C Hepatoduodenal ligament

○ D Lesser omentum

○ E Lienorenal ligament

4.11 **In the peritoneal cavity which of the following is normally the LEAST mobile structure?**

○ A Transverse colon

○ B Greater omentum

○ C Vermiform appendix

○ D Stomach

○ E Pancreas

abdomen

4.12 Which of the following structures is retroperitoneal?

O A Pancreas

O B Spleen

O C Transverse colon

O D Sigmoid colon

O E Vermiform appendix

4.13 The vagal trunks enter the abdomen through the:

O A Oesophageal hiatus

O B Inferior vena cava hiatus

O C Aortic hiatus

O D Medial arcuate ligament

O E Lateral arcuate ligament

4.14 Which of the following statements about the rectum is CORRECT?

O A It receives its blood supply from only one artery

O B It is an important anastomotic site for the portal and caval (systemic) venous systems

O C Its smooth muscle is innervated by somatic nerves

O D It has no circular smooth muscle in its wall

O E It is surrounded by peritoneum along its entire length (about 12 cm long, normally)

4.15 The ejaculatory duct opens into the:

O A Membranous urethra

O B Prostatic urethra

O C Spongy urethra

O D Lateral lobes of the prostate gland

O E Duct of the bulbourethral glands

abdomen

4.16   The inguinal ligament is formed by which of the deep fasciae located in the anterolateral abdominal wall?

○   A   Internal abdominal oblique aponeurosis
○   B   Transverse abdominal aponeurosis
○   C   Internal spermatic fascia
○   D   Transversalis fascia
○   E   External abdominal oblique aponeurosis

4.17   The cremasteric muscle is an extension of the:

○   A   External abdominal oblique muscle
○   B   Transverse abdominal muscle
○   C   Internal abdominal oblique muscle
○   D   Pyramidalis muscle
○   E   Dartos muscle

4.18   A builder falls from the second storey of a building under construction. The patient is conscious but complains of not feeling his 'legs'. Neurological assessment in A&E suggests that he has no cutaneous sensation from his umbilicus to his toes. The patient has sustained a spinal cord injury at which spinal cord level?

○   A   T6
○   B   T8
○   C   T10
○   D   L2
○   E   L4

abdomen

4.19 **A patient complains of dull discomfort in her abdomen that is accompanied by pain over her right shoulder and right scapula. Which of the following organ(s) is most likely to be the source of her complaints?**

○ A   Stomach
○ B   Liver, duodenum and gallbladder
○ C   Kidney and ureter
○ D   Spleen
○ E   Vermiform appendix

4.20 **Assuming that the gastrointestinal tract rotated normally, which of the following organs can be expected to lie within the right lower quadrant of the abdomen?**

○ A   Stomach, duodenum, spleen, pancreas and liver
○ B   Descending colon and sigmoid colon
○ C   Distal jejunum, caecum, vermiform appendix
○ D   Distal duodenum and proximal jejunum
○ E   Gallbladder

4.21 **Which of the following statements about the small intestine is CORRECT?**

○ A   The superior mesenteric artery courses between the body and uncinate process of the pancreas before the artery supplies the jejunum and ileum

○ B   The proximal jejunum has more arterial arcades than the distal ileum

○ C   The mesentery of the distal ileum has less fat that that of the proximal jejunum

○ D   Peyer's patches are more prominent in the proximal jejunum than the distal ileum

○ E   Postganglionic sympathetic fibres to the jejunum and ileum arise from synapses with preganglionic sympathetic fibres located in the coeliac ganglion

abdomen

4.22 **During an anatomy demonstration the medical students were told that the posterior wall of the rectus sheath ends in a thin curved margin, the concavity of which is directed downward. This inferior border of the rectus sheath posteriorly is called the:**

    A Falx inguinalis

    B Inguinal ligament

    C Internal inguinal ring

    D Arcuate line

    E Linea alba

4.23 **While examining a patient with an inguinal hernia the SHO passed his finger down the edge of the medial crus of the superficial inguinal ring and felt a bony protuberance deep to the lateral edge of the spermatic cord. This bony protuberance is the:**

    A Pecten pubis

    B Pubic symphysis

    C Pubic tubercle

    D Iliopubic eminence

    E Iliopectineal line

abdomen

4.24 **A medical student is about to witness a surgical operation on a young patient to treat an ulcer in the first part of the duodenum. The consultant surgeon asks the student to tell her the most appropriate site to make an incision on the anterior abdominal wall to approach this ulcer. The student replies, 'You should make the incision in the ...':**

    A Epigastric region

    B Left inguinal region

    C Left lumbar region

    D Right hypochondrial region

    E Hypogastric region

4.25 **Following an emergency appendicectomy the patient complained of having paraesthesia (numbness) of the skin at the pubic region. The most likely nerve that has been injured during the operation is:**

    A Genitofemoral

    B Iliohypogastric

    C Subcostal

    D Spinal nerve T10

    E Spinal nerve T9

4.26 **To retrieve a large stone from the urinary bladder the urologist makes a transverse suprapubic incision. Which of the following abdominal wall layers will not be encountered during this incision?**

    A Anterior rectus sheath

    B Posterior rectus sheath

    C Rectus abdominis muscle

    D Skin and subcutaneous tissue

    E Transversalis fascia, extraperitoneal fat and peritoneum

abdomen

4.27 **While performing a laparoscopic inguinal hernia repair the surgeon finds an artery in the extraperitoneal connective tissue (preperitoneal fat) running vertically just medial to the bowel as the bowel passes through the abdominal wall. This artery is the:**

○ A Deep circumflex iliac
○ B Inferior epigastric
○ C Superficial circumflex iliac
○ D Superficial epigastric
○ E Superficial external pudendal

4.28 **A 65-year-old man with suspected peritonitis due to a perforated colonic diverticulum was explored through a midline incision between the two rectus sheaths. This incision will be through the:**

○ A Linea aspera
○ B Arcuate line
○ C Semilunar line
○ D Iliopectineal line
○ E Linea alba

abdomen

4.29 A medical student was observing a specialist registrar harvest the left internal thoracic (mammary) artery so that it could be used as a graft for coronary artery bypass surgery. The left internal thoracic (mammary) artery was mobilised from the inside of the chest wall and divided near the caudal end of the sternum. After dividing the internal thoracic artery at its distal end the specialist registrar asked the student, 'Can you name the artery which will now have increased flow through it so that adequate blood flow is maintained to the rectus abdominis on the left side?' The student's reply should be the:

○ A Superficial epigastric artery
○ B Inferior epigastric artery
○ C Umbilical artery
○ D Superficial circumflex iliac artery
○ E Deep circumflex iliac artery

4.30 The normal pattern of venous and lymphatic drainage of the superficial tissues of the anterior abdominal wall is arranged around a horizontal plane. Above that plane, drainage is in a cranial direction; below the plane, drainage is in a caudal direction. This reference plane corresponds to the:

○ A Transpyloric plane
○ B Level of the anterior superior iliac spines
○ C Transtubercular line
○ D Level of the arcuate line
○ E Level of the umbilicus

abdomen

4.31 **While performing a laparoscopic inguinal hernia repair in a 68-year-old man with a direct inguinal hernia, the surgeon asked the specialist registrar to look at the medial inguinal fossa to identify the direct inguinal hernia. To do so, the specialist registrar would have to look at the area between the:**

○ A   Inferior epigastric artery and urachus

○ B   Medial umbilical ligament and urachus

○ C   Inferior epigastric artery and lateral umbilical fold

○ D   Medial umbilical ligament and inferior epigastric artery

○ E   Median umbilical ligament and medial umbilical ligament

4.32 **A specialist registrar while performing inguinal hernia repair made an incision parallel to and 5 cm (2 inches) above the inguinal ligament. The supervising consultant warned him to look out for the inferior epigastric vessels. The specialist registrar is most likely to find the inferior epigastric vessels between which layers of the abdominal wall?**

○ A   Camper's fascia and Scarpa's fascia

○ B   External abdominal oblique and internal abdominal oblique muscles

○ C   Internal abdominal oblique and transversus abdominis muscles

○ D   Skin and deep fascia of the abdominal wall

○ E   Transversus abdominis muscle and peritoneum

4.33 **A 45-year-old porter was admitted from the surgical outpatient clinic with a lump in the inguinal region. He underwent surgery next day and during the operation the surgeon opened the inguinal region and found a hernial sac with a small knuckle of intestine projecting through the abdominal wall, just above the inguinal ligament and lateral to the inferior epigastric vessels. The hernia was diagnosed as:**

- ○ A A congenital inguinal hernia
- ○ B A direct inguinal hernia
- ○ C A femoral hernia
- ○ D An incisional hernia
- ○ E An indirect inguinal hernia

4.34 **While performing inguinal hernia repair the specialist registrar injured a structure passing through the deep inguinal ring. Which of the following structures is most likely to be injured?**

- ○ A Iliohypogastric nerve
- ○ B Ilioinguinal nerve
- ○ C Inferior epigastric artery
- ○ D Medial umbilical ligament
- ○ E Round ligament of the uterus

4.35 **On inserting the laparoscope to repair an inguinal hernia, the surgeon visualised a loop of bowel protruding through the abdominal wall to form a direct inguinal hernia. When viewed from the abdominal side with a laparoscope, the hernial sac would be found in which region?**

- ○ A Deep inguinal ring
- ○ B Lateral inguinal fossa
- ○ C Medial inguinal fossa
- ○ D Superficial inguinal ring
- ○ E Supravesical fossa

abdomen

4.36 While repairing an indirect inguinal hernia in a female patient the surgeon noticed another structure lying alongside the herniated mass in the inguinal canal. Which of the following structures did the surgeon notice traversing the inguinal canal?

○ A Iliohypogastric nerve
○ B Inferior epigastric artery
○ C Ovarian artery and vein
○ D Pectineal ligament
○ E Round ligament of the uterus

4.37 A woman noticed a painful boil on the skin of the mons pubis. The skin of the mons pubis is supplied by which nerve?

○ A Anterior cutaneous
○ B Anterior labial
○ C Femoral branch of the genitofemoral
○ D Iliohypogastric
○ E Subcostal

4.38 A medical student was asked to examine a 19-year-old boy with a lump in the inguinal region. While performing a routine digital examination of the inguinal region the student felt that the lump was protruding from the superficial inguinal ring. He correctly concluded that it was:

○ A Definitely an indirect inguinal hernia
○ B Possibly an unusual femoral hernia
○ C Definitely a direct inguinal hernia
○ D Possibly an enlarged superficial inguinal lymph node
○ E Either a direct or an indirect inguinal hernia

abdomen

4.39 **An SHO scrubbed for the first time to assist the consultant with a repair of an indirect inguinal hernia. While performing dissection to repair the hernia, the consultant asked her to indicate the position of the deep inguinal ring. She would indicate the position of the deep inguinal ring to be:**

○ A Above the anterior superior iliac spine
○ B Above the midpoint of the inguinal ligament
○ C Above the pubic tubercle
○ D In the supravesical fossa
○ E Medial to the inferior epigastric artery

4.40 **A 69-year-old man with a long-standing, large indirect inguinal hernia came to your clinic complaining of pain in the scrotum. There was no evidence of obstruction or inflammation. You conclude that the hernial sac is most likely compressing the:**

○ A Femoral branch of the genitofemoral nerve
○ B Femoral nerve
○ C Iliohypogastric nerve
○ D Ilioinguinal nerve
○ E Subcostal nerve

4.41 **A newborn baby boy is diagnosed with right-sided cryptorchidism (undescended testis). Where is the undescended testis LEAST likely to be found?**

○ A At the deep inguinal ring
○ B Just outside the superficial inguinal ring
○ C Pelvic brim
○ D Perineum
○ E Somewhere in the inguinal canal

abdomen

4.42 **A 55-year-old man with a long-standing, left-sided indirect inguinal hernia underwent emergency surgery to relieve large bowel obstruction resulting from a segment of his large bowel becoming strangulated in his large left-sided indirect inguinal hernia. The most likely intestinal segment involved in this obstruction is the:**

A Ascending colon

B Caecum

C Descending colon

D Rectum

E Sigmoid colon

4.43 **A 55-year-old previously fit and healthy man underwent emergency appendicectomy for a perforated appendix. Six months later, he presented in the surgical outpatient clinic with a direct inguinal hernia on the right side. The specialist registrar examining him correlated the development of the hernia to iatrogenic nerve injury that happened during appendicectomy and weakened the falx inguinalis. Which nerve had been injured?**

A Femoral branch of the genitofemoral

B Genital branch of the genitofemoral

C Ilioinguinal

D Subcostal

E Ventral primary ramus of T10

4.44 **While performing dissection to repair an indirect inguinal hernia the consultant surgeon demonstrated the hernial sac protruding out of the superficial inguinal ring. The superficial inguinal ring is an opening in which structure?**

○ A External abdominal oblique aponeurosis

○ B Falx inguinalis

○ C Internal abdominal oblique muscle

○ D Scarpa's fascia

○ E Transversalis fascia

4.45 **While performing an inguinal hernia repair, a nerve that passes through the superficial inguinal ring sustained an iatrogenic injury. Which of the following nerves is it most likely to be?**

○ A Femoral branch of the genitofemoral

○ B Ilioinguinal

○ C Iliohypogastric

○ D Obturator

○ E Subcostal

4.46 **While performing exploratory laparotomy in a patient with suspected bowel obstruction, the surgeon identified a herniation of bowel between the lateral edge of the rectus abdominis muscle, the inguinal ligament and the inferior epigastric vessels. These boundaries defined the hernia as a(n):**

○ A Congenital inguinal hernia

○ B Direct inguinal hernia

○ C Femoral hernia

○ D Indirect inguinal hernia

○ E Umbilical hernia

abdomen

4.47 **In the human body veins usually run a course parallel to the artery of the same name. Which of the following veins does not run a course parallel to the artery of the same name?**

- A Superior epigastric
- B Superficial circumflex iliac
- C Inferior mesenteric
- D Superior rectal
- E Ileocolic

4.48 **An SHO was asked to distinguish small from large bowel on an X-ray with barium contrast. Which of the following features is the SHO most likely to mention that distinguishes small from large bowel on a barium contrast X-ray?**

- A Circular folds of the mucosa
- B Circular smooth muscle layer in the wall
- C Mucosal glands
- D Longitudinal smooth muscle layer in the wall
- E Serosa

4.49 **While reviewing the abdominal aortogram of a 67-year-old man with an abdominal aortic aneurysm, a radiologist noticed an occluded inferior mesenteric artery. However, on enquiry, the patient denied having any abdominal symptoms. Occlusion of the inferior mesenteric artery is seldom symptomatic because its territory may be supplied by branches of the:**

- A Gastroduodenal artery
- B Ileocolic artery
- C Middle colic artery
- D Right colic artery
- E Splenic artery

4.50 **An 18-year-old man complaining of right lower quadrant pain was diagnosed as having acute appendicitis and was listed for appendicectomy. The specialist registrar performing the operation initially saw no appendix on entering the peritoneal cavity but did not panic because he knew that he could quickly locate it by:**

○ A Looking at the confluence of the taenia coli

○ B Palpating the ileocaecal valve and looking just above it

○ C Following the course of the right colic artery

○ D Removing the right layer of the mesentery of the jejuno-ileum

○ E Palpating and inspecting the pelvic brim

4.51 **During exploratory laparotomy for acute abdomen the surgeon identified an inflamed Meckel's diverticulum. Meckel's diverticulum:**

○ A Is an abnormal persistence of the urachus

○ B Is a site of ectopic pancreatic tissue

○ C Is caused by a failure of the midgut loop to return to the abdominal cavity

○ D Is an abnormal connection of the midgut to the duodenum

○ E Is associated with polyhydramnios

4.52 **The spleen normally does not descend below the costal margin. However, it pushes downward and medially when pathologically enlarged. What structure limits the straight-vertical-downward movement?**

○ A Left colic flexure

○ B Left suprarenal gland

○ C Ligament of Treitz

○ D Pancreas

○ E Stomach

abdomen

4.53 **The coeliac branch of the posterior vagal trunk sustained iatrogenic injury during repair of a hiatus hernia. The damage to this nerve would affect the muscular movements, as well as some secretory activities, of the gastrointestinal tract. Which segment is LEAST likely to be affected by the nerve damage?**

○ A Ascending colon
○ B Caecum
○ C Jejunum
○ D Ileum
○ E Sigmoid colon

4.54 **While performing exploratory laparotomy in a patient with a firearm injury to the abdomen, the surgeon says, 'Oh the bullet has perforated the large bowel!' Which of the following characteristics of the bowel enabled the surgeon to identify it specifically as large bowel?**

○ A Serosa
○ B Circular folds
○ C Continuous longitudinal muscle layer
○ D Epiploic appendages
○ E Valvulae conniventes

abdomen

4.55 A 65-year-old woman with atrial fibrillation was brought to the emergency department complaining of acute abdominal pain. An abdominal angiogram revealed that her inferior mesenteric artery was occluded, most probably due to an embolus. On exploratory laparotomy, which of the following segments of large bowel is most likely to have preserved arterial supply?

- A Caecum
- B Descending colon
- C Rectum
- D Sigmoid colon
- E Splenic flexure

4.56 While performing repair of an infrarenal abdominal aortic aneurysm the consultant surgeon decided not to re-implant the inferior mesenteric artery into the repaired abdominal aorta. When asked by his specialist registrar, he said that the reason he has decided not to re-implant the inferior mesenteric artery was that in this patient the anastomotic artery running along the border of the large intestine is good enough to supply blood to the territory of the inferior mesenteric artery. To which anastomotic artery running along the border of the large intestine is the consultant referring?

- A Arcade
- B Arteriae rectae
- C Coronary
- D Ileocolic
- E Marginal

abdomen

4.57 Abdominal aortic angiography in a patient with an abdominal aortic aneurysm revealed that his inferior mesenteric artery was occluded although the patient was asymptomatic. In this patient, the normal area of distribution of the inferior mesenteric artery therefore must be supplied by collateral blood flow between which arteries?

○ A Ileocolic and right colic
○ B Left and middle colic
○ C Left colic and sigmoid
○ D Right and middle colic
○ E Sigmoid and superior rectal

4.58 During development of the human embryo the midgut bends around an artery to form the 'midgut loop'. Which of the following arteries does the midgut bend around?

○ A Coeliac trunk
○ B Inferior mesenteric
○ C Proper hepatic
○ D Splenic
○ E Superior mesenteric

4.59 A patient with massive haematemesis was diagnosed with a bleeding ulcer of the lesser curvature of the stomach. During exploratory laparotomy, which of the following arteries is most likely to be ligated in this patient to control the bleeding?

○ A Gastroduodenal
○ B Left gastric
○ C Left gastroepiploic
○ D Right gastroepiploic
○ E Short gastrics

abdomen

4.60 **In the developing human embryo, during the development of the gut, there are two mesogastria attaching to the developing stomach: the dorsal mesogastrium and the ventral mesogastrium. Which of the following is a derivative of the dorsal mesogastrium?**

○ A Falciform ligament
○ B Hepatoduodenal ligament
○ C Hepatogastric ligament
○ D Greater omentum
○ E Lesser omentum

4.61 **While delivering a lecture on the development of the spleen, which of the following facts is the embryology demonstrator most likely to tell the medical students?**

○ A It develops in the dorsal mesogastrium
○ B It develops in the ventral mesogastrium
○ C It develops in both the dorsal and ventral mesogastria
○ D It is always retroperitoneal
○ E It becomes retroperitoneal during its development

4.62 **A specialist registrar was about to perform his first splenectomy. The supervising consultant told the specialist registrar to pay special attention to locate and preserve the tail of the pancreas, which is closely associated with the spleen, to avoid a postoperative pancreatic fistula. Where is the specialist registrar most likely to find the tail of the pancreas?**

○ A Gastrocolic ligament
○ B Gastrosplenic ligament
○ C Phrenicocolic ligament
○ D Splenorenal ligament
○ E Transverse mesocolon

abdomen

4.63 **The structures that lie behind the peritoneum are termed 'retroperitoneal' and are not covered entirely by visceral peritoneum. Which of the following structures is completely invested by peritoneum?**

○ A Adrenal gland
○ B Kidney
○ C Pancreas
○ D Spleen
○ E Second part of the duodenum

4.64 **A 55-year-old male executive who had a history of a chronic duodenal ulcer was admitted to the casualty department exhibiting signs of a severe internal haemorrhage. He was quickly diagnosed with perforation of the posterior wall of the first part of the duodenum and erosion of an artery behind it by the gastric expellant. The involved artery is most likely to be the:**

○ A Common hepatic
○ B Gastroduodenal
○ C Left gastric
○ D Proper hepatic
○ E Superior mesenteric

abdomen

4.65 A 25-year-old man involved in a road traffic accident was brought to the emergency department in shock. Examination showed low blood pressure and tenderness on the left mid- and posterior axillary line. In addition, a large swelling was felt protruding downward and medially below the left costal margin. X-rays revealed that his 9th and 10th ribs were fractured near their angles on the left side. The abdominal organ most likely to be injured by these fractured ribs is the:

O   A   Descending colon
O   B   Left kidney
O   C   Pancreas
O   D   Spleen
O   E   Stomach

4.66 While performing an operation to remove the left suprarenal gland the surgeon mobilises the descending colon by cutting along its lateral attachment to the body wall and dissecting medialward in the fusion fascia behind it. Suddenly the operative field is filled with blood. The surgeon realises he has failed to cut a mesenteric attachment between the left colic flexure and another organ. As a result of the traction, the surface of the organ tore. Which organ was injured?

O   A   Duodenum
O   B   Kidney
O   C   Liver
O   D   Spleen
O   E   Suprarenal gland

abdomen

4.67 **During emergency surgery, it was found that a chronic gastric ulcer had perforated the posterior wall of the stomach and eroded a large artery running immediately posterior to the stomach. The artery is the:**

○   A   Gastroduodenal

○   B   Common hepatic

○   C   Left gastroepiploic

○   D   Splenic

○   E   Superior mesenteric

4.68 **Ligation of which of the following arteries is most likely to render the fundus of the stomach ischaemic?**

○   A   Common hepatic

○   B   Inferior phrenic

○   C   Left gastroepiploic

○   D   Right gastric

○   E   Splenic

4.69 **During an emergency splenectomy, the surgeon accidentally tore the gastrosplenic ligament and its contents. Which of the following arteries is most likely to be damaged as result of this iatrogenic injury?**

○   A   Left gastric

○   B   Splenic

○   C   Short gastric

○   D   Middle colic

○   E   Caudal pancreatic

abdomen

4.70 **While performing emergency surgery to control haemorrhage brought on by arterial erosion caused by a duodenal ulcer, surgeons ligated the badly damaged gastroduodenal artery near its origin, which affected all of its branches as well. Assuming 'average anatomy', in which of the following arteries would blood now flow in retrograde fashion (backwards) from collateral sources?**

   ◯ A Left hepatic
   ◯ B Right gastroepiploic
   ◯ C Short gastric
   ◯ D Left gastric
   ◯ E Omental branches

4.71 **A 45-year-old man with a long history of duodenal ulcer problems was brought in for emergency surgery to control severe haemorrhage into the peritoneal cavity. The surgeons found that erosion by the ulcer of a vessel passing behind the first part of the duodenum was the source of the haemorrhage. Which of the following vessels passes behind the first part of the duodenum and would need to be clamped off to control the bleeding?**

   ◯ A Coronary vein
   ◯ B Gastroduodenal artery
   ◯ C Inferior pancreaticoduodenal arcade
   ◯ D Proper hepatic artery
   ◯ E Splenic vein

abdomen

4.72 **During a cholecystectomy, the SHO accidentally jabbed a sharp instrument into the area immediately posterior to the epiploic foramen (its posterior boundary). He was horrified to see the surgical field immediately fill with blood, the source he knew to be the:**

- ○ A Aorta
- ○ B Inferior vena cava
- ○ C Portal vein
- ○ D Right renal artery
- ○ E Superior mesenteric vein

4.73 **The division between the true right and left lobes (internal lobes) of the liver may be visualised on the outside of the liver as a plane passing through the:**

- ○ A Gallbladder fossa and round ligament of the liver
- ○ B Falciform ligament and ligamentum venosum
- ○ C Gallbladder fossa and inferior vena cava
- ○ D Falciform ligament and right hepatic vein
- ○ E Gallbladder fossa and right triangular ligament

4.74 **In a road traffic accident victim, with evidence of intra-abdominal bleeding due to a ruptured spleen, the surgeon temporarily clamped the splenic artery near the coeliac trunk to stop the haemorrhage. The blood supply to which of the following structures is LEAST likely to be affected by this manoeuvre?**

- ○ A Duodenum
- ○ B Greater omentum
- ○ C Body of the pancreas
- ○ D Tail of the pancreas
- ○ E Stomach

abdomen

4.75 **A 58-year-old male patient with severe obstructive jaundice was diagnosed with pancreatic cancer. You suspect that the tumour is located in which portion of the pancreas?**

○ A Head
○ B Neck
○ C Body
○ D Tail
○ E Uncinate process

4.76 **A 38-year-old man was admitted with symptoms of bowel obstruction. Further examination revealed that the obstruction was caused by the nutcracker-like compression of the bowel between the superior mesenteric artery and the aorta. The compressed bowel is most likely the:**

○ A Duodenum
○ B Jejunum
○ C Ileum
○ D Ascending colon
○ E Transverse colon

4.77 **While performing laparoscopic cholecystectomy, the surgeon states that next he is going to expose the cystic artery in the 'triangle of Calot' to staple across it. What structures form this triangle and are the keys to finding the artery?**

○ A Common hepatic duct, liver and cystic duct
○ B Cystic duct, right hepatic artery and right hepatic duct
○ C Gallbladder, liver and common bile duct
○ D Left hepatic duct, liver and cystic duct
○ E Right branch of portal vein, liver and common bile duct

abdomen

4.78 **A 48-year-old patient was diagnosed with severe portal hypertension due to alcoholic cirrhosis of the liver. It was determined that a bypass between the vessels of the portal and caval systems was necessary. The plan most likely to be successful is:**

○ A Coronary vein to right gastroepiploic vein

○ B Left colic vein to sigmoid vein

○ C Inferior mesenteric vein to splenic vein

○ D Splenic vein to left renal vein

○ E Superior rectal vein to inferior rectal vein

4.79 **A 25-year-old man was admitted with symptoms of an upper bowel obstruction. Computed tomography showed that the third (transverse) portion of the duodenum was compressed by a large vessel causing the obstruction. The vessel involved is most likely to be the:**

○ A Inferior mesenteric artery

○ B Superior mesenteric artery

○ C Inferior mesenteric vein

○ D Portal vein

○ E Splenic vein

abdomen

4.80 **A 55-year-old man complains of intense chest pain, but tests rule out any cardiac pathology. It was determined that the patient suffers from an oesophageal (hiatal) hernia in which the stomach herniates through an enlarged oesophageal hiatus. Muscle fibres from which of the following parts of the diaphragm would border directly on this hernia?**

○   A   Left crus
○   B   Right crus
○   C   Central tendon
○   D   Costal fibres
○   E   Sternal fibres

4.81 **After successfully performing two adrenalectomies (removal of the adrenal gland), the specialist registrar was disappointed to learn that he would be merely assisting at the next one. The consultant surgeon told him: 'I'm doing this one because the one on the right side may be a little too difficult for you'. The difficulty he envisioned stems from the fact that the right suprarenal gland is partly overlaid anteriorly by the:**

○   A   Aorta
○   B   Inferior vena cava
○   C   Left hepatic vein
○   D   Right crus of the diaphragm
○   E   Right renal artery

abdomen

4.82 **A 26-year-old man was diagnosed with a rare tumour of the left suprarenal gland which had extended into the left suprarenal vein. Which of the following venous structures is most likely to be involved next by this tumour?**

○ A Inferior mesenteric vein
○ B Inferior vena cava
○ C Left renal vein
○ D Left testicular vein
○ E Portal vein

4.83 **While performing adrenalectomy on the left side the surgeon injured a vital structure which lies anterior to the suprarenal gland. Which of the following structures was most likely to have been injured by the surgeon?**

○ A Duodenum
○ B Inferior vena cava
○ C Kidney
○ D Liver
○ E Pancreas

4.84 **While performing a vascular procedure on the right common iliac artery the surgery injured an important vascular structure on the right side of the fifth lumbar vertebra, resulting in massive haemorrhage. Which of the following structures was most likely to have been injured?**

○ A Aorta
○ B Inferior vena cava
○ C Portal vein
○ D Right renal vein
○ E Right external iliac vein

4.85 **Ligation of which of the following arteries will not affect the blood supply to the stomach?**

○ A Hepatic
○ B Left gastroepiploic
○ C Short gastric
○ D Splenic
○ E Superior mesenteric

4.86 **While performing Kocher's manoeuvre to mobilise the duodenum the surgeon nicked a major artery near the upper margin of the superior part of the duodenum. This artery also forms the lower boundary of the epiploic foramen (foramen of Winslow). Which of the following arteries was most likely to be injured?**

○ A Coeliac
○ B Hepatic
○ C Left gastric
○ D Splenic
○ E Superior pancreaticoduodenal

4.87 **While performing Whipple's operation the surgeon ligated the superior pancreaticoduodenal artery. The superior pancreaticoduodenal artery is a branch of the:**

○ A Cystic artery
○ B Coeliac artery
○ C Gastroduodenal artery
○ D Splenic artery
○ E Superior mesenteric artery

abdomen

97

4.88 **While performing Whipple's operation the surgeon nicked the inferior pancreaticoduodenal artery accidentally. The inferior pancreaticoduodenal artery is a branch of the:**

○ A Coeliac artery

○ B Gastroduodenal artery

○ C Hepatic artery

○ D Splenic artery

○ E Superior mesenteric artery

4.89 **While mobilising the head of the pancreas as a part of Whipple's operation the surgeon must avoid injury to a vital structure that lies behind the head of pancreas, close to the right border. This vital structure is the:**

○ A Common bile duct

○ B Gastroduodenal artery

○ C Portal vein

○ D Splenic vein

○ E Superior mesenteric vein

4.90 **While mobilising the pancreas as a part of Whipple's operation the surgeon injured a vital structure lying immediately posterior to the neck of the pancreas, which flooded the operative field with blood. The structure most likely to be injured was the:**

○ A Abdominal aorta

○ B Coeliac artery

○ C Hepatic artery

○ D Portal vein

○ E Superior mesenteric artery

abdomen

4.91 **Ligation of which of the following arteries is most likely to affect the blood supply to the pancreas?**

○ A Inferior mesenteric
○ B Inferior phrenic
○ C Middle colic
○ D Ileocolic
○ E Superior mesenteric

4.92 **Ligation of which of the following arteries is most likely to affect the blood supply to the oesophagus?**

○ A Inferior mesenteric
○ B Left Inferior phrenic
○ C Right gastric
○ D Right suprarenal
○ E Superior mesenteric

4.93 **A 26-year-old man was brought to A&E after a road traffic accident. His spleen was shattered and therefore the splenic artery was ligated at its origin to perform splenectomy. Which of the following arteries will have reduced blood flow due to ligation of splenic artery at its origin?**

○ A Hepatic
○ B Inferior pancreaticoduodenal
○ C Left gastroepiploic
○ D Right gastroepiploic
○ E Superior pancreaticoduodenal

abdomen

4.94 **A 25-year-old man was brought to A&E in shock after sustaining a stab wound to the right iliac fossa. On exploratory laparotomy it was discovered that the ileocolic artery was severed and the knife had perforated the caecum. The ileocolic artery is a branch of the:**

O   A   Coeliac artery
O   B   Hepatic artery
O   C   Inferior mesenteric artery
O   D   Marginal artery
O   E   Superior mesenteric artery

4.95 **While performing gastrectomy the surgeon ligated short gastric arteries along the greater curvature of stomach. The short gastric arteries are branches of the:**

O   A   Hepatic artery
O   B   Left gastroepiploic artery
O   C   Right gastroepiploic artery
O   D   Splenic artery
O   E   Superior mesenteric artery

4.96 **While performing sigmoid colectomy the surgeon ligated sigmoid arteries. The sigmoid arteries are branches of the:**

O   A   Coeliac artery
O   B   Inferior mesenteric artery
O   C   Left colic artery
O   D   Middle colic artery
O   E   Superior mesenteric artery

abdomen

4.97 **While performing left adrenalectomy the surgeon ligated the left middle suprarenal artery. The left middle suprarenal artery is a branch of the:**

○ A Abdominal aorta
○ B Coeliac artery
○ C Inferior phrenic artery
○ D Splenic artery
○ E Superior mesenteric artery

4.98 **While performing left adrenalectomy the surgeon ligated the left superior suprarenal artery. The left superior suprarenal artery arises from the:**

○ A Left gastric artery
○ B Left gastroepiploic artery
○ C Left inferior phrenic artery
○ D Left renal artery
○ E Left testicular artery

4.99 **A 26-year-old man was brought to A&E after a fall from his motorcycle. He had fractured his pelvis and shattered his coccyx. The SHO looking after him in A&E mentioned that this man was likely to have a laceration of his middle sacral artery with this type of injury. The middle sacral artery is a branch of the:**

○ A Abdominal aorta
○ B Common iliac artery
○ C External iliac artery
○ D Fourth lumbar artery
○ E Superior haemorrhoidal artery

abdomen

4.100 While performing an abdominoperineal resection the surgeon ligated the superior haemorrhoidal (rectal) artery. The superior haemorrhoidal artery is a continuation of the:

O A Inferior mesenteric artery

O B Left colic artery

O C Marginal artery

O D Sigmoid artery

O E Superior mesenteric artery

abdomen

SECTION 5:
PELVIS – QUESTIONS

For each question given below choose the ONE BEST option.

5.1 **During a difficult vaginal delivery, the SHO on call was asked to come and make an episiotomy. She made a median episiotomy and in doing so cut too far through the perineal body into the structure immediately posterior. Which structure did she cut?**

○ A External anal sphincter
○ B Bulbospongiosus muscle
○ C Ischiocavernosus muscle
○ D Sphincter urethrae
○ E Sacrospinous ligament

5.2 **While consenting a patient for prostatectomy the surgeon explained to the patient that he could have loss of penile erection after the operation due to injury to the prostatic plexus of nerves that contains nerve fibres that innervate penile tissue to cause erection. From which nerves do these fibres originate?**

○ A Deep perineal
○ B Pelvic splanchnics
○ C Pudendal
○ D Genitofemoral
○ E Dorsal nerve of penis

5.3 **A young man developed a boil on his scrotum. Which of the following lymph nodes are most likely to enlarge in this patient due to lymphatic spread of infection?**

O   A   Internal iliac nodes
O   B   Sacral nodes
O   C   Superficial inguinal nodes
O   D   Lumbar nodes
O   E   External iliac nodes

5.4 **The pelvic diaphragm is formed by the:**

O   A   Levator ani and piriformis muscles
O   B   Piriformis and internal obturator muscles
O   C   Levator ani and coccygeus muscles
O   D   Obturator internus and coccygeus muscles
O   E   Levator ani and obturator internus muscles
O

5.5 **Which of the following nerves is the principal motor and sensory nerve of the perineum?**

O   A   Lateral femoral cutaneous
O   B   Pudendal
O   C   Superior gluteal
O   D   Femoral
O   E   Genitofemoral

pelvis

5.6   Which of the following structures lies between the layers of the mesosalpinx?

○   A   Ovary
○   B   Fallopian tube
○   C   Uterus
○   D   Vaginal artery
○   E   Round ligament of the uterus

5.7   A patient complains of dull pain in her pelvis, along the midline from the pubic bone in front to the sacrum at the back. Which organ or organs, from the options provided, would be the most likely cause of this patient's pain?

○   A   Vermiform appendix
○   B   Sigmoid colon, left ureter
○   C   Spleen
○   D   Transverse colon, pylorus of the stomach, duodenum, pancreas
○   E   Urinary bladder, uterus/cervix/vagina, rectum

5.8   What is the root value of the pudendal nerve?

○   A   S2, S3, S4
○   B   L4, L5, S1
○   C   L5, S1, S2
○   D   S1
○   E   S5

pelvis

5.9   The perineum is divided into two triangles by a line connecting the:

O   A Anterior superior iliac crests

O   B Pubic tubercles

O   C Inferior pubic rami

O   D Sacral promontory to the pubic symphysis

O   E Ischial tuberosities

5.10   The inferior fascia of the urogenital diaphragm is called the:

O   A Colles' fascia

O   B Fascia lata

O   C Obturator fascia

O   D Perineal membrane

O   E Scarpa's fascia

5.11   Which list of muscles correctly identifies all of the components of the pelvic diaphragm?

O   A Coccygeus and piriformis muscles

O   B Coccygeus, iliococcygeus, pubococcygeus and puborectalis muscles

O   C Obturator internus, coccygeus, iliococcygeus and pubococcygeus muscles

O   D Iliococcygeus, pubococcygeus and puborectalis muscles

O   E Psoas and iliacus muscles

pelvis

5.12 **The levator ani muscle arises from the tendinous arch of the fascia of which pelvic wall muscle?**

○ A Obturator internus
○ B Piriformis
○ C Puborectalis
○ D Psoas major
○ E Iliacus

5.13 **Unless the surgeon is careful, the ureter is most likely to be ligated during hysterectomy while the surgeon is clamping the:**

○ A Broad ligaments
○ B Uterine tubes
○ C Uterine arteries
○ D Bleeding vessel in the anterior abdominal wall
○ E Ovarian ligaments

5.14 **A patient with ovarian cancer has spread of tumour from the ovaries to the first group of lymph nodes around the aorta that directly drains the ovaries. Where are these lymph nodes located?**

○ A The origin of the inferior phrenic arteries
○ B The origin of the ovarian arteries
○ C The origin of the superior mesenteric artery
○ D The origin of the lumbar arteries
○ E The origin of the renal arteries

pelvis

5.15 **A 32-year-old woman opted for bilateral pudendal nerve block at the time of her second delivery. To inject the anaesthetic agent near the pudendal nerve the anaesthetic consultant inserted a finger into the vagina and pressed laterally to palpate which landmark?**

○ A Arcus tendineus levator ani

○ B Coccyx

○ C Ischial spine

○ D Lateral fornix

○ E Obturator foramen

5.16 **During a vaginal delivery the SHO noticed that the baby's head was stuck. To avoid serious damage to the perineal structures she decided to perform a median episiotomy. However, her incision cut through the perineal body into the structure immediately posterior to it. Which perineal structure did she cut?**

○ A Bulbospongiosus muscle

○ B External anal sphincter muscle

○ C Ischiocavernosus muscle

○ D Sacrospinous ligament

○ E Sphincter urethrae

pelvis

5.17 While consenting a patient for abdominoperineal
resection the consultant surgeon told the patient
that during the operation he would try his best
to protect the prostatic plexus of nerves, which
contains nerve fibres that innervate penile tissue
to cause erection. However, there is a risk that if
these nerve fibres are injured the patient may not
have an erection after the operation. From which
of the following nerves do these fibres originate?

   ○ A Deep perineal
   ○ B Dorsal nerve of the penis
   ○ C Genitofemoral
   ○ D Pelvic splanchnics
   ○ E Pudendal

5.18 A 38-year-old woman was seen in the outpatient
clinic complaining of a boil located on her labia
majora. Lymphatic spread of the infection would
most likely enlarge which nodes?

   ○ A Lumbar
   ○ B Sacral
   ○ C External iliac
   ○ D Superficial inguinal
   ○ E Internal iliac

pelvis

5.19 **If the venous drainage of the anal canal above the pectinate line is impaired in a patient with portal hypertension, there may be an increase in blood flow downward to the systemic venous system via anastomoses with the inferior rectal vein, which is a tributary of the:**

- ○ A External iliac vein
- ○ B Inferior gluteal vein
- ○ C Inferior mesenteric vein
- ○ D Internal iliac vein
- ○ E Internal pudendal vein

5.20 **While performing a hysterectomy the surgeon ligated the uterine artery on either side. The uterine artery arises from the:**

- ○ A Abdominal aorta
- ○ B External iliac artery
- ○ C Inferior rectal artery
- ○ D Internal iliac artery
- ○ E Ovarian artery

5.21 **A 36-year-old woman is to undergo excision of her right ovary for a malignant tumour. Which of the following structures lying posterior to it is at risk if the surgeon is not careful?**

- ○ A External iliac artery
- ○ B External iliac vein
- ○ C Obliterated umbilical artery
- ○ D Ureter
- ○ E Uterine tube

pelvis

5.22 **Which of the following structures directly related to the base of the prostate is likely to be involved by a malignant growth in the base of the prostate?**

○ A Anus
○ B Levator ani
○ C Superior fascia of the urogenital diaphragm
○ D Rectum
○ E Urinary bladder

5.23 **The seminal vesicles are found between the:**

○ A Base of the bladder and prostate
○ B Base of the bladder and rectum
○ C Ductus deferens and ureter
○ D Ejaculatory ducts and ductus deferens
○ E Prostate and rectum

5.24 **Ligation of which of the following arteries is most likely to affect the blood supply to the seminal vesicles?**

○ A Inferior rectal
○ B Middle rectal
○ C Superior rectal
○ D Superior vesical
○ E Renal

pelvis

5.25 The ductus deferens unites with the duct of the seminal vesicle to form the:

○ A Ampulla
○ B Aberrant ductules
○ C Ejaculatory duct
○ D Paradidymis
○ E Prostatic utricle

5.26 A 46-year-old male homosexual presented in the surgical outpatient clinic with a malignant growth involving his anus. Which of the following groups of lymph nodes is likely to be enlarged in this patient?

○ A Internal iliac
○ B Lateral aortic
○ C Pararectal
○ D Preaortic
○ E Superficial inguinal

5.27 A 52-year-old man presented with a carcinoma involving the anal canal. Which of the following lymph nodes are likely to be enlarged in this patient?

○ A Internal iliac
○ B Lateral aortic
○ C Pararectal
○ D Preaortic
○ E Superficial inguinal

pelvis

5.28 **A 38-year-old woman with an extensive malignant growth in the anterior wall of the vagina is most likely to have involvement of which adjacent structure?**

○ A   Anal canal

○ B   Fundus of the bladder

○ C   Perineal body

○ D   Rectum

○ E   Rectovesical fascia

5.29 **While performing a repair of an inguinal hernia the surgeon had to ligate a branch of the external iliac artery near the deep inguinal ring to gain better exposure. Which of the following arteries did the surgeon ligate?**

○ A   Iliolumbar

○ B   Inferior epigastric

○ C   Inferior gluteal

○ D   Internal pudendal

○ E   Superior vesical

5.30 **Which of the following plexuses of veins is most likely to dilate in a patient with portal hypertension?**

○ A   Haemorrhoidal plexus

○ B   Prostatic plexus

○ C   Uterine plexus

○ D   Vaginal plexus

○ E   Vesical plexus

pelvis

SECTION 6:
HEAD AND NECK – QUESTIONS

For each question given below choose the ONE BEST option.

6.1   A 22-year-old man was received in A&E with a stab wound involving the left side of the neck. He was bleeding profusely and was rushed to the operating theatre for exploration of the neck injury. On exploration, a posterior branch of the external carotid artery was severed that was then suture-ligated. Which of the following arteries was injured?

    A Superior thyroid

    B Lingual

    C Facial

    D Occipital

    E Superficial temporal

6.2   During a street fight a young man was slashed on the face with a broken glass bottle. He received a laceration on the right side of his face that transected the facial artery. Both cut ends of the facial artery were ligated. Which of the following statements about the facial artery is true?

    A It arises in the digastric triangle a little above the lingual artery

    B It runs a very straight course both in the neck and on the face

    C It is crossed by the branches of the facial nerve from behind forward

    D It terminates as the submental artery

    E It supplies the parotid gland

6.3 **During thyroidectomy, the inferior laryngeal branch of the right recurrent laryngeal nerve was injured. The action of which of the following laryngeal muscles is most likely to be affected?**

○ A   Thyroarytenoid

○ B   Arytenoid

○ C   Lateral cricoarytenoid

○ D   Posterior cricoarytenoid

○ E   Cricothyroid

6.4 **The vocal ligaments:**

○ A   Are formed by the superior free edge of the conus elasticus

○ B   Are formed by the junction of the aryepiglottic and thyroepiglottic ligaments

○ C   Are formed by the inferior free edge of the thyrohyoid ligament

○ D   Contain the cricothyroid muscle

○ E   Are attached to the superior margin of the epiglottis

6.5 **The neck is divided into two large triangles by which muscle?**

○ A   Anterior scalene

○ B   Sternocleidomastoid

○ C   Strap

○ D   Subclavius

○ E   Trapezius

head and neck

6.6 **The phrenic nerves course over which muscles in the neck?**

O A Anterior scalene

O B Middle scalene

O C Posterior scalene

O D Sternocleidomastoid

O E Trapezius

6.7 **The carotid sheath extends from the base of the skull to the root of the neck. The inferior part of this sheath contains the:**

O A Common carotid artery, inferior jugular vein, sympathetic chain

O B Common carotid artery, external jugular vein, sympathetic chain

O C Internal carotid artery, external jugular vein, vagus nerve

O D Internal carotid artery, internal jugular vein, phrenic nerve

O E Common carotid artery, internal jugular vein, vagus nerve

head and neck

6.8   The boundaries of the anterior triangle of the neck are the:

◯   A   Inferior border of the mandible, anterior of border of the sternocleidomastoid muscle, anterior midline of the neck

◯   B   Inferior border of the mandible, anterior border of the omohyoid muscle and anterior midline of the neck

◯   C   Inferior border of the mandible, superior border of the digastric muscle and anterior midline of the neck

◯   D   Inferior border of the mandible, anterior border of the sternocleidomastoid muscle and anterior border of the omohyoid muscle

◯   E   Inferior border of the mandible, superior border of the omohyoid muscle and anterior midline of the neck

6.9   From superficial to deep, identify the CORRECT order of the visceral layers of the neck:

◯   A   Pharynx/oesophagus, larynx/trachea, thyroid/parathyroids

◯   B   Larynx/trachea, pharynx/oesophagus, thyroid/parathyroids

◯   C   Thyroid/parathyroids, larynx/trachea, pharynx/oesophagus

◯   D   Thyroid/parathyroids, pharynx/oesophagus, larynx/trachea

◯   E   Larynx/trachea, thyroid/parathyroids, pharynx/trachea

head and neck

6.10 **The hyoid muscles steady or move the hyoid bone and larynx. Which of the following statements about the hyoid muscles is CORRECT?**

O   A   The four suprahyoid muscles are the mylohyoid, geniohyoid, stylohyoid and omohyoid muscles

O   B   The four infrahyoid muscles are the sternohyoid, omohyoid, sternothyroid and digastric muscles

O   C   All of the hyoid muscles (suprahyoid and infrahyoid muscles) are innervated exclusively by the cervical plexus of nerves

O   D   The two bellies of the digastric muscle arise from two separate pharyngeal arches

O   E   The action of all four infrahyoid muscles is to steady the hyoid bone and larynx or to depress the hyoid bone and larynx

6.11 **The pterygomandibular raphé serves as a point of attachment for the:**

O   A   Superior pharyngeal constrictor muscle
O   B   Middle pharyngeal constrictor muscle
O   C   Lateral pterygoid muscle
O   D   Medial pterygoid muscle
O   E   Tensor veli palatini muscle

head and neck

6.12 The CORRECT boundaries of the posterior triangle of the neck are the:

○ A   Anterior border of the sternocleidomastoid muscle, inferior border of the mandible and anterior midline of the neck

○ B   Posterior border of the sternocleidomastoid muscle, the clavicle and anterior border of the trapezius muscle

○ C   Anterior borders of both sternocleidomastoid muscles, inferior border of the mandible, suprasternal notch of the manubrium

○ D   Anterior borders of both trapezius muscles, the occipital bone and the posterior midline of the neck

○ E   Both bellies of the digastric muscle and inferior border of the mandible

6.13 Which of the following statements about the arteries of the neck is CORRECT?

○ A   The thyrocervical trunk typically gives rise to the inferior thyroid artery, transverse cervical artery and suprascapular artery

○ B   Arterial branches to the face arise from the internal carotid artery

○ C   The carotid sinus is located at the origin of the external carotid artery

○ D   The facial artery courses superficial to the submandibular salivary gland

○ E   The vertebral arteries arise from the external carotid arteries

head and neck

6.14 **The action of the posterior cricoarytenoid muscles is to:**

○ A Adduct the arytenoid cartilages

○ B Abduct the vocal processes of the arytenoid cartilages

○ C Relax the vocal ligaments

○ D Assist in closure of the vestibule

○ E Elevate the vocal ligaments

6.15 **A patient with a boil on the upper lip developed septic thrombophlebitis of the cavernous sinus resulting in the development of acute meningitis. What is the usual superficial venous connection through which an infected blood clot courses to the cavernous sinus?**

○ A Lingual vein

○ B Superficial temporal vein

○ C Facial vein

○ D Inferior alveolar vein

○ E Retromandibular vein

6.16 **Which arteries unite to form the basilar artery?**

○ A Internal carotid

○ B Middle meningeal

○ C Anterior ethmoidal

○ D Ophthalmic

○ E Vertebral

head and neck

6.17 **The pterion is an important clinical landmark because it overlies the:**

○ A Superior sagittal sinus
○ B Anterior branches of the middle meningeal artery
○ C Confluence of sinuses
○ D Anterior cerebral arteries
○ E Straight sinus

6.18 **In which bone of the base of the skull are located the optic foramen, superior orbital fissure, foramen rotundum, foramen ovale and foramen spinosum?**

○ A Frontal
○ B Ethmoid
○ C Sphenoid
○ D Temporal
○ E Occipital

6.19 **The direct branch of the facial nerve that carries the special sense of taste from the anterior two-thirds of the tongue:**

○ A Passes through the superior orbital fissure
○ B Also carries parasympathetic fibres to the palate
○ C Exits the skull through the stylomastoid foramen
○ D Eventually joins with fibres of the inferior alveolar nerve
○ E Can be injured by erroneous placement of a tympanic membrane shunt

head and neck

6.20 **Cessation of parasympathetic innervation to the lacrimal gland (and subsequently a chief complaint of dry eye) could result from which of the following?**

○ A Increased pressure in the cavernous sinus

○ B Compression at the superior orbital fissure

○ C A tumour in the optic nerve

○ D Compression at the internal acoustic meatus

○ E Severing of the lingual nerve during 3rd molar surgery

6.21 **The supratrochlear nerve is a terminal branch of which nerve?**

○ A Ophthalmic

○ B Frontal

○ C Nasociliary

○ D Lacrimal

○ E Maxillary

6.22 **Which of the following statements is CORRECT regarding the muscles of facial expression?**

○ A The digastric muscle is a muscle of facial expression

○ B Some muscles of facial expression are innervated by the long buccal nerve

○ C They are in the same subcutaneous plane as the platysma muscle

○ D Some muscles of facial expression receive their motor supply via the zygomaticofacial nerve

○ E All muscles of facial expression are attached to bone

head and neck

6.23 Acting together, the lateral pterygoid muscles:

O A Protrude the mandible

O B Retract the mandible

O C Close the mandible

O D Open the mandible

O E Have no effect on the mandible

6.24 The mental foramen is found:

O A In the maxilla

O B In the mandible

O C In the zygomatic bone

O D Immediately inferior to the orbit

O E In the infratemporal fossa

6.25 Which statement is CORRECT regarding the parasympathetic innervation to the nose?

O A It is supplied by the oculomotor nerve

O B Preganglionic fibres exit the cranial cavity through the jugular foramen

O C Preganglionic fibres synapse in the pterygopalatine ganglion

O D Postganglionic fibres run along with cranial nerve V1

O E There is no need for parasympathetic innervation to the nose

6.26 To gain access into the frontal sinus via the nasal cavity, one would enter through the:

O A Sphenoethmoidal recess

O B Middle meatus

O C Inferior meatus

O D Superior meatus

O E Nasolacrimal duct

head and neck

6.27 The olfactory foramina:

○ A Are located in the middle cranial fossa

○ B Are located in the anterior cranial fossa

○ C Are located immediately inferior to the optic foramen

○ D Have motor neurones running through them

○ E Are located in the sphenoid bone

6.28 The inferior sagittal sinus:

○ A Drains directly into the confluence of sinuses

○ B Is found in the falx cerebelli

○ C Is formed between two layers of meningeal dura

○ D Drains into the superior petrosal sinus

○ E Contains valves, unlike the other venous dural sinuses

6.29 The ciliary ganglion:

○ A Is a sympathetic ganglion

○ B Is used for parasympathetic innervation to the lacrimal gland

○ C Is used by the facial nerve (cranial nerve VII)

○ D Would be affected by severance of the oculomotor nerve (cranial nerve III)

○ E Is a sensory ganglion

6.30 During a plastic surgical procedure on the face the inferior palpebral nerve on the right side was transected accidentally. The inferior palpebral nerve is a terminal branch of the:

○ A Infraorbital nerve

○ B Nasociliary nerve

○ C Lacrimal nerve

○ D Zygomatic nerve

○ E Facial nerve

head and neck

6.31 Motor innervation of the orbicularis oculi muscle is by:

○ A A branch of a nerve that exits through the infraorbital foramen

○ B A branch of a nerve that exits through the stylomastoid foramen

○ C A branch of the same nerve that innervates the temporalis muscle

○ D A branch of a nerve that would be affected by increased pressure in the cavernous venous sinus

○ E A branch of the same nerve that innervates the levator palpebrae superioris muscle

6.32 Ligation of the facial artery at the inferior border of the mandible will:

○ A Decrease blood flow to some parts of the nasal septum

○ B Decrease blood flow to the mandibular teeth

○ C Eliminate blood flow to the lower eyelid

○ D Decrease the blood flow to the cornea

○ E Eliminate blood flow to the lower lip

6.33 The left lateral pterygoid muscle, acting alone, will shift the mandible:

○ A Laterally, to the right

○ B Laterally, to the left

○ C Anteriorly

○ D Posteriorly

○ E Down

head and neck

6.34 Which of the following statements regarding the mouth and pharynx is CORRECT?

○ A The hard palate is formed mostly by the maxillary and sphenoid bones

○ B Elevation of the soft palate is achieved by a muscle innervated by the glossopharyngeal nerve

○ C A muscle that both elevates the pharynx and depresses the soft palate is innervated by cranial nerve XII

○ D A muscle that both opens the auditory tube and tenses the palate is innervated by cranial nerve V

○ E The nerves that contribute to the pharyngeal plexus are cranial nerve IX, cranial nerve X, preganglionic sympathetic fibres and cranial nerve XII

6.35 The muscle whose action is to tense the tympanic membrane is innervated by the:

○ A Chorda tympani nerve
○ B Trigeminal nerve
○ C Facial nerve
○ D Vagus nerve
○ E Glossopharyngeal nerve

6.36 Which of the following structures separates the anterior and posterior chambers in the eyeball?

○ A The lens
○ B The cornea
○ C The iris
○ D The pupil
○ E The ciliary processes

head and neck

6.37 **Injury to which of the following nerves will paralyse the lateral rectus muscle of the eyeball?**

○ A Oculomotor
○ B Trigeminal
○ C Abducent
○ D Trochlear
○ E Optic

6.38 **Which of the following muscles hooks around the pterygoid hamulus?**

○ A Salpingopharyngeus
○ B Tensor veli palatini
○ C Palatopharyngeus
○ D Levator veli palatini
○ E Palatoglossus

6.39 **A patient presents with a large, bilateral swelling in the middle of her throat (anterior neck). You diagnose a goitre (enlarged thyroid gland). The thyroid gland is located in which part of the neck?**

○ A Visceral space
○ B Submandibular triangle
○ C Carotid sheath
○ D Posterior triangle
○ E Retropharyngeal space

head and neck

6.40 A patient presents with a large, bilateral swelling in the anterior neck. You diagnose a goitre. Which of the following statements about the thyroid gland is CORRECT?

○ A Its arterial supply is exclusively via the superior thyroid arteries

○ B Its venous drainage is via the inferior thyroid veins only

○ C Its isthmus lies posterior to the trachea

○ D The recurrent laryngeal nerves run along its posterior surface

○ E Normally, the thyroid gland is immobile

6.41 A patient presents with a large, bilateral swelling in the middle anterior neck. You diagnose a goitre. While performing thyroidectomy in this patient, what is the CORRECT order of anatomical structures encountered, from superficial to deep?

○ A Skin, investing fascia, pretracheal fascia, thyroid gland, parathyroid glands

○ B Skin, pretracheal fascia, investing fascia, thyroid gland, parathyroid glands

○ C Skin, pretracheal fascia, investing fascia, parathyroid glands, thyroid gland

○ D Skin, investing fascia, pretracheal fascia, thyroid gland, parathyroid glands

○ E Skin, thyroid gland, parathyroid glands, investing fascia, pretracheal fascia

head and neck

6.42 **A patient who had surgery in the left carotid triangle complained to his physician that he has little sense of touch to the skin over the left side of his neck and difficulty swallowing. The patient's hyoid bone is deviated to the right side. The patient's tongue is not affected. The physician suspects that the cervical plexus of nerves to the left side of this patient's neck was harmed during the surgical procedure. Loss of touch sensation to the skin over the anterior triangle would result from injury to which nerve?**

    A Lateral supraclavicular

    B Spinal accessory

    C Hypoglossal

    D Medial supraclavicular

    E Transverse cervical

6.43 **A patient who had surgery in the left carotid triangle complained to his physician that he has little sense of touch to the skin over the left side of his neck and difficulty swallowing. The patient's hyoid bone is deviated to the right side. The patient's tongue is not affected. The physician suspects that the cervical plexus of nerves to the left side of this patient's neck was harmed during the surgical procedure. Of the following nerves, which is embedded in the carotid sheath and therefore vulnerable to injury during surgical procedures to the carotid artery?**

    A Spinal accessory nerve

    B Ansa cervicalis

    C Cervical sympathetic chain

    D Phrenic nerve

    E Suprascapular nerve

6.44 **A young patient sustained fractures to the base of his skull in a high-speed car crash. The patient was ejected from the vehicle because he was not wearing a seat belt. The skull fractures are primarily located along the base of the middle cranial fossa. Neurological examination reveals that the patient has no sense of touch to the skin over his cheek (maxilla) and chin (mandible). What are the names of the foramina through which the two affected sensory branches leave the cranial cavity?**

○ A Superior orbital fissure and foramen rotundum

○ B Foramen rotundum and foramen ovale

○ C Foramen ovale and foramen spinosum

○ D Inferior orbital fissure and foramen rotundum

○ E Foramen ovale and the hiatus for the greater petrosal nerve

6.45 **A young patient sustained a head injury in a high-speed car crash. The patient was ejected from the vehicle because he was not wearing a seat belt. His head hit the tarmac and he sustained a sharp blow to the side of the head, over the temporal region, which resulted in rupture of the principal artery that supplies the meninges. What is the name of the artery?**

○ A Basilar artery

○ B Anterior cerebral artery

○ C Cavernous sinus

○ D Middle meningeal artery

○ E Posterior meningeal artery

head and neck

6.46 Aqueous humour:

○ A Is the only source of nutrients for the ciliary body

○ B Is the only source of nutrients for the iris

○ C Is produced in the posterior chamber

○ D Replaces spent vitreous humour

○ E Is the only source of nutrients for the lens of the eye

6.47 Postganglionic sympathetic fibres innervating the dilator pupillae muscle begin in the:

○ A Ciliary ganglion

○ B Superior cervical ganglion

○ C Brain

○ D Trigeminal ganglion

○ E Spinal cord (T1–L2)

6.48 The ophthalmic artery emerges through which of the following foramina to reach the eye?

○ A Optic canal

○ B Foramen spinosum

○ C Superior orbital fissure

○ D Foramen rotundum

○ E Inferior orbital fissure

6.49 Care must be taken during surgery of the parotid gland so as not to damage the:

○ A External carotid artery

○ B Chorda tympani nerve

○ C Greater petrosal nerve

○ D Main trunk of cranial nerve VIII

○ E Levator labii alaeque nasi muscle

6.50 Inability of a patient to gaze directly to the right with both eyes simultaneously could indicate deficits in which of the following combinations:

O   A   The medial rectus muscle of the right eye and cranial nerve VI on the left side

O   B   The lateral rectus muscle of the left eye and the inferior rectus muscle of the right eye

O   C   The medial rectus muscle of the right eye and cranial nerve IV on the left side

O   D   The lateral rectus muscle of the right eye and cranial nerve III on the left side

O   E   Left cranial nerve VI and right cranial nerve V

6.51 General sensory innervation of the cornea:

O   A   Is supplied by cranial nerve VIII

O   B   Is supplied by the ophthalmic nerve

O   C   Is supplied by the oculomotor nerve

O   D   Is supplied by the facial nerve

O   E   Enters the eyeball exclusively through short ciliary nerves

6.52 The lingual artery is usually a direct branch of which artery?

O   A   Maxillary

O   B   Internal carotid

O   C   External carotid

O   D   Facial

O   E   Sphenopalatine

head and neck

6.53 A patient has an aneurysm associated with the lingual artery in the floor of the mouth. By ligating the artery with the aneurysm for surgical repair, what structure will experience decreased blood flow?

○ A The mandibular teeth

○ B The skin of the lower lip

○ C The parotid gland

○ D The sublingual gland

○ E The masseter muscle

6.54 The sphenopalatine artery:

○ A Accompanies the infraorbital nerve to its termination

○ B Enters the infratemporal fossa through the pterygomaxillary fissure

○ C Supplies blood to the lateral nasal wall and nasal septum

○ D Is a terminal branch of the middle superior alveolar artery

○ E Sends a branch into the pharyngeal canal

6.55 The submandibular duct opens:

○ A Near the maxillary second molar

○ B Near the mandibular first molar

○ C From the incisive foramen

○ D Near the midline in the anterior aspect of the floor of the mouth

○ E Into the buccal vestibule near the mandibular ramus

head and neck

6.56 Which of the following is associated with the tensor veli palatini muscle?

○ A The middle pharyngeal constrictor

○ B The hamulus of the lateral pterygoid plate

○ C The hamulus of the medial pterygoid plate

○ D Cranial nerve V1

○ E The greater petrosal nerve

6.57 Which of the following statements regarding the muscle contained in the anterior palatal arch is CORRECT?

○ A It acts on the pharynx

○ B It is innervated by the hypoglossal nerve

○ C It is innervated by the glossopharyngeal nerve

○ D It is considered a muscle of facial expression

○ E It acts on the tongue

6.58 Which of the following statements about the lingual artery is CORRECT?

○ A It is a branch of the maxillary artery

○ B It gives rise to the submental artery

○ C It is crossed by the hypoglossal nerve

○ D Its branches provide blood supply to the mandibular teeth

○ E It lies superficial to the hyoglossal muscle

head and neck

6.59 The lingual nerve supplies which of the following?

O   A Motor innervation to the mylohyoid muscle

O   B Taste to the posterior third of the tongue

O   C Motor innervation to the genioglossus muscle

O   D General sensation to the posterior third of the tongue

O   E General sensation to the anterior two-thirds of the tongue

6.60 Which of the following cranial nerves supply the interior of the tympanic membrane?

O   A Facial

O   B Glossopharyngeal

O   C Hypoglossal

O   D Oculomotor

O   E Vestibulocochlear

6.61 A patient has an aneurysm associated with the lingual artery in the floor of the mouth. The patient is to undergo surgical repair of this vascular defect. If the surgical approach was from inside the mouth, which muscle would you have to go through to reach the main portion of the lingual artery?

O   A Styloglossus

O   B Hyoglossus

O   C Geniohyoid

O   D Mylohyoid

O   E Anterior belly of the digastric

head and neck

6.62 **For what anatomical reason can infections in the skin of the face, scalp or diploic bone of the neurocranium reach the dural venous sinuses?**

○　A　Valves do not exist in the veins of the face, scalp or diploic bone and they communicate directly with the dural venous sinuses

○　B　Arteries to the face, scalp and diploic bone communicate directly with arteries to the brain

○　C　Capillaries of the face, scalp and diploic bone communicate directly with capillaries of the brain

○　D　Arteries to the face, scalp and diploic bone communicate directly with veins from the brain

○　E　Valves exist in the arteries of the face, scalp or diploic bone that function to direct blood to the dural venous sinuses

6.63 **Inability to move the mandible to the left would indicate paralysis of the:**

○　A　Right lateral pterygoid muscle
○　B　Left medial pterygoid muscle
○　C　Left lateral pterygoid muscle
○　D　Right medial pterygoid muscle
○　E　Right temporalis muscle

head and neck

6.64 **A child with a history of a cold and sore throat, a bulging, inflamed tympanic membrane and a severe earache probably is suffering from an infection of the middle ear (otitis media). What is the most probable path that the infection took to arrive in the middle ear?**

○　A　External acoustic meatus, through tympanic membrane, middle ear

○　B　Mastoid air cells, through tympanic membrane, middle ear

○　C　Cavernous sinus, internal acoustic meatus, inner ear, through oval window, middle ear

○　D　Pharynx, pharyngotympanic tube, through tympanic membrane, middle ear

○　E　Pharynx, pharyngotympanic tube, middle ear

6.65 **The dural venous sinuses are located between which matched structures listed below?**

○　A　Neurocranium and the periosteal layer of the dura mater

○　B　Periosteal and meningeal layers of the arachnoid mater

○　C　Carotid sheath and prevertebral fascia

○　D　Meningeal and periosteal layers of the dura mater

○　E　Pia mater and the brain

6.66 **The malleus:**

○　A　Is in direct contact with the oval window

○　B　Is in direct contact with the tympanic membrane

○　C　Lies between the incus and the oval window

○　D　Provides a point of insertion for the stapedius muscle

○　E　Is a feature of the external acoustic meatus

head and neck

6.67   The sphincter pupillae muscle:

O   A   Contracts when it receives signals from postganglionic sympathetic fibres

O   B   Contracts when it receives signals originating from the otic ganglion

O   C   Contracts when it receives postganglionic parasympathetic fibres that originate in the ciliary ganglion

O   D   Dilates when it receives signals from the facial nerve

O   E   Is an extension of the sclera of the eyeball

6.68   The middle meningeal artery is a branch of the:

O   A   Occipital artery

O   B   Maxillary artery

O   C   Sphenopalatine artery

O   D   Internal carotid artery

O   E   Lingual artery

6.69   Of the following intrinsic muscles of the larynx, which tenses (stretches) the vocal folds?

O   A   Posterior cricoarytenoid

O   B   Lateral cricoarytenoid

O   C   Thyroarytenoid

O   D   Transverse arytenoid

O   E   Cricothyroid muscle

6.70   The nasolacrimal duct empties into the:

O   A   Sphenoethmoidal recess

O   B   Inferior meatus

O   C   Middle meatus

O   D   Maxillary sinus

O   E   Infundibulum

head and neck

6.71 The palatoglossus and levator veli palatini muscles are both innervated by:

O A Mandibular nerve

O B Cranial nerve X

O C Cranial nerve XII

O D Cranial nerve IX

O E Cranial nerve XI

6.72 Fibres running in the nerve of the pterygoid canal are:

O A Purely sensory

O B Preganglionic sympathetic and preganglionic parasympathetic

O C Preganglionic sympathetic and postganglionic parasympathetic

O D Postganglionic sympathetic and preganglionic parasympathetic

O E Destined to synapse in the otic ganglion

6.73 A sharp blow to the side of the head, over the temporal region, is frequently associated with rupture of the principal artery that supplies the meninges. What is the name of this vessel?

O A Basilar artery

O B Anterior cerebral artery

O C Cavernous sinus

O D Middle meningeal artery

O E Posterior meningeal artery

head and neck

6.74 General sensory innervation of the lacrimal gland is:

O   A   Supplied by the ophthalmic nerve

O   B   Supplied by the maxillary nerve

O   C   Supplied by the oculomotor nerve

O   D   Supplied by the facial nerves

O   E   Contained in the short ciliary nerves

6.75 The rectus capitis anterior muscle is innervated by ventral rami from which cervical spinal levels?

O   A   C1, C2

O   B   C3, C4

O   C   C4, C5

O   D   C1, C2, C3, C4

O   E   C3, C4, C5

6.76 The recurrent laryngeal nerves are vulnerable to injury during surgical procedures in the neck. If a recurrent laryngeal nerve is severed, which intrinsic muscle of the larynx will be spared on the same side as the cut?

O   A   Cricothyroid

O   B   Oblique arytenoid

O   C   Thyroarytenoid

O   D   Posterior cricoarytenoid

O   E   Lateral cricoarytenoid

head and neck

6.77 The descending palatine artery arises within the:

○ A Pterygopalatine fossa

○ B Infratemporal fossa

○ C Infraorbital canal

○ D Temporal fossa

○ E Cranial cavity

6.78 Which of the following statements about the carotid body is CORRECT?

○ A It is located at the bifurcation of the maxillary and superficial temporal arteries

○ B It senses changes in blood pressure

○ C It is innervated by the glossopharyngeal nerve

○ D It is a swelling in the wall of the carotid artery

○ E It is an aggregate of lymphoid tissue

6.79 A muscle that is contained exclusively in the anterior triangle of the neck is the:

○ A Sternocleidomastoid

○ B Platysma

○ C Omohyoid

○ D Digastric

○ E Trapezius

6.80 Sensory innervation to the mandibular teeth and bone is supplied by the:

○ A Posterior superior alveolar nerve

○ B Greater palatine nerve

○ C Buccal nerve

○ D Inferior alveolar nerve

○ E Auriculotemporal nerve

6.81 **The lateral cricoarytenoid and arytenoid muscles have a similar action on the vocal folds. What is the common action?**

○ A Adduction
○ B Abduction
○ C Relaxation
○ D Stretch
○ E Twist

6.82 **The ciliary muscle:**

○ A Relaxes when it receives parasympathetic innervation from cranial nerve VII

○ B Contracts when it receives parasympathetic innervation from cranial nerve VII

○ C Contracts when it receives parasympathetic innervation from cranial nerve III

○ D Tenses the suspensory ligaments of the lens when it contracts

○ E Causes the lens to become more round when it relaxes

6.83 **The anterior chamber of the eye:**

○ A Is filled with vitreous humour
○ B Is where the lens is located
○ C Is separated from the posterior chamber by the iris
○ D Contains the optic disc
○ E Is where aqueous humour is secreted

head and neck

6.84 The arterial pulse that is found in front of the upper part of the ear is from the:

◯   A   Transverse facial artery
◯   B   Facial artery
◯   C   Superficial temporal artery
◯   D   Posterior auricular artery
◯   E   Maxillary artery

6.85 In surgery of the thyroid gland, the external laryngeal nerve may be injured and must be identified before ligating the:

◯   A   Inferior thyroid artery
◯   B   Superior thyroid artery
◯   C   Superior pharyngeal artery
◯   D   Inferior laryngeal artery
◯   E   Ascending palatine artery

6.86 The parotid duct reaches the oral vestibule by piercing the:

◯   A   Masseter muscle
◯   B   Buccinator muscle
◯   C   Levator anguli oris muscle
◯   D   Superior pharyngeal constrictor muscle
◯   E   Middle pharyngeal constrictor muscle

6.87 The mucosa of the larynx inferior to the true vocal folds receives its innervation from the:

◯   A   Recurrent laryngeal nerve
◯   B   Superior laryngeal nerve
◯   C   External branch of the superior laryngeal nerve
◯   D   Internal branch of the superior laryngeal nerve
◯   E   Facial nerve

head and neck

6.88 The piriform recess is located:

○ A Above the palatine tonsil

○ B Beneath the middle nasal concha

○ C On either side of the larynx, within the laryngopharynx

○ D Posterior to the salpingopharyngeal folds, within the nasopharynx

○ E Between the glossoepiglottic folds

6.89 Which of the following structures cannot be easily palpated in a live subject?

○ A Hyoid bone

○ B Sternocleidomastoid muscle

○ C Pulse of the common carotid artery

○ D Styloid process of the temporal bone

○ E Thyroid cartilage

6.90 You have a patient with an infection in the mastoid air cells. The infection could probably be transmitted to the middle ear directly through the:

○ A Torus tubarius

○ B Umbo

○ C Semicircular canals

○ D External auditory canal

○ E Epitympanic recess

head and neck

6.91 Directing the gaze downward when the eye is abducted requires the:

   ○ A Lateral rectus muscle

   ○ B Inferior rectus muscle

   ○ C Superior oblique muscle

   ○ D Inferior oblique muscle

   ○ E Medial rectus muscle

6.92 Which artery is the sole supply for the retina:

   ○ A Lacrimal artery

   ○ B Ophthalmic artery

   ○ C Central artery of the retina

   ○ D Anterior ciliary artery

   ○ E Posterior ethmoidal artery

6.93 The occipital artery, as it arises from the external carotid artery, normally has which nerve associated with it laterally?

   ○ A Hypoglossal nerve (cranial nerve XII)

   ○ B Glossopharyngeal nerve (cranial nerve IX)

   ○ C Carotid nerve

   ○ D Vagus nerve (cranial nerve X)

   ○ E Auriculotemporal branch of the trigeminal nerve (cranial nerve V3)

head and neck

6.94 The pterygoid venous plexus drains the infratemporal fossa via the:

○ A External jugular vein
○ B Internal jugular vein
○ C Posterior auricular vein
○ D Maxillary vein
○ E Superficial temporal vein

6.95 The ostium of the maxillary sinus opens into the:

○ A Sphenoethmoidal recess
○ B Superior meatus
○ C Middle meatus
○ D Inferior meatus
○ E Bulla ethmoidalis

6.96 The medial boundary of the infratemporal fossa is formed by the:

○ A Styloid process of the temporal bone
○ B Medial pterygoid plate of the sphenoid bone
○ C Lateral pterygoid plate of the sphenoid bone
○ D Infratemporal surface of the maxillary bone
○ E Zygomatic arch

6.97 The duct of the submandibular gland empties into the oral cavity:

○ A At the base of the tongue via the foramen caecum
○ B Opposite the lower second molar tooth
○ C Via several small openings along the sublingual fold
○ D Beside the lingual frenulum through the sublingual caruncle
○ E Opposite the maxillary second molar tooth

head and neck

6.98 **The muscle whose action is to dampen movement of the stapes is innervated by the:**

○ A Chorda tympani nerve
○ B Trigeminal nerve
○ C Facial nerve
○ D Vagus nerve
○ E Cranial nerve VIII

6.99 **Damage to the facial nerve after it emerges from the stylomastoid foramen would affect:**

○ A Facial expression
○ B Taste from the anterior two-thirds of the tongue
○ C Salivation
○ D Sensation from the eyebrows
○ E Lacrimation

6.100 **The hyoid bone serves as attachment for which of the following muscles?**

○ A Middle pharyngeal constrictor
○ B Inferior pharyngeal constrictor
○ C Sternothyroid
○ D Genioglossus
○ E Trapezius

head and neck

6.101 Which of the following statements regarding the ophthalmic division of the trigeminal nerve is CORRECT?

○ A It provides sensory innervation for most of the globe and motor innervation to smooth muscle in the globe

○ B The ophthalmic nerve as a single structure does not reach the interior of the globe

○ C It passes through the inferior orbital fissure

○ D It follows the optic nerve and enters the bony orbit with it

○ E One of its branches gives motor innervation to the lacrimal gland

6.102 What structure divides the posterior triangle of the neck further into an upper and lower triangle?

○ A Anterior belly of the digastric

○ B Inferior belly of the omohyoid

○ C Posterior belly of the digastric

○ D Scalenus anterior muscle

○ E Superior belly of the omohyoid

6.103 The common carotid artery usually bifurcates into the external and internal carotids at which one of the following levels?

○ A C2

○ B C4

○ C C6

○ D C7

○ E C8

head and neck

6.104 The fascial plane enclosing the muscles forming the borders of the posterior triangle of the neck is the:

○ A Retropharyngeal fascia
○ B Prevertebral fascia
○ C Investing fascia
○ D Pretracheal fascia
○ E Superficial fascia

6.105 Which of the following structures forms the posterior boundary of the carotid triangle?

○ A Anterior belly of the digastric
○ B Posterior belly of the digastric
○ C Sternocleidomastoid
○ D Stylohyoid
○ E Superior belly of the omohyoid

6.106 Injury to the sympathetic efferent fibres of the oculomotor nerve will affect the:

○ A Ciliary muscle
○ B Parotid gland
○ C Sublingual nerve
○ D Submandibular gland
○ E Uvula

6.107 The nerves and blood vessels to the scalp are found in which layer?

○ A Skin
○ B Connective tissue
○ C Aponeurosis
○ D Loose areolar connective tissue
○ E Pericranium

head and neck

6.108 The thyroid gland in some cases can have a thyroidea ima artery that supplies the isthmus of the thyroid. If present, it would take origin:

○ A From the inferior thyroid artery
○ B Directly from the thyrocervical trunk
○ C From the superior thyroid artery
○ D From the brachiocephalic trunk
○ E Directly from the external carotid artery

6.109 Which of the following foramina transmits the vertebral artery?

○ A Jugular foramen
○ B Foramen spinosum
○ C Foramen magnum
○ D Internal acoustic meatus
○ E Foramen ovale

6.110 Which of the following foramina transmits the facial nerve?

○ A Jugular foramen
○ B Foramen spinosum
○ C Foramen magnum
○ D Internal acoustic meatus
○ E Foramen ovale

6.111 Which of the following foramina transmits the vagus nerve?

○ A Jugular foramen
○ B Foramen spinosum
○ C Foramen magnum
○ D Internal acoustic meatus
○ E Foramen ovale

head and neck

6.112 Which of the following foramina transmits the vestibulocochlear nerve?

O A Jugular foramen
O B Foramen spinosum
O C Foramen magnum
O D Internal acoustic meatus
O E Foramen ovale

6.113 Which of the following foramina transmits the dura mater?

O A Jugular foramen
O B Foramen spinosum
O C Foramen magnum
O D Internal acoustic meatus
O E Foramen ovale

6.114 Which of the following foramen transmits the accessory meningeal artery?

O A Jugular foramen
O B Foramen spinosum
O C Foramen magnum
O D Internal acoustic meatus
O E Foramen ovale

6.115 The mandibular nerve exits the cranial cavity by way of the:

O A Foramen magnum
O B Foramen ovale
O C Foramen rotundum
O D Foramen hallucidum
O E Foramen spinosum

6.116 A patient's eyelid was drooping and the pupil was dilated. Which nerve could be involved in this lesion?

○ A Oculomotor nerve
○ B Trochlear nerve
○ C Abducens nerve
○ D Long ciliary nerve
○ E Frontal nerve

6.117 The ganglion that is found on the medial side of the mandibular trunk of the trigeminal nerve receives its preganglionic sympathetic fibres from the:

○ A Chorda tympani nerve
○ B Optic nerve
○ C Vagus nerve
○ D Trigeminal nerve
○ E Glossopharyngeal nerve

6.118 The bone of the skull that contains the foramen ovale is the:

○ A Sphenoid
○ B Ethmoid
○ C Frontal
○ D Temporal
○ E Zygomatic

head and neck

6.119 The cell bodies of the parasympathetic preganglionic nerve fibres to the ciliary muscle of accommodation are located in the:

○ A Thoracic spinal cord segments

○ B Superior cervical ganglion

○ C Edinger–Westphal nucleus

○ D Ciliary ganglion

○ E Facial nerve

6.120 The two vessels that are connected by the superior petrosal sinus are the:

○ A Inferior petrosal and cavernous sinuses

○ B Sphenoparietal and transverse sinuses

○ C Sigmoid and superior sagittal sinuses

○ D Cavernous and transverse sinuses

○ E Superior sagittal and inferior petrosal sinuses

6.121 The artery off the thyrocervical trunk that passes medially over the first portion of the vertebral artery is the:

○ A Suprascapular

○ B Transverse cervical

○ C Inferior thyroid

○ D Internal thoracic

○ E Deep cervical

head and neck

154

6.122 **The ocular muscle on whose superior surface the frontal nerve is situated has the following action:**

○ A Elevation of the eyeball
○ B Elevation of the upper eyelid
○ C Temporal rotation of the eyeball
○ D Nasal rotation of the eyeball
○ E Adduction of the eyeball

6.123 **Which cervical spinal nerves give rise to the motor nerve over which the suprascapular artery passes to enter the posterior triangle of the neck?**

○ A C2 and C3
○ B C1, C2 and C3
○ C C2, C3, C4 and C5
○ D C3, C4 and C5
○ E C6, C7 and C8

6.124 **Into what larger vessel does the vein usually empty which drains the inferior pole of the thyroid gland?**

○ A Internal jugular vein
○ B Brachiocephalic vein
○ C Subclavian vein
○ D External jugular vein
○ E Vertebral vein

head and neck

6.125 The name of the bone that the internal carotid artery enters to reach the intracranial cavity is the:

○ A   Frontal
○ B   Occipital
○ C   Sphenoid
○ D   Temporal
○ E   Maxillary

SECTION 7:
BRAIN AND CRANIAL NERVES
– QUESTIONS

For each question given below choose the ONE BEST option.

7.1 **During a boxing match, a boxer is hit on the right side of the head, between the eye and the ear. He immediately loses consciousness, wakes up momentarily and then becomes comatose. He is rushed to A&E and undergoes immediate computed tomography. The scan shows a skull fracture and an accumulation of blood between the dura and the cranial bone on the side of his head, compressing his cerebrum. He is rushed to surgery where a hole is bored into his skull to relieve the pressure. After a few tense hours, he regains consciousness and has an uneventful recovery. What type of haemorrhage did this patient have?**

- A Subdural
- B Epidural
- C Intracerebral
- D Subaponeurotic
- E Subarachnoid

brain

7.2 **A 6-month-old baby was seen in the neurosurgical outpatient clinic with a gradually progressive hydrocephalus. Computed tomography of the brain suggested a blockage in the ventricular system of the baby's brain, between the third and fourth ventricles. Which of the following structures is most likely to be blocked?**

- A Cerebral aqueduct
- B Central canal
- C Interventricular foramen
- D Foramen of Luschka
- E Foramen of Magendie

7.3 **Which of the following cranial nerves is considered to be purely motor?**

- A Oculomotor
- B Abducens
- C Facial
- D Trigeminal
- E Optic

7.4 **Which cranial nerve would be affected by a bone tumour at the stylomastoid foramen?**

- A VII
- B X
- C IX
- D XII
- E V

7.5   Lesions of the glossopharyngeal nerve would:

O   A   Affect the sympathetic innervation to the parotid gland

O   B   Affect the parasympathetic innervation to the submandibular gland

O   C   Affect taste to the anterior third of the tongue

O   D   Result in general sensory deficit to the pharynx

O   E   Result in loss of motor innervation to the risorius muscle

7.6   A young patient sustained fractures to the base of his skull from a high-speed car crash. The patient was ejected from the vehicle because he was not wearing a seat belt. The skull fractures are primarily located along the base of the middle cranial fossa. Neurological examination reveals that the patient has no sense of touch to the skin over his cheek (maxilla) and chin (mandible). Which cranial nerve is normally responsible for sensation to both areas of the face that are affected in this patient?

O   A   Abducens

O   B   Trigeminal

O   C   Facial

O   D   Glossopharyngeal

O   E   Hypoglossal

brain

7.7 **A young patient sustained fractures to the base of his skull from a high-speed car crash. The patient was ejected from the vehicle because he was not wearing a seat belt. The skull fractures are primarily located along the base of the middle cranial fossa. Neurological examination reveals that the patient has no sense of touch to the skin over his cheek (maxilla) and chin (mandible). Where are the cell bodies of the affected general sensory nerves located?**

○ A Cranial nerve I ganglion
○ B Cranial nerve VII ganglion
○ C Cranial nerve VIII ganglion
○ D Cranial nerve X ganglion
○ E Cranial nerve V ganglion

7.8 **Which cranial nerve innervates a muscle that is contained in the palatoglossal arch?**

○ A XII
○ B X
○ C VIII
○ D IX
○ E VII

7.9 **The posterior communicating artery of the cerebral arterial circle (of Willis) directly connects the posterior cerebral artery to the:**

O A Anterior communicating artery
O B Ophthalmic artery
O C Internal carotid artery
O D Anterior cerebral artery
O E Vertebral artery

7.10 **To test for trochlear nerve (cranial nerve IV) damage, have the patient gaze:**

O A In (medially), then down
O B In, then up
O C Out (laterally), then down
O D Out, then up
O E In, then out

7.11 **Which of the following muscles is innervated by cranial nerve XII?**

O A Geniohyoid
O B Mylohyoid
O C Palatoglossus
O D Hyoglossus
O E Stylopharyngeus

brain

7.12 **A computed tomographic scan of a 45-year-old man with a 3-weeks history of headache showed a mass in the roof of the posterior horn of the lateral ventricle. Which structure is likely to be compressed by this mass?**

○ A Caudate nucleus

○ B Ependyma

○ C Fibres of the corpus callosum

○ D Frontal lobe

○ E Thalamus

7.13 **A tumour in the medial wall of the body of the lateral ventricle will involve which of the following structures?**

○ A Caudate nucleus of the corpus striatum

○ B Stria terminalis

○ C Posterior part of the septum pellucidum

○ D Terminal vein

○ E Undersurface of the corpus callosum

7.14 **A 48-year-old woman with a history of persistent headache and occasional vomiting for 4 weeks underwent a computed tomographic scan, which showed a tumour in the floor of the inferior cornu of the lateral ventricle. Which of the following structures is most likely to be compressed by this tumour?**

○ A Inferior surface of the tapetum of the corpus callosum

○ B Hippocampus

○ C Putamen

○ D Stria terminalis

○ E Tail of the caudate nucleus

7.15 A 63-year-old man with long-standing, poorly controlled diabetes and hypertension suddenly suffered a stroke. On clinical examination he had features suggestive of lateral medullary syndrome and a computed tomographic scan showed that he had an extensive infarction of the entire dorsolateral part of the rostral medulla oblongata. Occlusion of which of the following arteries is most likely to affect the entire dorsolateral part of the rostral medulla and produce the lateral medullary syndrome?

- A Anterior inferior cerebellar
- B Anterior spinal
- C Posterior inferior cerebellar
- D Posterior spinal
- E Superior cerebellar

7.16 A 65-year-old man developed a homonymous hemianopia following the stroke. This visual field defect is caused by a lesion of the:

- A Abducent nucleus
- B Oculomotor nucleus
- C Optic chiasma
- D Optic nerve
- E Optic radiation

7.17 A patient with headache was found to have aneurysmal dilatation of the great cerebral vein on computed tomography. The great cerebral vein is formed by the union of the two:

- A Inferior sagittal sinuses
- B Internal cerebral veins
- C Middle cerebral veins
- D Striate veins
- E Superficial cerebral veins

7.18   The superior cerebral veins drain into the:

○ A   Cavernous sinus

○ B   Great cerebral vein

○ C   Inferior petrosal sinus

○ D   Superior petrosal sinus

○ E   Superior sagittal sinus

7.19   A 70-year-old man was brought to A&E following a stroke. A computed tomographic scan showed a cerebral infarction due to right middle cerebral artery thrombosis. Which of the following clinical defects is most likely to be found in this patient?

○ A   Bitemporal hemianopia

○ B   Complete blindness

○ C   Contralateral hemiplegia

○ D   Ipsilateral hemiplegia

○ E   Sensory loss in the ipsilateral face, arm and leg

7.20   A 48-year-old man with a 3-week history of persistent headache and signs of raised intracranial pressure had a computed tomographic scan that showed a tumour in the floor of the fourth ventricle. Which of the following cranial nerve nuclei is most likely to be compressed by this tumour?

○ A   Abducent

○ B   Oculomotor

○ C   Optic

○ D   Spinal accessory

○ E   Trigeminal

SECTION 8:
BACK AND SPINAL CORD – QUESTIONS

For each question given below choose the ONE BEST option.

8.1 **A 25-year-old woman with history of high-grade fever, gradual-onset loss of consciousness and a petechial rash is suspected of having bacterial meningitis. As part of the diagnostic procedure, a lumbar puncture is to be performed. To avoid injury to the spinal cord and nerves you must insert the spinal needle just below the spine of the fourth lumbar vertebra. What anatomical landmark would you use to identify the spine of the fourth lumbar vertebra?**

○ A Pubic symphysis
○ B Iliac crest
○ C Xiphoid process
○ D Iliac tuberosity
○ E Umbilicus

8.2 **An 85-year-old man with prostatic cancer is most likely to have metastatic spread of cancer through which of the following veins?**

○ A Testicular vein
○ B Cephalic vein
○ C Basilic vein
○ D External iliac vein
○ E Internal vertebral venous plexus

8.3 While wandering around in the dark in an unfamiliar home, a visitor accidentally walks into a plate-glass door. The door shatters and a shard of glass severs the posterolateral aspect of the woman's neck. Examination reveals that she is unable to elevate the tip of her shoulder on the injured side. The nerve injured is the:

O   A   Accessory
O   B   Dorsal scapular
O   C   Greater occipital
O   D   Spinal nerve C4
O   E   Thoracodorsal

8.4 A person receives a laceration along the anterior border of the trapezius muscle in the neck and subsequently the point of his shoulder (scapula) sags and he has some difficulty fully abducting his arm. Which nerve appears to have been severed?

O   A   Accessory (cranial nerve XI)
O   B   Axillary
O   C   Dorsal scapular
O   D   Greater occipital
O   E   Suprascapular

8.5 Itching sensation from the skin immediately over the base of the spine of your scapula is mediated through the:

O   A   Accessory nerve
O   B   Dorsal primary ramus of C7
O   C   Dorsal root of T2
O   D   Ventral primary ramus of C7
O   E   Ventral root of T2

8.6 **A patient complains of pain on the lower left side of her back. An X-ray confirms a hernia passing posterolaterally, immediately superior to the iliac crest. This hernia passes through the:**

○ A Lumbar triangle
○ B Triangle of auscultation
○ C Inguinal triangle
○ D Triangle of Calot
○ E Greater sciatic foramen

8.7 **Which of the following effects is most likely to be seen if the right dorsal scapular nerve is injured near its origin?**

○ A Skin of the upper back on the right side would be numb
○ B The point of the right shoulder would droop
○ C Scapular retraction on the right would be weakened
○ D Extension of the right arm would be weakened
○ E Inability to adduct the right arm

8.8. **The transverse cervical artery is severed in a road traffic accident. Which muscle would be affected the most?**

○ A Levator scapulae
○ B Rhomboideus minor
○ C Rhomboideus major
○ D Trapezius
○ E Latissimus dorsi

back and spine

8.9 The cutaneous branch of the posterior primary ramus of C2 is called the:

O   A   Accessory nerve

O   B   Great auricular nerve

O   C   Greater occipital nerve

O   D   Lesser occipital nerve

O   E   Superior ramus of the ansa cervicalis

8.10 Which of the following statements regarding the vertebral column is CORRECT?

O   A   The vertebral column is a rigid column, formed from a series of bones called vertebrae

O   B   The vertebrae are 35 in number

O   C   The vertebrae in the upper three regions of the column are known as true vertebrae

O   D   The vertebrae in the sacral and coccygeal regions are true vertebrae

O   E   The common characteristics of true vertebrae are best studied by examining the first or second cervical vertebrae

8.11 A 25-year-old man fractured his fourth thoracic vertebra following a fall from a 3-m (10-ft) ladder. Which of the following statements regarding a typical thoracic vertebra is CORRECT?

O   A   The anterior segment of a typical thoracic vertebra is called the vertebral arch

O   B   The vertebral arch consists of a pair of pedicles and a pair of laminae

O   C   The body of a typical vertebra supports seven processes

O   D   The spinous processes of adjacent typical thoracic vertebrae enclose the vertebral foramen

O   E   The intervertebral foramina transmit the spinal cord

8.12 **A 62-year-old man with back pain was noted to have metastatic deposits in the bodies of the upper six thoracic vertebrae on computed tomography. The body of a thoracic vertebra:**

○ A Is more or less triangular in shape

○ B Gives attachment to intervertebral fibrocartilages on its sides

○ C In front is concave from side to side and convex from above downward

○ D Has a few small apertures for the passage of nutrient vessels on its anterior surface

○ E Has a single large, irregular aperture on its anterior surface for the exit of the basivertebral veins

8.13 **A rugby player sustained fractures of the transverse and spinous processes of middle three thoracic vertebrae following a rash tackle. Which of the following statements regarding the vertebral processes is CORRECT?**

○ A The spinous process serves for the attachment of muscles and ligaments

○ B There is one superior and one inferior articular process in each typical thoracic vertebra

○ C The articular surfaces on the articular processes are covered with fibrocartilage

○ D The transverse processes provide attachment to intervertebral discs

○ E The transverse processes are lined with hyaline cartilage

back and spine

8.14   A young man suffered a fractured seventh cervical vertebra following a street fight. The seventh cervical vertebra:

○   A   Is called the axis

○   B   Is best identified by the presence of a large body

○   C   Has a shallow sulcus on its transverse process for the seventh cervical nerve

○   D   Has a foramen transversarium for the passage of the vertebral artery

○   E   Sometimes gives rise to a cervical rib from its spinous process

8.15   A disease process has selectively affected the medial group of nuclei in the anterior horn of the spinal cord. The function of which of the following muscles will be affected by this disease process?

○   A   Axial

○   B   Forearm

○   C   Gluteal

○   D   Hand

○   E   Leg

8.16   A disease process has selectively affected cells in a nucleus of the posterior grey column, resulting in loss of pain and temperature sensations. Which of the following nuclei is affected?

○   A   Intermediolateral nucleus

○   B   Nucleus dorsalis

○   C   Nucleus proprius

○   D   Posteromarginal nucleus

○   E   Substantia gelatinosa

8.17 **Which of the following statements regarding the spinal arachnoid mater is CORRECT?**

○ A It is very thick compared with the cranial part
○ B It is separated from the dura by the subarachnoid space
○ C It forms the denticulate ligaments
○ D It invests the cauda equina
○ E It has a rich plexus of nerves derived from the vagus

8.18 **Which of the following statements regarding the ligamentum denticulatum is CORRECT?**

○ A It is a narrow fibrous band situated on either side of the spinal cord limited to the cervical region
○ B It is formed from the dura mater
○ C It separates the anterior from the posterior nerve roots
○ D It has ten tooth-like processes on either side
○ E It is a narrow fibrous band situated on either side of the spinal cord in the lumbar region

8.19 **The arterial circle of Willis is contained in the:**

○ A Cisterna basalis
○ B Cisterna chiasmatis
○ C Cisterna magna
○ D Cisterna pontis
○ E Cisterna venae magnae cerebri

back and spine

8.20 Which of the following statements regarding the subarachnoid cavity (space) is CORRECT?

○   A   It is the interval between the arachnoid and the dura mater

○   B   It is largest at the upper part of the vertebral canal

○   C   It is separated from the cranial subarachnoid cavity by the subarachnoid septum

○   D   It communicates with the general ventricular cavity of the brain by three openings

○   E   The spinal part of the subarachnoid cavity is a very narrow interval

SECTION 9:
DEVELOPMENTAL ANATOMY
– QUESTIONS

For each question given below choose the ONE BEST option.

9.1 Meiosis is essential for sexual reproduction. It therefore occurs in most eukaryotes, including single-celled organisms. In meiosis:

○ A Bivalents, each composed of two chromatids, align at the metaphase plate

○ B Chiasmata separate during anaphase I

○ C Nuclear envelopes may reform during anaphase I

○ D One kinetochore forms per chromatid during prometaphase I

○ E The nuclear membrane disappears during prophase I

9.2 The ovum is the largest cell in the human body, typically visible to the naked eye without the aid of a microscope or other magnification device. The ova:

○ A Are developed from the primitive germ cells which are embedded in the substance of the ovaries

○ B Are released by the rupture of the corona radiata at the time of ovulation

○ C Give rise to oögonia

○ D Measure about 2 mm in diameter

○ E Undergo routine further development after liberation

development

9.3 **A 26-year-old primigravida gave birth to a normal healthy male baby weighing 3 kg (6.5 lbs). Which of the following circulatory changes would normally occur immediately at birth in this baby?**

○ A Decreased blood flow through the lungs

○ B Increased flow through the ductus arteriosus

○ C Increased left atrial pressure

○ D Increased right atrial pressure

○ E Reversal of flow through the foramen ovale

9.4 **A 28-year-old primigravida is 36 weeks pregnant. A 20-week anomaly scan suggested that the fetus was normal. Which of the following peculiarities is most likely to be found in the cardiovascular system in the fetus?**

○ A In early fetal life, the heart lies immediately below the mandibular arch and is relatively large

○ B Just before birth, the walls of the ventricles are of equal thickness

○ C There is a direct communication between the atria through the foramen primum

○ D The Eustachian valve of the inferior vena cava is small

○ E The proportion of the heart size compared with the rest of the body at the second month is 1 to 160

9.5 **Mesonephric tubules are genital ridges next to the developing mesonephros in a fetus. Mesonephric tubules give rise to:**

○ A Appendix of epididymis

○ B Appendix of testis

○ C Efferent ductules

○ D Rete testis

○ E Seminiferous tubules

development

9.6 **In the development of humans, the branchial arches develop during the fourth and fifth week in utero as a series of mesodermal outpouchings on the either sides of the developing pharynx. The second branchial arch gives rise to the:**

○ A Anterior belly of the digastric muscle
○ B Incus
○ C Lesser horn of the hyoid bone
○ D Malleus
○ E Mylohyoid

9.7 **The sinus venosus is the large quadrangular cavity located between the two vena cava vessels in the embryonic human heart. In the adult heart the sinus venosus gives rise to the:**

○ A Aortic vestibule of the left ventricle
○ B Coronary sinus
○ C Fossa ovalis
○ D Trabeculated part of the right ventricle
○ E Trabeculated portion of the right atrium

9.8 **The human embryonic heart rate is nearly twice that of the adult. Which of the following statements regarding the development of the human heart is CORRECT?**

○ A In the second week, the endocardial tubes begin to fuse to form a single tube
○ B The septum primum appears in the eighth week
○ C The heart begins to beat in the fourth week
○ D The primordium of the heart forms in the cardiogenic plate located at the caudal end of the embryo
○ E The bulboventricular loop is formed in the sixth week

development

175

9.9   **Horseshoe kidney is a congenital disorder, affecting about 1 in 500 to 1 in 600 people, in which a person's two kidneys fuse together to form a horseshoe shape. This is the most common type of fusion anomaly in the kidneys. Which of the following statements regarding the development of the kidney is CORRECT?**

○   A   Metanephric glomeruli are derived from a distal (caudal) dorsal region of the mesoderm

○   B   The kidney is derived from the inner embryonic layer or endoderm

○   C   The metanephros is a rudimentary kidney that develops first during vertebrate embryogenesis

○   D   The pronephros evolves from the mid-dorsal region of the mesoderm

○   E   The metanephric ureters, renal pelvis, renal calyces and renal tubules develop as outpouchings of paramesonephric duct remnants

9.10   **The ectoderm is the outermost of the germ layers of the embryo. Which of the following organs is a derivative of the ectoderm?**

○   A   Adrenal cortex
○   B   Adrenal medulla
○   C   Gonads
○   D   Kidney
○   E   Mesothelium

development

9.11 **In human development, week 3 to week 8 is known as the embryonic period. Which of the following changes occur during the fourth week of intrauterine life?**

O   A   Hair follicles are formed

O   B   The heart tube is formed

O   C   The lungs are formed

O   D   Spontaneous limb movements can be detected by ultrasound

O   E   The hands and feet have digits

9.12 **Endoderm is one of the germ layers formed during embryogenesis. Which of the following organs is a derivative of the endoderm?**

O   A   Adrenal medulla

O   B   Dermis of the skin

O   C   Epithelial part of the tympanic cavity

O   D   Gonads

O   E   Lens

9.13 **Each branchial (pharyngeal) arch has a cartilaginous bar, a muscle component that differentiates from the cartilaginous tissue, an artery and a cranial nerve. The first pharyngeal (branchial) arch:**

O   A   Gives rise to the styloid process and hyoid bone

O   B   Gives rise to the palatine tonsil

O   C   Gives rise to the muscles of facial expression

O   D   Gives rise to the sphenomandibular ligament

O   E   Is innervated by the glossopharyngeal nerve

development

9.14 **In the embryo, the midgut bends around the superior mesenteric artery to form the 'midgut loop'. Which of the following organs is a derivative of the midgut?**

○ A Biliary system

○ B Caecum

○ C Liver

○ D Pancreas

○ E Sigmoid colon

9.15 **The circulatory system of a human fetus works differently from that of born humans. In the fetal circulation:**

○ A The ductus arteriosus receives blood from the pulmonary artery

○ B The ductus venosus receives blood from the pulmonary artery

○ C Oxygenated blood is mostly in the inferior vena cava

○ D The pulmonary artery carries oxygenated blood

○ E Right ventricular blood passes through the left ventricle

9.16 **The circulatory system of a human fetus works differently from that of born humans, mainly because the lungs are not in use. Which of the following peculiarities is most likely to be found in the cardiovascular system in the fetus?**

○ A The foramen ovale, situated at the upper part of the atrial septum, forms a free communication between the atria until the end of fetal life

○ B The valve of the inferior vena cava serves to direct the blood from that vessel through the foramen ovale into the left atrium

○ C The ductus arteriosus is a long tube, about 3 cm in length at birth

○ D The ductus arteriosus conducts the greater amount of the blood from the left ventricle into the aorta

○ E The hypogastric arteries convey blood from the placenta to the fetus

9.17 **Which of the following statements regarding the development of the neural groove and tube is CORRECT?**

○ A The coalescence of the neural folds occurs first in the region of the forebrain

○ B The endodermal wall of the neural tube forms the rudiment of the nervous system

○ C The neurenteric canal is a transitory communication between the neural tube and the primitive digestive tube

○ D The neuroglial elements of the medulla spinalis are developed from mesoderm

○ E The rhombencephalon is a primary brain vesicle that develops into the forebrain

9.18 **The branchial arches (or pharyngeal arches) develop during the fourth and fifth week in utero as a series of mesodermal outpouchings on either side of the developing pharynx. The first branchial arch:**

○ A Lies between the first branchial groove and the proctodeum

○ B Gives rise to the medial part of the upper lip

○ C Gives rise to the muscles of facial expression

○ D Gives rise to the anterior part of the tongue

○ E Gives rise to the stapes

development

9.19 Which of the following statements regarding the branchial arches is CORRECT?

○ A The cartilage of the third arch gives origin to the greater cornu of the hyoid bone

○ B The cartilage of the fifth arch gives origin to the cricoid and arytenoid cartilages

○ C The second arch gives rise to the incus

○ D The stapes arises in the upper part of the third arch

○ E The ventral portions of the cartilages of the fourth and fifth arches unite to form the thyroid cartilage

9.20 The yolk sac is the first element seen in the gestational sac during pregnancy, usually at 5 weeks' gestation. The yolk sac:

○ A Is situated on the dorsal aspect of the embryo

○ B Is lined by ectoderm, outside of which is a layer of mesoderm

○ C Is filled with amniotic fluid

○ D Opens into the digestive tube by a long narrow tube, the vitelline duct

○ E Persists as Meckel's diverticulum in about 3% of cases

9.21 The allantois:

○ A Arises as a tubular diverticulum of the anterior part of the yolk sac

○ B Assumes the form of a vesicle outside the embryo in man

○ C Grows out into the body stalk, which is an ectodermal structure

○ D Is absent in reptiles and birds

○ E Is carried backward with the development of the hind-gut and then opens into the cloaca or terminal part of the hindgut

development

9.22 **The amnion is a membranous sac that surrounds and protects the embryo. The amnion:**

O   A   Contains liquor amnii by about the fourth week of development

O   B   Contains fluid which contains 20% solids

O   C   Contains about 2 litres of fluid at the end of pregnancy

O   D   Is well developed in fish and amphibia

O   E   Is a closed sac lined by endoderm

9.23 **The umbilicus is a scar on the abdomen caused when the umbilical cord is removed from a newborn baby. The umbilical cord:**

O   A   Attaches the fetus to the allantois

O   B   Contains a pair of umbilical arteries and a pair of umbilical veins at birth

O   C   Is contained inside the body stalk

O   D   Is covered by a layer of endoderm

O   E   Is filled with jelly of Wharton

9.24 **The placenta has a fetal and a maternal portion. The fetal portion of the placenta:**

O   A   Consists of the villi of the chorion laeve

O   B   Contains villi which are covered with endoderm

O   C   Contains villi the vessels of which are surrounded by a thin layer of mesoderm consisting of gelatinous connective tissue

O   D   Contains villi that only have cytotrophoblast after the third month of pregnancy

O   E   Contains villi that only have syncytiotrophoblast after the second month of pregnancy

development

9.25 A 26-year-old primigravida aborted a 4-week-old embryo. On gross examination:

◯   A   Differentiation of the limbs into their segments has occurred

◯   B   The cerebral hemispheres appear as hollow buds

◯   C   The cloacal tubercle is evident

◯   D   The embryo is less curved and the head is relatively large

◯   E   The nose forms a short, flattened projection

9.26 A 26-year-old primigravida aborted a 5-week-old embryo. On gross examination:

◯   A   The embryo is markedly curved on itself

◯   B   The elevations that form the rudiments of the auricula are visible

◯   C   The primitive segments number about 30

◯   D   The limbs appear as oval flattened projections

◯   E   The cloacal tubercle is evident

9.27 A 25-year-old primigravida aborted a 2-month-old embryo. On gross examination:

◯   A   The eyelids are present in the shape of folds above and below the eye

◯   B   The different parts of the auricula are not distinguishable

◯   C   The lower lip is completed

◯   D   The neck is fully developed

◯   E   The palate is completely developed

development

9.28 A 26-year-old primigravida aborted a 4-month-old fetus secondary to massive antepartum haemorrhage. Normally during the fourth month of development of the human fetus:

○ A The first movements of the fetus are usually observed

○ B The hair on the head are fully formed

○ C The loop of gut that projected into the umbilical cord is withdrawn within the fetus

○ D The total length of the fetus, including the legs, is from 25 to 27 cm

○ E The vernix caseosa begins to be deposited

9.29 A 36-year-old diabetic primigravida gave birth to a 7-month-old premature baby. Normally during the seventh month of fetal development:

○ A The skin assumes a pink colour

○ B The testis descends with the vaginal sac of the peritoneum

○ C The lanugo begins to disappear

○ D The total length from head to heels is about 40 cm

○ E The weight varies between 2 kg and 2.5 kg (4.5–5.5 lb)

9.30 In a baby born during the ninth month of gestation:

○ A The baby measures from head to heels about 90 cm

○ B The baby weighs from 3 kg to 3.5 kg (6.5–8 lb)

○ C The trunk is covered by lanugo hair

○ D The testes are in the abdomen

○ E The umbilicus is in the lower half of the body

development

9.31 **The branchial arches (or pharyngeal arches) develop during the fourth and fifth week in utero as a series of mesodermal outpouchings on either side of the developing pharynx. The second pharyngeal arch gives rise to the:**

    ○ A Anterior belly of the digastric

    ○ B Genioglossus muscle

    ○ C Geniohyoid muscle

    ○ D Stylohyoid muscle

    ○ E Stylopharyngeus muscle

9.32 **Which of the following statements regarding the aortic arches is CORRECT?**

    ○ A The dorsal end of the first aortic arch gives origin to the stapedial artery

    ○ B The fourth left aortic arch constitutes the left subclavian artery

    ○ C The fourth right aortic arch forms the right subclavian as far as the origin of its internal mammary branch

    ○ D The left fifth aortic arch gives rise to the ductus arteriosus

    ○ E The third aortic arch constitutes the commencement of the external carotid artery

9.33 **Which of the following statements regarding the development of the tongue is CORRECT?**

    ○ A The copula and hypobranchial eminence give rise to the oral part of the tongue

    ○ B The epithelial and mucosal tissues of the tongue develop from the occipital cervical somites

    ○ C The median tongue bud appears in the fifth week of development

    ○ D The mesenchyme of the pharyngeal arches forms connective tissue, and lymphatic and blood vessels of the tongue

    ○ E The tongue is fully covered with ectodermal epithelium

development

9.34 **Which of the following statements regarding the development of the pancreas is CORRECT?**

O   A   The dorsal pancreatic bud arises as a diverticulum from the dorsal aspect of the duodenum a short distance below the hepatic diverticulum

O   B   The duct of the dorsal part opens with the common bile duct

O   C   The pancreas develops between the two layers of the ventral mesogastrium

O   D   The pancreas is ectodermal in origin

O   E   The ventral pancreatic bud forms part of the head and uncinate process of the pancreas

9.35 **Which of the following statements regarding the development of the pituitary gland is CORRECT?**

O   A   The anterior pituitary gland develops from endoderm of the roof of the mouth

O   B   The stroma of the anterior pituitary gland is endodermal in origin

O   C   The posterior lobe of the pituitary is neuroectodermal in origin

O   D   The posterior lobe of the pituitary develops as a downward diverticulum of the floor of the midbrain

O   E   The pouch of Rathke is the rudiment of the posterior lobe of the hypophysis

development

9.36 Which of the following statements regarding the development of the liver is CORRECT?

O A The liver arises as a diverticulum from the dorsal surface of the descending part of the duodenum

O B The parenchyma of the liver is mesodermal in origin

O C The hepatic sinusoids are derived from the umbilical arteries

O D The anterior part of the ventral mesogastrium forms the falciform and coronary ligaments

O E Near the end of fetal life the left and right lobes of the liver are almost equal in size

9.37 Which of the following statements regarding the development of the thyroid gland is CORRECT?

O A The stroma of the thyroid gland is endodermal in origin

O B The parenchyma of the thyroid gland is ectodermal in origin

O C The thyroid diverticulum appears about the sixth week

O D The thyroid hormone-secreting cells are derived from the ultimobranchial bodies

O E The thyroid gland is developed from a median diverticulum that appears on the summit of the tuberculum impar

9.38 Normal herniation of the gut in fetus:

O A Involves only small intestine

O B Involves only large intestine

O C Is accompanied by anticlockwise rotation of the herniated gut loop

O D Occurs during the fourth to sixth months of intrauterine life

O E Results in rotation of the stomach

9.39 **A full-term baby boy is born with incomplete fusion of the embryonic endocardial cushions in the heart. The baby is most likely to have:**

○ A An atrioventricular septal defect

○ B Coarctation of the aorta

○ C Pulmonary stenosis

○ D Tetralogy of Fallot

○ E Transposition of the great arteries

9.40 **A 2-year-old boy is brought to the paediatric emergency department because he has had several episodes of rectal bleeding. On evaluation he is diagnosed to have a 3-cm ileal outpouching located 0.6 m (2 ft) from the ileocaecal valve. This structure most commonly contains which type of ectopic tissue?**

○ A Duodenal

○ B Gastric

○ C Hepatic

○ D Jejunal

○ E Oesophageal

development

ANSWERS

SECTION 1:
UPPER LIMB AND BREAST –
ANSWERS

1.1

Answer: C   Serratus anterior

Serratus anterior is innervated by the long thoracic nerve. Serratus anterior keeps the scapula held forward, balancing trapezius and the rhomboids, which retract the scapula. If the long thoracic nerve is injured (which is common in surgery, because the long thoracic nerve is on the superficial side of serratus anterior), you may see a 'winged scapula' protruding posteriorly. The anterior scalene muscle is innervated by C5–C7 and the middle scalene muscle is innervated by C3–C8. Teres major is innervated by the lower subscapular nerve from the posterior cord of the brachial plexus. Subscapularis is innervated by the upper and lower subscapular nerves from the posterior cord of the brachial plexus.

1.2

Answer: B   The top of the shoulder and the lateral side of the arm

The C5 and C6 dermatomes cover the top of the shoulder and lateral side of the arm. The T1 and C8 dermatomes cover the medial side of the arm, with C8 extending to the tip of the little finger. The back of the shoulder is covered by numerous dermatomes, including C6, C7, C8 and T1. Finally, the pectoral region is covered by T1, T2 and T3 dermatomes.

1.3

Answer: E   Triceps brachii

The olecranon process is a large, thick, curved prominence, situated at the posterosuperior aspect of the ulna. It is bent forward at the summit so as to present a prominent lip that lodges into the olecranon fossa of the humerus when the forearm is extended. Its base is narrowed where it joins the body and the narrowest part of the upper end of the ulna. It has a subcutaneous triangular posterior surface, which is smooth and covered by a bursa. Its quadrilateral superior surface has a rough impression for the insertion of the triceps brachii posteriorly and a slight transverse groove for the attachment of part of the posterior ligament of the elbow joint anteriorly. It has a smooth, concave anterior surface that forms the upper part of the semilunar notch. Its medial border provides attachment to the back part of the ulnar collateral ligament and a part of the flexor carpi ulnaris. The posterior ligament and the anconeus are attached to the lateral border.

The brachialis is inserted into the coronoid process of ulna while pronator teres, flexor digitorum profundus and flexor pollicis longus take origin from the coronoid process.

1.4

Answer: D   Thoracodorsal nerve

The thoracodorsal nerve, a branch of the posterior cord of the plexus, derives its fibres from the fifth, sixth and seventh cervical nerves. It follows the course of the subscapular artery, along the posterior wall of the axilla to the latissimus dorsi, in which it can be traced as far as the lower border of the muscle. Latissimus dorsi is responsible for extension of the humerus and in this scenario it is the affected muscle due to injury to the thoracodorsal nerve.

1.5

Answer: A   Encircles the head of the radius

The annular ligament is a strong band of fibres, which encircles the head of the radius and retains it in contact with the radial notch of the ulna. It forms about four-fifths of the osseofibrous ring and is attached to the anterior and posterior margins of the radial notch. A few of its lower fibres are continued around below the radial notch and form at this level a complete fibrous ring. Its upper border blends with the anterior and posterior ligaments of the elbow, while from its lower border a thin, loose membrane passes to be attached to the neck of the radius. A thickened band that extends from the inferior border of the annular ligament below the radial notch to the neck of the radius is known as the 'quadrate ligament'. The superficial surface of the annular ligament is strengthened by the radial collateral ligament of the elbow and affords origin to part of the supinator. Its deep surface is smooth and lined by synovial membrane, which is continuous with that of the elbow joint.

1.6

Answer: B   Elbow joint

The branches of the brachial artery are:

- Profunda brachii
- Superior ulnar collateral
- Inferior ulnar collateral
- Muscular
- Nutrient.

The vessels engaged in the anastomosis around the elbow joint can be conveniently divided into those situated in front of and those behind the medial and lateral epicondyles of the humerus. The branches anastomosing in front of the medial epicondyle are the anterior branch of the inferior ulnar collateral, the anterior ulnar recurrent and the anterior branch of the superior ulnar collateral. Those behind the medial epicondyle are the inferior ulnar collateral, the posterior ulnar recurrent and the posterior branch of the superior

upper limb

ulnar collateral. The branches anastomosing in front of the lateral epicondyle are the radial recurrent and the terminal part of the profunda brachii. Those behind the lateral epicondyle (perhaps more properly described as being situated between the lateral epicondyle and the olecranon) are the inferior ulnar collateral, the interosseous recurrent and the radial collateral branch of the profunda brachii. There is also an arch of anastomosis above the olecranon, formed by the interosseous recurrent joining with the inferior ulnar collateral and posterior ulnar recurrent.

1.7

Answer: D   Initiation of abduction of the humerus

The supraspinatus occupies the whole of the supraspinatus fossa, arising from its medial two-thirds and from the strong supraspinatus fascia. The muscular fibres converge to a tendon, which crosses the upper part of the shoulder joint and is inserted into the highest of the three impressions on the greater tubercle of the humerus. The tendon is intimately adherent to the capsule of the shoulder joint. The supraspinatus is supplied by the fifth and sixth cervical nerves through the suprascapular nerve. The supraspinatus assists the deltoid in raising the arm from the side of the trunk (initiating abduction of the humerus) and fixes the head of the humerus in the glenoid cavity.

1.8

Answer: C   Accompanies the long thoracic nerve to the serratus anterior muscle

The lateral thoracic artery, accompanied by the long thoracic nerve, follows the lower border of the pectoralis minor to the side of the chest, supplying the serratus anterior and the pectoralis and sending branches across the axilla to the axillary glands and subscapularis. It anastomoses with the internal mammary, subscapular and intercostal arteries and with the pectoral branch of the thoracoacromial. In women, it supplies an external mammary branch, which turns round the free edge of the pectoralis major and supplies the breast.

1.9

Answer: A   Pectoralis minor

The pectoralis minor is a thin, triangular muscle, situated at the upper part of the thorax, beneath the pectoralis major. It arises from the upper margins and outer surfaces of the third, fourth and fifth ribs, near their cartilage and from the aponeurosis covering the intercostals. The fibres pass upward and lateralward and converge to form a flat tendon, which is inserted into the medial border and upper surface of the coracoid process of the scapula. The pectoralis minor receives its fibres from the eighth cervical and first thoracic nerves through the medial anterior thoracic nerve. The pectoralis minor depresses the point of the shoulder (glenoid fossa), drawing the scapula downward and medialward toward the thorax and throwing the inferior angle backward.

1.10

Answer: A   Flexor digitorum superficialis

The superficial group of muscles of the forearm takes origin from the medial epicondyle of the humerus by a common tendon. They receive additional fibres from the deep fascia of the forearm near the elbow and from the septa, which pass from this fascia between the individual muscles. These muscles include pronator teres, palmaris longus, flexor carpi radialis, flexor carpi ulnaris and flexor digitorum superficialis.

1.11

Answer: C   Extensor carpi radialis brevis and flexor carpi radialis

Abduction (radial flexion) at the wrist joint is brought about by the abductor pollicis longus, the extensors of the thumb and the extensors carpi radialis longus and brevis and the flexor carpi radialis.

upper limb

1.12

Answer: D   All of the adductors of the digits take at least part of their attachments from metacarpal bones

The four palmar interossei are smaller than the dorsal interossei. They lie on the palmar surfaces of the metacarpal bones rather than between them. Each palmar interosseous arises from the entire length of the metacarpal bone of one finger, and is inserted into the side of the base of the first phalanx and the aponeurotic expansion of the extensor digitorum communis tendon to the same finger. All the interossei are innervated by the eighth cervical nerve, through the deep palmar branch of the ulnar nerve. The palmar interossei adduct the fingers to an imaginary line drawn longitudinally through the centre of the middle finger.

1.13

Answer: A   Ulnar nerve

The ulnar nerve arises from the medial cord of the brachial plexus and derives its fibres from the eighth cervical and first thoracic nerves. It supplies all the palmar interossei, which adduct the fingers to an imaginary line drawn longitudinally through the centre of the middle finger.

1.14

Answer: D   Lateral pectoral

The lateral pectoral nerve arises from the lateral cord of the brachial plexus and through it from the fifth, sixth and seventh cervical nerves. It passes across the axillary artery and vein, pierces the coracoclavicular fascia and is distributed to the deep surface of the pectoralis major. It sends a filament to join the medial pectoral nerve and form with it a loop in front of the first part of the axillary artery.

upper limb

1.15

Answer: C   The hypothenar muscles would be completely paralysed

The hypothenar muscles include the palmaris brevis, opponens digiti minimi, abductor digiti minimi and flexor digiti minimi brevis. All the muscles of this group are supplied by the eighth cervical nerve through the ulnar nerve and will be completely paralysed in a lesion at spinal level C8.

1.16

Answer: E   Tendon of the long head of the biceps brachii muscle

The greater and lesser tubercles are separated from each other by a deep groove, the intertubercular groove (bicipital groove), which lodges the long tendon of the biceps brachii and transmits a branch of the anterior humeral circumflex artery to the shoulder joint. It runs obliquely downward and ends near the junction of the upper with the middle third of the bone. In the fresh state, its upper part is covered with a thin layer of cartilage, lined by a prolongation of the synovial membrane of the shoulder joint. Its lower portion gives insertion to the tendon of the latissimus dorsi. It is deep and narrow above and becomes shallow and a little broader as it descends. Its lips are called the crests of the greater and lesser tubercles (bicipital ridges) and form the upper parts of the anterior and medial borders of the body of the bone.

1.17

Answer: C   Brachial

The superior ulnar collateral artery, of small size, arises from the brachial artery a little below the middle of the arm. It pierces the medial intermuscular septum and descends on the surface of the medial head of the triceps brachii to the space between the medial epicondyle and the olecranon, accompanied by the ulnar nerve, and ends under the flexor carpi ulnaris by anastomosing with the posterior ulnar recurrent and inferior ulnar collateral. It sometimes sends a branch in front of the medial epicondyle to anastomose with the anterior ulnar recurrent.

1.18

Answer: D   Form the trunks of the brachial plexus

The brachial plexus is formed by the union of the anterior divisions (primary ventral rami) of the lower four cervical nerves and the greater part of the anterior division of the first thoracic nerve. The fourth cervical usually gives a branch to the fifth cervical and the first thoracic frequently receives one from the second thoracic. The plexus extends from the lower part of the side of the neck to the axilla. The nerves that form it are nearly equal in size, but their mode of communication is subject to some variation. The following is, however, the most constant arrangement. The fifth and sixth cervical unite soon after their exit from the intervertebral foramina to form a trunk. The eighth cervical and first thoracic also unite to form one trunk, while the seventh cervical runs out alone. Three trunks – upper, middle and lower – are so formed and, as they pass beneath the clavicle, each splits into an anterior and a posterior division. The anterior divisions of the upper and middle trunks unite to form a cord, which is situated on the lateral side of the second part of the axillary artery and is called the lateral cord or fasciculus of the plexus. The anterior division of the lower trunk passes down on the medial side of the axillary artery and forms the medial cord or fasciculus of the brachial plexus. The posterior divisions of all three trunks unite to form the posterior cord or fasciculus of the plexus, which is situated behind the second portion of the axillary artery.

1.19

Answer: B   Pronator teres

Pronator teres has two heads of origin. The larger and more superficial humeral head has a wider origin. It arises immediately above the medial epicondyle, and from the tendon common to the origin of the other muscles; it also arises from the intermuscular septum between it and the flexor carpi radialis and from the antebrachial fascia. The ulnar head, much smaller than the humeral head, arises from the medial side of the coronoid process of the ulna, and joins the humeral head at an acute angle. The median nerve enters the forearm between the two heads of the muscle, and is separated from the ulnar artery by the ulnar head. The muscle passes obliquely across the forearm, and ends in a flat tendon, which is inserted into a rough impression at the middle of the lateral surface of the body of the radius. The lateral border of the muscle forms the medial boundary of the cubital fossa, which contains the brachial artery, the median nerve, and the tendon of the biceps brachii muscle. Pronator teres is supplied by the median nerve, primarily from the sixth cervical nerve. Pronator teres rotates the radius on the ulna at the proximal radioulnar joint, moving the hand into a prone position; when the radius is fixed, it assists in flexing the forearm.

1.20

Answer: E   It prevents the tendons of the posterior compartment of the forearm from 'bowstringing' when the hand is extended at the wrist

The extensor tendons are held closely applied to the dorsal surface of the distal radius and ulna by the extensor retinaculum. This is a ribbon-like fascial band, 2.5 cm wide, that extends obliquely from the anterolateral surface of the radius across the dorsum of the wrist, inserting into the pisiform and triquetral bones, but not directly into the ulna. The radius and carpus are free to rotate about the ulna without affecting tension in the extensor retinaculum. The extensor retinaculum prevents bowstringing of the extensor tendons with wrist extension, and bony attachments of the retinaculum produce six extensor compartments that control the tendons with wrist movement.

1.21

Answer: D   Anterior aspect of the elbow

The veins of the arm carry blood from the extremities of the limb, as well as drain the arm itself. The two main veins are the basilic and the cephalic veins. There is a connecting vein between the two, the median cubital vein, which passes through the cubital fossa on the anterior aspect of the elbow and is clinically important for venepuncture (withdrawing blood). The median nerve and brachial artery are the deep relations of the median cubital vein and can be damaged during venous access.

1.22

Answer: C   Olecranon process of the ulna

The olecranon is a large, thick, curved eminence, situated at the upper and back part of the ulna. It is bent forward at the summit to present a prominent lip, which is received into the olecranon fossa of the humerus in extension of the forearm. Its base is contracted where it joins the body and the narrowest part of the upper end of the ulna. Its posterior surface, directed backward, is triangular, smooth, subcutaneous and covered by a bursa. Its superior surface is of quadrilateral form, marked behind by a rough impression for the insertion of the triceps brachii. In front, near the margin, it is marked by a slight transverse groove for the attachment of part of the posterior ligament of the elbow joint. Its anterior surface is smooth, concave and forms the upper part of the semilunar notch. Its borders present continuations of the groove on the margin of the superior surface; they serve as ligament attachments, viz. the back part of the ulnar collateral ligament medially and the posterior ligament laterally. Part of the flexor carpi ulnaris arises from the medial border, while the anconeus is attached to the lateral border (see also *Answer* to **1.3**).

1.23

Answer: D   Teres minor

The rotator cuff is an anatomical term given to the group of muscles and their tendons that act to stabilise the shoulder. These muscles arise from the scapula and connect to the head of the humerus, forming a cuff at shoulder joint. They are important because they hold the head of the humerus in the small and shallow glenoid fossa of the scapula. The shoulder joint (glenohumeral joint) is often compared to a golf ball sitting on a golf tee. During elevation of the arm, the rotator cuff compresses the glenohumeral joint to allow the large deltoid muscle to elevate the arm further. In other words, without the rotator cuff, the humeral head would partially ride up out of the glenoid fossa and the efficiency of the deltoid muscle would be much reduced. The four muscles that comprise this group are:

- Supraspinatus, originating from the supraspinous fossa of the scapula, which abducts the arm

- Infraspinatus, originating from the infraspinous fossa of the scapula, which laterally rotates the arm

- Teres minor, originating in the lateral border of the scapula, which laterally rotates the arm

- Subscapularis, originating from the subscapular fossa of the scapula, which medially rotates the humerus.

A mnemonic to help remember which muscles form the rotator cuff is SITS (supraspinatus, infraspinatus, teres minor, subscapularis) – someone with a rotator cuff injury SITS out.

1.24

Answer: C   Scaphoid

The scaphoid bone is the largest bone in the proximal row of carpal bones. Its name is derived from its fancied resemblance to a boat. It is situated at the radial side of the wrist. Its long axis is directed from above downward, laterally and forward. Its convex, triangular superior surface is smooth, and articulates with the lower end of the radius. The inferior surface, directed downward, laterally and backward, is also smooth, convex, and triangular. It is divided by a slight ridge into two parts, the lateral articulating with the trapezium, the medial with the trapezoid. On the dorsal surface is a narrow, rough groove, which runs the entire length of the bone, and serves for the attachment of ligaments. The palmar surface is concave above, and elevated at its lower and lateral part into a rounded projection, the tubercle, which is directed forward and gives attachment to the transverse carpal ligament and sometimes gives origin to a few fibres of the abductor pollicis brevis. The lateral surface is rough and narrow. It gives attachment to the radial collateral ligament of the wrist. The medial surface presents two articular facets; of these, the semilunar, superior or smaller, flattened facet articulates with the lunate bone; the concave, inferior or larger facet forms with the lunate a concavity for the head of the capitate bone. It articulates with five bones: the radius proximally, the trapezium and trapezoid distally, and the capitate and lunate medially. It is commonly fractured in falls on the outstretched hand.

1.25

Answer: B   Hinge

The elbow joint is a ginglymus or hinge joint. The trochlea of the humerus is received into the semilunar notch of the ulna and the capitulum of the humerus articulates with the fovea on the head of the radius. The articular surfaces are connected by a capsule, which is thickened medially and laterally and, to a lesser extent, in front and behind. These thickened portions are usually described as distinct ligaments under the following names: anterior ligament, posterior ligament, ulnar collateral ligament and radial collateral ligament.

1.26

Answer: D   Lower subscapular

The lower subscapular nerve supplies the lower part of the subscapularis, which inserts onto the crest of the lesser tubercle of the humerus and ends in the teres major. The latter muscle is sometimes supplied by a separate branch.

1.27

Answer: B   Flexion in the distal interphalangeal joint of digit 5

The ulnar nerve runs along the medial side of the limb and is distributed to the muscles and skin of the forearm and hand. It arises from the medial cord of the brachial plexus and derives its fibres from the eighth cervical and first thoracic nerves. It is smaller than the median nerve and lies at first behind it, but diverges from it in its course down the arm. At its origin, it lies medial to the axillary artery and bears the same relation to the brachial artery as far as the middle of the arm. Here it pierces the medial intermuscular septum, runs obliquely across the medial head of the triceps brachii and descends to the groove between the medial epicondyle and the olecranon, accompanied by the superior ulnar collateral artery. At the elbow, it lies on the back of the medial epicondyle and enters the forearm between the two heads of the flexor carpi ulnaris. Injury at the level of the medial epicondyle will damage the supply to flexor carpi ulnaris and the ulnar half of the flexor digitorum profundus as well as the palmar interossei and hypothenar muscles in the hand. Of the options given in the vignette, flexion in the distal interphalangeal joint of digit 5 will be affected by this injury (see also *Answer* to **1.13**).

1.28

Answer: A   Latissimus dorsi

The latissimus dorsi is a triangular, flat muscle, which covers the lumbar region and the lower half of the thoracic region and is gradually contracted into a narrow fasciculus at its insertion into the humerus. It forms the posterior wall of the axilla along with the scapula. It arises by tendinous fibres from the spinous processes of the lower six thoracic vertebrae and from the posterior layer of the lumbodorsal fascia, by which it is attached to the spines of the lumbar and sacral vertebrae, to the supraspinal ligament and to the posterior part of the crest of the ilium. It also arises by muscular fibres from the external lip of the crest of the ilium lateral to the margin of the sacrospinalis and from the three or four lower ribs by fleshy digitations, which are interposed between similar processes of the external oblique. From this extensive origin, the fibres pass in different directions, the upper ones horizontally, the middle fibres obliquely upward and the lower fibres vertically upward, to converge and form a thick fasciculus, which crosses the inferior angle of the scapula and usually receives a few fibres from it. The muscle curves around the lower border of the teres major and is twisted upon itself, so that the superior fibres become at first posterior and then inferior and the vertical fibres at first anterior and then superior. It ends in a quadrilateral tendon, about 7 cm long, which passes in front of the tendon of the teres major and is inserted into the bottom of the intertubercular groove of the humerus. Its insertion extends higher on the humerus than that of the tendon of the pectoralis major. The lower border of its tendon is united with that of the teres major, the surfaces of the two being separated near their insertions by a bursa. Another bursa is sometimes interposed between the muscle and the inferior angle of the scapula. The tendon of the muscle gives off an expansion to the deep fascia of the arm. It is supplied by the sixth, seventh and eighth cervical nerves through the thoracodorsal (long subscapular) nerve. When the latissimus dorsi acts on the humerus,

upper limb

it depresses and draws it backward and at the same time rotates it inward. It is the muscle that is principally employed in giving a downward blow, as in felling a tree or in sabre practice. If the arm is fixed, the muscle can act in various ways on the trunk. It can raise the lower ribs and assist in forcible inspiration or, if both arms are fixed, the two muscles can assist the abdominal muscles and intercostal in suspending and drawing the trunk forward, as in climbing.

1.29

Answer: C   C5, C6, C7, C8 and T1

The posterior divisions of all three trunks – upper, middle, lower – of the brachial plexus unite to form the posterior cord or fasciculus of the plexus, which is situated behind the second portion of the axillary artery. The posterior cord of the brachial plexus contains nerve fibres from C5, C6, C7, C8 and T1. The posterior cord gives rise to thoracodorsal nerve (C5, 6, 7), axillary nerve (C5, 6) and radial nerve (C5, 6, 7, 8, T1).

1.30

Answer: A   Subclavian – axillary – subscapular –thoracodorsal

The artery that supplies the upper extremity continues as a single trunk from its commencement down to the elbow. Different portions are called different names, depending on the regions through which they pass. That part of the vessel that extends from its origin to the outer border of the first rib is termed the subclavian. Beyond this point to the lower border of the axilla it is named the axillary and from the lower margin of the axillary space to the bend of the elbow it is termed brachial. Here the trunk ends by dividing into two branches, the radial and ulnar. The subscapular artery, the largest branch of the axillary artery, arises at the lower border of the subscapularis, which it follows to the inferior angle of the scapula, where it anastomoses with the lateral thoracic and intercostal arteries and with the descending branch of the transverse cervical and ends in the neighbouring muscles. The latissimus dorsi muscle blood supply is via the subscapular artery. The subscapular sends off a circumflex scapular branch posteriorly and then distributes a serratus branch before it enters the substance of the muscle on its undersurface as the thoracodorsal artery.

1.31

Answer: B   It contains nerve fibres from C5 and C6 spinal cord segments

The suprascapular nerve arises from the trunk formed by the union of the fifth and sixth cervical nerves. It runs lateralward beneath the trapezius and the omohyoid and enters the supraspinatus fossa through the suprascapular notch, below the superior transverse scapular ligament. It then passes beneath the supraspinatus and curves around the lateral border of the spine of the scapula to the infraspinatus fossa. In the supraspinatus fossa, it gives off two branches to the supraspinatus muscle and an articular filament to the shoulder joint; and in the infraspinatus fossa it gives off two branches to the infraspinatus muscle, as well as some filaments to the shoulder joint and scapula.

1.32

Answer: B   Radial

Radial nerve compression or injury can occur at any point along the anatomical course of the nerve and can have various causes. The most frequent site of compression is in the proximal forearm in the area of the supinator muscle and involves the posterior interosseous branch. However, problems can occur proximally in relation to fractures of the humerus at the junction of the middle and proximal thirds, as well as distally on the radial aspect of the wrist.

Symptoms depend on the site of the lesion. The most common complaint is wrist drop. If the lesion is high above the elbow, then numbness of the forearm and hand may be an additional complaint. If the lesion is in the forearm, sensation typically is spared despite the wrist drop. Pain in the forearm resembling tennis elbow may be prominent. This presentation is initially acute, lasting for several days to weeks.

If the lesion is at the wrist, patients complain of isolated sensory

upper limb

changes and paresthesias over the back of the hand without motor weakness. Radial neuropathy typically presents with weakness of wrist dorsiflexion (ie, wrist drop) and finger extension. If the lesion is in the axilla, all radial-innervated muscles are involved. The triceps and brachioradialis reflexes are decreased. Sensation is decreased occur over the triceps, the posterior part of the forearm and dorsum of the hand. Acute compression of the radial nerve commonly occurs at the spiral groove. If the lesion is at this level, all radial-innervated muscles distal to the triceps are weak. Triceps reflex is preserved, but brachioradialis is decreased. Sensory loss is over the radial dorsal part of the hand and the posterior part of the forearm. Numbness over the triceps area is variable.

In isolated posterior interosseous lesions, sensation is spared and motor involvement occurs in radial muscles distal to the supinator. Brachioradialis reflex is intact. The extensor carpi radialis sometimes is also spared, resulting in radial deviation with wrist extension. Pain may occur with palpation at the proximal forearm and with forceful supination. In distal radial sensory lesions at the wrist, no motor weakness occurs. Numbness of the dorsal hand is noted, sparing the fifth digit.

1.33

Answer: A   Superior ulnar collateral

The superior ulnar collateral artery, of small size, arises from the brachial artery a little below the middle of the arm. It pierces the medial intermuscular septum and descends on the surface of the medial head of the triceps brachii to the space between the medial epicondyle and the olecranon, accompanied by the ulnar nerve, and ends under the flexor carpi ulnaris by anastomosing with the posterior ulnar recurrent and inferior ulnar collateral. It sometimes sends a branch in front of the medial epicondyle to anastomose with the anterior ulnar recurrent.

1.34

Answer: C   Posterior circumflex humeral artery

The long head of the triceps brachii descends between the teres minor and teres major, dividing the triangular space between these two muscles and the humerus into two smaller spaces, one triangular, the other quadrangular. The triangular space contains the scapular circumflex vessels. It is bounded by the teres minor above, the teres major below and the scapular head of the triceps laterally. The quadrangular space transmits the posterior circumflex humeral vessels and the axillary nerve. It is bounded by the teres minor and the capsule of the shoulder joint above, the teres major below, the long head of the triceps brachii medially and the humerus laterally.

1.35

Answer: B   Musculocutaneous

The musculocutaneous nerve arises from the lateral cord of the brachial plexus, opposite the lower border of the pectoralis minor, its fibres derived from the fifth, sixth and seventh cervical nerves. It pierces the coracobrachialis muscle and passes obliquely between the biceps brachii and the brachialis, to the lateral side of the arm. A little above the elbow it pierces the deep fascia lateral to the tendon of the biceps brachii and is continued into the forearm as the lateral antebrachial cutaneous nerve. In its course through the arm, it supplies the coracobrachialis, biceps brachii and the greater part of the brachialis. The branch to the coracobrachialis is given off from the nerve close to its origin and in some instances as a separate filament from the lateral cord of the plexus. It is derived from the seventh cervical nerve. The branches to the biceps brachii and brachialis arise after the musculocutaneous has pierced the coracobrachialis. The branch that supplies the brachialis gives a filament to the elbow joint. The nerve also sends a small branch to the bone, which enters the nutrient foramen with the accompanying artery.

1.36

Answer: B   Rhomboid major

The rhomboid major arises by tendinous fibres from the spinous processes of the second, third, fourth and fifth thoracic vertebrae and the supraspinal ligament and is inserted into a narrow tendinous arch, attached above to the lower part of the triangular surface at the root of the spine of the scapula. Below it is inserted on the inferior angle, the arch being connected to the vertebral border by a thin membrane. When the arch extends, as it occasionally does, only a short distance, the muscular fibres are inserted directly into the scapula. The rhomboid major is supplied by the dorsal scapular nerve from the fifth cervical segment. The rhomboids carry the inferior angle backward and upward, so producing a slight rotation of the scapula on the side of the chest, the rhomboid major acting especially on the inferior angle of the scapula, through the tendinous arch by which it is inserted. The rhomboids, acting together with the middle and inferior fibres of the trapezius, also retract the scapula.

1.37

Answer: E   Long thoracic nerve

The long thoracic nerve (external respiratory nerve of Bell; posterior thoracic nerve) supplies the serratus anterior. It usually arises by three roots from the fifth, sixth and seventh cervical nerves (C5–C7) but the root from C7 may be absent. The roots from C5 and C6 pierce the scalenus medius, while the C7 root passes in front of the muscle. The nerve descends behind the brachial plexus and the axillary vessels, resting on the outer surface of the serratus anterior. It extends along the side of the thorax to the lower border of that muscle, supplying filaments to each of its digitations. Due to its long, relatively superficial course, it is susceptible to injury, either through direct trauma or stretch. Injury has been reported in almost all sports, typically occurring from a blow to the ribs underneath an outstretched arm. Surgically, the long thoracic nerve can also be damaged in breast surgery, for example in a mastectomy. Injuries can also result from carrying heavy bags over the shoulder for a prolonged time. There are also reports of isolated damage to this nerve as a variant of Parsonage–Turner syndrome, an autoimmune disease. Symptoms are often minimal – if symptomatic, a posterior shoulder or scapular burning type of pain may be reported. A lesion of the nerve paralyses the serratus anterior to produce winging of the scapula, which is most prominent when the arm is lifted forward or when the patient pushes the outstretched arm against a wall. However, even winging may not be evident until the trapezius stretches enough to reveal an injury that occurred several weeks before.

1.38

Answer: B   Supination

The movements allowed at the proximal radioulnar articulation are limited to rotatory movements of the head of the radius within the ring formed by the annular ligament and the radial notch of the ulna. A rotation of the forearm that moves the palm from an anterior-facing position to a posterior-facing position, or palm facing down is called pronation. This is not medial rotation as this must be performed when the arm is half-flexed. The opposite of pronation, the rotation of the forearm so that the palm faces anteriorly, or palm facing up is called supination. Supination is performed by the biceps brachii and supinator, assisted to a slight extent by the extensor muscles of the thumb. Pronation is performed by the pronator teres and pronator quadratus.

1.39

Answer: E   Thoracodorsal

The thoracodorsal nerve innervates latissimus dorsi, which is an important muscle for adducting, medially rotating and extending the arm. This is the muscle that is used when swimming the crawl. Because she cannot perform these movements, the triathlete must have injured her thoracodorsal nerve. Another indication of this injury is that the thoracodorsal nerve is particularly vulnerable following trauma to the axilla.

The accessory nerve innervates trapezius. If this nerve was injured, the patient could not raise the tip of her shoulder. The dorsal scapular nerve innervates the rhomboids and levator scapulae. If this nerve was injured, the patient would have problems elevating or retracting her scapula. The lateral and medial pectoral nerves innervate pectoralis major, a medial rotator and flexor of the arm. An injury to this nerve would cause a problem with flexion, not extension, of the arm.

1.40

Answer: A Latissimus dorsi

Latissimus dorsi makes the posterior axillary fold, so it is easy to see why that should be the muscle injured following a wound to the posterior axillary fold. Latissimus dorsi is the muscle important for medial rotation, extension and adduction of the arm. The patient's symptoms fit with an injury to this structure.

Pectoralis major medially rotates and flexes the arm – this muscle makes the anterior axillary fold. Levator scapulae elevates the scapula, while rhomboideus major retracts the scapula. Trapezius elevates and depresses the scapula (depending on which part of the muscle contracts), rotates the scapula superiorly and retracts the scapula. It also helps raise the tip of the shoulder, or acromion (see also *Answer* to **1.28**).

1.41

Answer: E Posterior interosseous nerve

The aetiology of posterior interosseous nerve syndrome is similar to that of radial tunnel syndrome. Compression is thought to occur after takeoff of the branches to the radial wrist extensors and the radial sensory nerve. After emerging from the supinator, the nerve may be compressed before it bifurcates into medial and lateral branches, causing a complete paralysis of the digital extensors and dorsoradial deviation of the wrist secondary to paralysis of the extensor carpi ulnaris. If compression occurs after the nerve bifurcates, selective paralysis of muscles occurs, depending on which branch is involved. Compression of the medial branch causes paralysis of the extensor carpi ulnaris, extensor digiti quinti and extensor digitorum communis. Compression of the lateral branch causes paralysis of the abductor pollicis longus, extensor pollicis brevis, extensor pollicis longus and extensor indicis proprius. Most commonly, entrapment occurs at the proximal edge of the supinator. Other possible causes of posterior interosseous nerve dysfunction include trauma (Monteggia fractures), synovitis (rheumatoid), tumours and iatrogenic injuries.

Patients with posterior interosseous nerve syndrome present with weakness or paralysis of the wrist and digital extensors. Pain may be present, but it usually is not a primary symptom. Attempts at active wrist extension often result in weak dorsoradial deviation due to preservation of the radial wrist extensors but involvement of the extensor carpi ulnaris and extensor digitorum communis. These patients do not have a sensory deficit. Rarely, compression of the posterior interosseous nerve may occur after bifurcation into medial and lateral branches. Selective medial branch involvement causes paralysis of the extensor carpi ulnaris, extensor digiti quinti and extensor digitorum communis. With compression of the lateral branch, paralysis of the abductor pollicis longus, extensor pollicis brevis, extensor pollicis longus and extensor indicis proprius is noted.

1.42

Answer: A   Median nerve

The median nerve runs into the hand to supply sensation to the thumb, index finger, long finger and half of the ring finger. The nerve also supplies a branch to the muscles of the thumb, the thenar muscles. An isolated lesion of the motor supply to thenar muscles can result in the clinical picture presented in this vignette.

1.43

Answer: D   Musculocutaneous

The biceps brachii is a flexor of the elbow and, to a less extent, of the shoulder. It is also a powerful supinator and serves to render tense the deep fascia of the forearm by means of the lacertus fibrosus given off from its tendon. The brachialis is a flexor of the forearm and forms an important defence to the elbow joint. Both of these muscles are supplied by the musculocutaneous nerve and injury to this nerve will produce the features described in this vignette.

1.44

Answer: E   Suprascapular nerve

Let us take the findings of the neurological assessment one by one to break down this question. If the diaphragm is functioning normally, you know that the phrenic nerve is probably uninjured, which means that the C5 root has not been damaged. Because the scapula is not winged, there was no damage to the long thoracic nerve or the C5–C7 nerve roots. Finally, because the patient cannot initiate abduction of the arm, you know that the suprascapular nerve is injured and supraspinatus has been denervated. Nevertheless, the patient can abduct the arm once it is lifted to 45°, so the deltoid muscle and the axillary nerve must be intact.

Taking the answer choices one by one: the axillary nerve is intact, because deltoid is functioning. The posterior cord of the brachial plexus must also be intact, because this cord gives off the axillary nerve. The roots of the brachial plexus are intact, as the phrenic nerve and long thoracic nerve (which are derived from the roots) are still functioning. The superior trunk of the brachial plexus must also be undamaged, because this trunk contributes to the posterior cord, which is intact. Therefore, this means that the injury must be to the suprascapular nerve.

1.45

Answer: B   Abduction

Injuries to the upper roots of the brachial plexus (C5 and C6) are the most common types of injuries – resulting in a condition known as Erb–Duchenne's palsy. It affects especially the suprascapular, axillary and musculocutaneous nerves, causing paralysis of the rotator cuff muscles, biceps, brachialis, coracobrachialis and deltoid. It also knocks out the upper and lower subscapular nerves, denervating subscapularis and teres major. It knocks out most of the lateral pectoral nerve, but the majority of pectoralis major is innervated by medial pectoral nerve, so it is only weakened. After this injury, the upper limb hangs limply, medially rotated by an unopposed latissimus and pectoralis major muscles and pronated due to a loss of biceps. Therefore, the limb is constantly adducted and medially rotated. However, the limb can no longer be abducted because both supraspinatus, which initiates abduction, and deltoid, which allows for complete abduction, have been denervated. As far as extension and flexion go, extension occurs through the actions of the triceps, which is innervated by the radial nerve. This nerve should still be intact. Flexion of the arm is not totally lost if biceps brachii and coracobrachialis are denervated, because pectoralis major is not completely lost.

1.46

Answer: A Apical

The axillary glands or lymph nodes are of large size, vary from 20 to 30 in number and may be arranged in the following groups:

- A lateral group of from four to six glands lies in relation to the medial and posterior aspects of the axillary vein. The afferents of these glands drain the whole arm with the exception of that portion whose vessels accompany the cephalic vein. The efferent vessels pass partly to the central and subclavicular groups of axillary glands and partly to the inferior deep cervical glands.

- An anterior or pectoral group consists of four or five glands along the lower border of the pectoralis minor, in relation with the lateral thoracic artery. Their afferents drain the skin and muscles of the anterior and lateral thoracic walls and the central and lateral parts of the breast. Their efferents pass partly to the central and partly to the subclavicular groups of axillary glands.

- A posterior or subscapular group of six or seven glands is found along the lower margin of the posterior wall of the axilla in the course of the subscapular artery. The afferents of this group drain the skin and muscles of the lower part of the back of the neck and of the posterior thoracic wall. Their efferents pass to the central group of axillary glands.

upper limb

- A central or intermediate group of three or four large glands is embedded in the adipose tissue near the base of the axilla. Its afferents are the efferent vessels of all the preceding groups of axillary glands. Its efferents pass to the subclavicular group.

- A medial, apical or subclavicular group of six to twelve glands is situated partly posterior to the upper portion of the pectoralis minor and partly above the upper border of this muscle. Its only direct territorial afferents are those that accompany the cephalic vein and one that drains the upper peripheral part of the breast, but it receives the efferents of all the other axillary glands.

If all the lymph nodes lateral to the medial edge of pectoralis minor are removed, the central, lateral, pectoral and subscapular nodes will be removed. The central nodes are found directly under pectoralis minor, while the other three groups of nodes are lateral to the entire muscle. The apical nodes, which are medial to the medial edge of pectoralis minor, will not be removed.

1.47

Answer: C   Median

The median nerve provides sensory innervation to the palmar skin of the radial three and a half fingers of the palm. Therefore, the patient's loss of cutaneous sensation is suggestive of a median nerve injury. The location of the injury also implies that there has been an injury to the median nerve – this nerve enters the hand by crossing over the anterior side of the wrist. The lateral and medial antebrachial cutaneous nerves provide cutaneous innervation to the anterior side of the forearm – the symptoms here are not consistent with an injury to these nerves. The radial nerve innervates the radial side of the dorsum of the hand but does not innervate the palmar side of the hand. The ulnar nerve innervates the medial (ulnar) side of both the dorsum and palm of the hand (see also *Answer* to **1.42**).

1.48

Answer: B   Posterior humeral circumflex

The posterior humeral circumflex artery arises from the axillary artery at the lower border of the subscapularis and runs backward with the axillary nerve through the quadrangular space bounded by the subscapularis and teres minor above, the teres major below, the long head of the triceps brachii medially and the surgical neck of the humerus laterally. It winds around the neck of the humerus and is distributed to the deltoid muscle and shoulder joint, anastomosing with the anterior humeral circumflex and profunda brachii. As the posterior and anterior circumflex arteries wrap around the humerus near its surgical neck, a fracture to the surgical neck could damage either of these arteries or the axillary nerve. (Remember: the posterior circumflex humeral artery and the axillary nerve cross through the quadrangular space together.) The subscapular artery is a branch of the third part of the axillary artery − it branches to form the thoracodorsal artery and the circumflex scapular artery. The radial recurrent artery is a branch of the radial collateral artery − it contributes to collateral circulation around the elbow. The deep brachial artery is an artery in the deep arm − it is close to the humerus, so fracturing the humerus mid-arm level might result in damage to this vessel.

1.49

Answer: A   Infraspinatus

Infraspinatus and teres minor are the two lateral rotators of the arm. These were probably the muscles that this patient had strained. The infraspinatus is a thick triangular muscle, which occupies the chief part of the infraspinatus fossa. It arises by fleshy fibres from its medial two-thirds and by tendinous fibres from the ridges on its surface. It arises from the infraspinatus fascia, which covers it and separates it from the teres major and minor. The fibres converge to a tendon, which glides over the lateral border of the spine of the scapula and, passing across the posterior part of the capsule of the shoulder joint, is inserted into the middle impression on the greater tubercle of the humerus. The tendon of this muscle is sometimes separated from the capsule of the shoulder joint by a bursa, which

upper limb

215

may communicate with the joint cavity. The teres minor is a narrow, elongated muscle, which arises from the dorsal surface of the axillary border of the scapula for the upper two-thirds of its extent and from two aponeurotic laminae, one of which separates it from infraspinatus, the other from teres major. Its fibres run obliquely upward and lateralward. The upper ones end in a tendon which is inserted into the lowest of the three impressions on the greater tubercle of the humerus. The lowest fibres are inserted directly into the humerus immediately below this impression. The tendon of this muscle passes across and is united with the posterior part of the capsule of the shoulder joint.

Infraspinatus is supplied by the fifth and sixth cervical nerves through the suprascapular nerve, while the teres minor is supplied by the fifth cervical through the axillary nerve. Latissimus dorsi, teres major, subscapularis and pectoralis major are all important medial rotators of the arm. Supraspinatus is the muscle that initiates abduction of the arm through the first 15°.

1.50

Answer: A   Basilic

There are two large cutaneous veins running up the forearm. Both veins take origin from the dorsal venous arch of the hand and run up the lateral and medial sides of the forearm. On the medial side (near the fifth digit) there is the basilic vein. On the lateral side, there is the cephalic vein. The infection is on the medial side, so the correct answer is the basilic vein. (Remember that the hands are supinated in the anatomical position – this comes in handy when you are thinking about the medial and lateral sides of the forearm.)

The basilic vein originates from the medial side of the dorsal venous network. It ascends along the posterior surface of the medial side of the forearm and inclines forward to the anterior surface below the elbow, where it is joined by the median cubital vein. It ascends obliquely in the groove between the biceps brachii and pronator teres and crosses the brachial artery, from which it is separated by the lacertus fibrosus. Here it is accompanied by filaments of the medial cutaneous nerve of the forearm. It then runs upward along the medial border of the biceps brachii muscle. It perforates the deep fascia a little below the middle of the arm, and, runs forward on the medial side of the brachial artery to the lower border of teres major. From here on it continues as the axillary vein.

The brachial vein runs with the brachial artery – it is a deep vein that ends at the level of the elbow. The ulnar vein runs with the ulnar artery, draining the ulnar side of the forearm. Neither of these veins are located in superficial tissue. The median cubital vein is a cutaneous vein, but it is short and only found in the median cubital fossa. It provides a connection between the cephalic vein and basilic vein.

1.51

Answer: A   Anterior humeral circumflex

The branches of the axillary artery are:

- from the first part: superior thoracic artery

- from the second part: thoracoacromial artery, lateral thoracic artery, subscapular artery

- from the third part: anterior humeral circumflex artery, posterior humeral circumflex artery.

The anterior humeral circumflex artery, considerably smaller than the posterior, arises nearly opposite it, from the lateral side of the axillary artery. It runs horizontally, beneath the coracobrachialis and short head of the biceps brachii, in front of the neck of the humerus. On reaching the intertubercular sulcus, it gives off a branch that ascends in the sulcus to supply the head of the humerus and the shoulder joint. The trunk of the vessel is then continued onward beneath the long head of the biceps brachii and the deltoid and anastomoses with the posterior humeral circumflex artery.

1.52

Answer: C   Radial artery

The arteria princeps pollicis arises from the radial artery just as it turns medially to the deep part of the hand. It descends along the ulnar side of the metacarpal bone of the thumb to the base of the first phalanx, between the first dorsal interosseous and adductor pollicis muscles. At the base of the first phalanx it lies beneath the tendon of the flexor pollicis longus and divides into two branches. These make their appearance between the medial and lateral insertions of the adductor pollicis, and run along the sides of the thumb, forming on the palmar surface of the last phalanx an arch, from which branches are distributed to the skin and subcutaneous tissue of the thumb.

1.53

Answer: E   Radial recurrent artery

The radial recurrent artery arises from the radial artery immediately below the elbow. It ascends between the branches of the radial nerve, lying on the supinator and then between the brachioradialis and brachialis, supplying these muscles and the elbow joint and anastomosing with the terminal part of the profunda brachii.

1.54

Answer: E   Trapezium

The carpal bones, eight in number, are arranged in two rows. Those of the proximal row, from the radial to the ulnar side, are named the scaphoid, lunate, triquetral and pisiform; those of the distal row, in the same order, are named the trapezium, trapezoid, capitate and hamate. Each bone (excepting the pisiform) presents six surfaces. Of these, the volar or anterior and the dorsal or posterior surfaces are rough, for ligamentous attachment, the dorsal surfaces being the broader, except in the navicular and lunate. The superior or proximal and inferior or distal surfaces are articular, the superior generally convex, the inferior concave; the medial and lateral surfaces are also articular where they are in contact with contiguous bones, otherwise they are rough and tuberculated. The structure in all is similar, viz. cancellous tissue enclosed in a layer of compact bone. A mnemonic to remember the carpal bones: (She Looks Too Pretty, Try To Catch Her).

1.55

Answer: C   Triquetral

The pisiform bone (a sesamoid bone) is recognisable by its small size and by its presenting a single articular facet. It is situated on a plane anterior to the other carpal bones and is spheroidal in form. Its dorsal surface presents a smooth, oval facet, for articulation with the triquetral (hence triquetral is the correct option): this facet approaches the superior, but not the inferior border of the bone. The volar surface is rounded and rough and gives attachment to the transverse carpal ligament and to the flexor carpi ulnaris and the abductor digiti quinti. The lateral and medial surfaces are also rough, the former being concave, the latter usually convex.

upper limb

SECTION 2:
LOWER LIMB – ANSWERS

2.1

Answer: E   The medial compartment is called the femoral canal

The femoral sheath (crural sheath) is formed by a prolongation downward, behind the inguinal ligament, of the fasciae, which line the abdomen, the transversalis fascia being continued down in front of the femoral vessels and the iliac fascia behind them. The sheath assumes the form of a short funnel, the wide end of which is directed upward, while the lower, narrow end fuses with the fascial investment of the vessels, about 4 cm below the inguinal ligament. It is strengthened in front by a band called the deep crural arch. The lateral wall of the sheath is vertical and is perforated by the femoral branch of the genitofemoral nerve (lumboinguinal nerve); the medial wall is directed obliquely downward and lateralward and is pierced by the great saphenous vein and by some lymphatic vessels. The sheath is divided by two vertical partitions, which stretch between its anterior and posterior walls. The lateral compartment contains the femoral artery and the intermediate compartment the femoral vein, while the medial and smallest compartment is called the femoral canal and contains some lymphatic vessels and a lymph gland embedded in a small amount of areolar tissue. The femoral canal is conical and measures about 1.25 cm in length. Its base, directed upward and called the femoral ring, is oval in form, its long diameter directed transversely and measuring about 1.25 cm.

2.2

Answer: D   Has nine to twelve valves

The small saphenous vein (external or short saphenous vein) begins behind the lateral malleolus as a continuation of the lateral marginal vein; it first ascends along the lateral margin of the tendocalcaneus and then crosses it to reach the middle of the back of the leg. Running directly upward, it perforates the deep fascia in the lower part of the popliteal fossa and ends in the popliteal vein, between the heads of the gastrocnemius muscle. It communicates with the deep veins on the dorsum of the foot and receives numerous large tributaries from the back of the leg. Before it pierces the deep fascia, it gives off a branch which runs upward and forward to join the great saphenous vein. The small saphenous vein possesses from nine to twelve valves, one of which is always found near its termination in the popliteal vein. In the lower third of the leg the small saphenous vein is in close relation with the sural nerve, in the upper two-thirds with the medial sural cutaneous nerve. The saphenous nerve accompanies the great saphenous vein.

2.3

Answer: C   Deep peroneal

Tibialis anterior and peroneus tertius are the direct flexors of the foot at the ankle joint. Tibialis anterior, acting with tibialis posterior, raises the medial border of the foot, inverting the foot. Peroneus tertius, acting with peroneus brevis and longus, raises the lateral border of the foot, everting the foot. The extensor digitorum longus and extensor hallucis longus muscles extend the phalanges of the toes, and, continuing their action, flex the foot on the leg. These muscles are supplied by the fourth and fifth lumbar nerves and the first sacral nerve through the deep peroneal nerve. The deep peroneal nerve begins at the bifurcation of the common peroneal nerve, between the fibula and the upper part of the peroneus longus. On the basis of the clinical presentation of this patient, this is the nerve that is most likely to be injured.

The tibial nerve supplies gastrocnemius, plantaris, soleus, and popliteus. The femoral nerve supplies the quadriceps femoris muscle. The superficial peroneal nerve supplies the peronei longus and brevis and the skin over the greater part of the dorsum of the foot. The medial plantar nerve supplies the abductor hallucis, the flexor digitorum brevis, the flexor hallucis brevis and the first lumbrical.

lower limb

2.4

Answer: D   Great saphenous

The great saphenous vein, the longest vein in the body, begins in the medial marginal vein of the dorsum of the foot and ends in the femoral vein about 3 cm below the inguinal ligament. It ascends in front of the tibial malleolus and along the medial side of the leg in relation with the saphenous nerve. It runs upward behind the medial condyles of the tibia and femur and along the medial side of the thigh and, passing through the fossa ovalis, ends in the femoral vein. At the ankle it receives branches from the sole of the foot through the medial marginal vein. In the leg it anastomoses freely with the small saphenous vein, communicates with the anterior and posterior tibial veins and receives many cutaneous veins. In the thigh it communicates with the femoral vein and receives numerous tributaries; those from the medial and posterior parts of the thigh frequently unite to form a large accessory saphenous vein that joins the main vein at a variable level. Near the fossa ovalis it is joined by the superficial epigastric, superficial iliac circumflex and superficial external pudendal veins. A vein, named the thoracoepigastric, runs along the lateral aspect of the trunk between the superficial epigastric vein below and the lateral thoracic vein above and establishes an important communication between the femoral and axillary veins. The valves in the great saphenous vein vary from ten to 20 in number; they are more numerous in the leg than in the thigh.

2.5

Answer: B   L2, L3

The lateral femoral cutaneous nerve arises from the posterior divisions of the second and third lumbar nerves, and a spinal lesion at this level will affect it. It emerges from the middle of the lateral border of the psoas major muscle and crosses the iliacus obliquely, toward the anterior superior iliac spine. It then passes under the inguinal ligament and over the sartorius muscle into the thigh. It divides into an anterior and a posterior branch here. The anterior branch becomes superficial about 10 cm below the inguinal ligament, and divides into branches which are distributed to the skin of the anterior and lateral parts of the thigh, as far as the knee. It participates in the

lower limb

formation of the patellar plexus, along with the anterior cutaneous branches of the femoral nerve and the infrapatellar branch of the saphenous nerve. The posterior branch pierces the fascia lata, and subdivides into filaments which pass backward across the lateral and posterior surfaces of the thigh, supplying the skin from the level of the greater trochanter to the middle of the thigh.

2.6

Answer: A   Extension of the leg

The quadriceps femoris is the great extensor muscle of the leg, forming a large fleshy mass which covers the front and sides of the femur. It is subdivided into separate portions, which have received distinctive names. One, occupying the middle of the thigh and connected above with the ilium, is called from its straight course the rectus femoris. The other three lie in immediate connection with the body of the femur, which they cover from the trochanters to the condyles. The portion on the lateral side of the femur is the vastus lateralis; that covering the medial side, the vastus medialis; and that in front, the vastus intermedius.

2.7

Answer: B   skin, fibular collateral ligament, popliteus muscle tendon, lateral meniscus

The correct order of superficial to deep structures on the lateral aspect of the knee joint is skin, fibular collateral ligament, popliteus muscle tendon and lateral meniscus.

2.8

Answer: D   Innervates the medial compartment of the thigh

The obturator nerve arises from the anterior divisions of the second, third and fourth lumbar nerves; the branch from the third is the largest, while that from the second is often very small. It descends through the fibres of the psoas major muscle, and appears at its medial border near the brim of the pelvis. It then passes behind the common iliac vessels and runs along the lateral wall of the lesser pelvis to reach the upper part of the obturator foramen, anterosuperior to the obturator vessels. During this course it is on the lateral side of the hypogastric vessels and ureter, with the hypogastric vessels separating it from the ureter. From the upper part of the obturator foramen it enters the thigh, and divides into anterior and posterior branches, which are separated at first by some of the fibres of the obturator externus muscle, and lower down by adductor brevis.

The anterior branch leaves the pelvis anterior to the obturator externus. It descends anterior to the adductor brevis and posterior to the pectineus and adductor longus. It forms a plexus with the anterior cutaneous and saphenous branches of the femoral nerve at the lower border of the adductor longus. It then descends on the femoral artery, to which it is finally distributed. Near the obturator foramen the nerve gives off an articular branch to the hip joint. Behind pectineus it distributes branches to adductor longus and gracilis, usually to adductor brevis and, in rare cases, to the pectineus muscle. When the accessory obturator nerve is present it gives a communicating branch to the obturator nerve. Occasionally the communicating branch to the anterior cutaneous and saphenous branches of the femoral nerve is continued down, as a cutaneous branch, to the thigh and leg. When this is so, it emerges from beneath the lower border of the adductor longus, descends along the posterior margin of sartorius to the medial side of the knee, where it pierces the deep fascia, communicates with the saphenous nerve, and is distributed to the skin of the tibial side of the leg, as low down as its middle part.

The posterior branch pierces the anterior part of obturator externus, and supplies this muscle. It then passes behind adductor brevis, anterior to the adductor magnus, and divides into numerous muscular branches, which are distributed to the adductor magnus and the adductor brevis when the latter does not receive a branch from the anterior division of the nerve. It usually gives off an articular filament to the knee-joint.

lower limb

2.9

Answer: C   Calcaneus

The muscles of the back of the leg are subdivided into two groups – superficial and deep. Those of the superficial group constitute a powerful muscular mass, forming the calf of the leg. Their large size is one of the most characteristic features of the muscular apparatus in man and bears a direct relation to his erect attitude and his mode of progression. The muscles of the superficial posterior compartment of leg include gastrocnemius, soleus and plantaris. Gastrocnemius and soleus together form a muscular mass which is occasionally described as the triceps surae; its tendon of insertion is the tendo calcaneus. The tendo calcaneus, the common tendon of gastrocnemius and soleus, is the thickest and strongest in the body. It is about 15 cm long and begins near the middle of the leg, but receives fleshy fibres on its anterior surface, almost to its lower end. Gradually becoming contracted below, it is inserted into the middle part of the posterior surface of the calcaneus, a bursa being interposed between the tendon and the upper part of this surface. The tendon spreads out somewhat at its lower end, so that its narrowest part is about 4 cm above its insertion. It is covered by the fascia and the skin and is separated from the deep muscles and vessels by a considerable space filled up with areolar and adipose tissue. Along its lateral side, but superficial to it, is the small saphenous vein.

Plantaris is placed between the gastrocnemius and soleus muscles. It arises from the lower part of the lateral prolongation of the linea aspera and from the oblique popliteal ligament of the knee joint. It forms a small fusiform belly, from 7 to 10 cm long, ending in a long slender tendon, which crosses obliquely between the two muscles of the calf and runs along the medial border of the tendo calcaneus, to be inserted with it into the posterior part of the calcaneus. This muscle is sometimes double and at other times missing. Occasionally, its tendon is lost in the laciniate ligament, or in the fascia of the leg. The gastrocnemius and soleus are supplied by the first and second sacral nerves and the plantaris by the fourth and fifth lumbar and first sacral nerves, through the tibial nerve.

lower limb

2.10

Answer: C   Profunda femoris artery

The profunda femoris artery (deep femoral artery) is a large vessel arising from the lateral and back part of the femoral artery, from 2 to 5 cm below the inguinal ligament. At first it lies lateral to the femoral artery; it then runs behind it and the femoral vein to the medial side of the femur and, passing downward behind the adductor longus, ends at the lower third of the thigh in a small branch which pierces the adductor magnus and is distributed on the back of the thigh to the hamstring muscles. The terminal part of the profunda is sometimes known as the fourth perforating artery.

2.11

Answer: A   The common peroneal part of the sciatic nerve

The short head of biceps femoris arises from the lateral lip of the linea aspera, between the adductor magnus and vastus lateralis, extending up almost as high as the insertion of the gluteus maximus; from the lateral prolongation of the linea aspera to within 5 cm of the lateral condyle; and from the lateral intermuscular septum. The fibres of the short head merge into the aponeurosis formed by the long head; this aponeurosis becomes gradually contracted into a tendon, which is inserted into the lateral side of the head of the fibula and by a small slip into the lateral condyle of the tibia. At its insertion, the tendon of biceps femoris divides into two portions, which embrace the fibular collateral ligament of the knee joint. From the posterior border of the tendon, a thin expansion is given off to the fascia of the leg. The tendon of insertion of this biceps forms the lateral hamstring; the common peroneal nerve descends along its medial border. The nerve to the short head of the biceps femoris is derived from the common peroneal part of the sciatic nerve.

2.12

Answer: E   Base of the fifth metatarsal

The fifth metatarsal bone is recognised by a rough eminence, the tuberosity, on the lateral side of its base. The base articulates behind, by a triangular surface cut obliquely in a transverse direction, with the cuboid; and medially with the fourth metatarsal. On the medial part of its dorsal surface is inserted the tendon of the peroneus tertius and on the dorsal surface of the tuberosity that of the peroneus brevis. A strong band of the plantar aponeurosis connects the projecting part of the tuberosity with the lateral process of the tuberosity of the calcaneus. The plantar surface of the base is grooved for the tendon of the abductor digiti quinti and gives origin to the flexor digiti quinti brevis.

2.13

Answer: D Extension of the thigh would be the action most affected

The inferior gluteal nerve arises from the dorsal divisions of the fifth lumbar and first and second sacral nerves: it leaves the pelvis through the greater sciatic foramen, below the piriformis, and divides into branches that enter the deep surface of the gluteus maximus. When the gluteus maximus takes its fixed point from the pelvis, it extends the femur and brings the bent thigh into line with the body. A complete transection of the inferior gluteal nerve will affect extension of the thigh.

2.14

Answer: B It emerges from the pelvis through the lesser sciatic foramen

The obturator internus is situated partly within the lesser pelvis and partly at the back of the hip joint. It arises from the inner surface of the anterolateral wall of the pelvis, where it surrounds the greater part of the obturator foramen, being attached to the inferior rami of the pubis and ischium and at the side to the inner surface of the hip bone below and behind the pelvic brim, reaching from the upper part of the greater sciatic foramen above and behind to the obturator foramen below and in front. It also arises from the pelvic surface of the obturator membrane except in the posterior part, from the tendinous arch, which completes the canal for the passage of the obturator vessels and nerve and to a slight extent from the

lower limb

obturator fascia, which covers the muscle. The fibres converge rapidly toward the lesser sciatic foramen and end in four or five tendinous bands, which are found on the deep surface of the muscle. These bands are reflected at a right angle over the grooved surface of the ischium between its spine and tuberosity. This bony surface is covered by smooth cartilage, which is separated from the tendon by a bursa and presents one or more ridges corresponding to the furrows between the tendinous bands. These bands leave the pelvis through the lesser sciatic foramen and unite into a single flattened tendon, which passes horizontally across the capsule of the hip joint and, after receiving the attachments of the gemellae, is inserted into the forepart of the medial surface of the greater trochanter above the trochanteric fossa. A bursa, narrow and elongated in form, is usually found between the tendon and the capsule of the hip joint; it occasionally communicates with the bursa between the tendon and the ischium. Obturator internus is supplied by the first, second and third sacral nerves, sharing innervation with superior gemellus. It rotates the thigh laterally and also helps abduct the thigh when it is flexed.

2.15

Answer: A It gives rise to the nerve that supplies the anterior compartment leg muscles

The common peroneal nerve, about half the size of the tibial, is derived from the dorsal branches of the fourth and fifth lumbar and the first and second sacral nerves. It descends obliquely along the lateral side of the popliteal fossa to the head of the fibula, close to the medial margin of the biceps femoris muscle. It lies between the tendon of the biceps femoris and lateral head of the gastrocnemius muscle, winds around the neck of the fibula, between the peroneus longus and the bone, and divides beneath the muscle into the superficial and deep peroneal nerves. Before its division, it gives off articular and lateral sural cutaneous nerves. In the leg, the deep peroneal nerve supplies muscular branches to the tibialis anterior, extensor digitorum longus, peroneus tertius and extensor hallucis longus, all of which are anterior compartment leg muscles.

lower limb

2.16

Answer: B   Sartorius

Sartorius, the longest muscle in the body, is narrow and ribbon-like; it arises by tendinous fibres from the anterior superior iliac spine and the upper half of the notch below it. It passes obliquely across the upper and anterior part of the thigh, from the lateral to the medial side of the limb, then descends vertically, as far as the medial side of the knee, passing behind the medial condyle of the femur to end in a tendon. This curves obliquely forward and expands into a broad aponeurosis, which is inserted in front of the gracilis and semitendinosus, into the upper part of the medial surface of the body of the tibia, nearly as far forward as the anterior crest. The upper part of the aponeurosis is curved backward over the upper edge of the tendon of the gracilis to be inserted behind it. An offset from its upper margin blends with the capsule of the knee joint and another from its lower border with the fascia on the medial side of the leg. It supplied by the second, third and fourth lumbar nerves, through the femoral nerve. The sartorius flexes the leg on the thigh and, continuing to act, flexes the thigh on the pelvis; it next abducts and rotates the thigh outward. When the knee is bent, the sartorius assists the semitendinosus, semimembranosus and popliteus in rotating the tibia inward. Taking its fixed point from the leg, it flexes the pelvis on the thigh and assists in rotating the pelvis.

2.17

Answer: E   S3

The inferior gluteal nerve arises from the dorsal divisions of the fifth lumbar and first and second sacral nerves and hence will be spared any deficit if a spinal cord injury occurs at or below the level of S3 (see also *Answer* to **2.13**).

2.18

Answer: E   Pudendal

The arteries supplying the joint are derived from the obturator, medial femoral circumflex, lateral circumflex, femoral and superior and inferior gluteals.

2.19

Answer: A   Lateral compartment

The femoral sheath (crural sheath) is formed by a prolongation downward, behind the inguinal ligament, of the fasciae which line the abdomen, the transversalis fascia being continued down in front of the femoral vessels and the iliac fascia behind them. The sheath assumes the form of a short funnel, the wide end of which is directed upward, while the lower, narrow end fuses with the fascial investment of the vessels, about 4 cm below the inguinal ligament. It is strengthened in front by a band called the deep crural arch. The lateral wall of the sheath is vertical and is perforated by the lumboinguinal nerve; the medial wall is directed obliquely downward and lateralward and is pierced by the great saphenous vein and by some lymphatic vessels. The sheath is divided by two vertical partitions that stretch between its anterior and posterior walls. The lateral compartment contains the femoral artery and the intermediate compartement the femoral vein, while the medial and smallest compartment is called the femoral canal and contains some lymphatic vessels and a lymph gland embedded in a small amount of areolar tissue.

2.20

Answer: C   Extensor hallucis muscle

The deep fascia of the leg forms a complete investment to the muscles and is fused with the periosteum over the subcutaneous surfaces of the bones. It is continuous above with the fascia lata and is attached around the knee to the patella, the ligamentum patellae, the tuberosity and condyles of the tibia and the head of the fibula. Behind, it forms the popliteal fascia, covering in the popliteal fossa;

lower limb

here it is strengthened by transverse fibres and perforated by the small saphenous vein. It receives an expansion from the tendon of the biceps femoris laterally and from the tendons of the sartorius, gracilis, semitendinosus and semimembranosus medially. In front, it blends with the periosteum covering the subcutaneous surface of the tibia and with that covering the head and malleolus of the fibula; below, it is continuous with the transverse crural and laciniate ligaments. It is thick and dense in the upper and anterior part of the leg and gives attachment, by its deep surface, to the tibialis anterior and extensor digitorum longus; but thinner behind, where it covers the gastrocnemius and soleus. It gives off from its deep surface, on the lateral side of the leg, two strong intermuscular septa, the anterior and posterior peroneal septa, which enclose the peronei longus and brevis and separate them from the muscles of the anterior and posterior crural regions, and several more slender processes that enclose the individual muscles in each region. A broad transverse intermuscular septum, called the deep transverse fascia of the leg, intervenes between the superficial and deep posterior crural muscles.

The muscles in the anterior crural compartment include tibialis anterior, extensor digitorum longus, extensor hallucis longus and peroneus tertius. The muscles of the back of the leg are subdivided into two groups – superficial and deep. Those of the superficial group constitute a powerful muscular mass, forming the calf of the leg. Their large size is one of the most characteristic features of the muscular apparatus in man and bears a direct relation to his erect attitude and his mode of progression. The superficial muscles include gastrocnemius, soleus and plantaris. The deep muscles include tibialis posterior, flexor hallucis longus, flexor digitorum longus and popliteus.

2.21

Answer: E   Will flex the leg at the knee joint

Sartorius, the longest muscle in the body, is narrow and ribbon-like; it arises by tendinous fibres from the anterior superior iliac spine and the upper half of the notch below it. It passes obliquely across the upper and anterior part of the thigh, from the lateral to the medial side of the limb and then descends vertically, as far as the medial side of the knee, passing behind the medial condyle of the femur to end in a tendon. This curves obliquely forward and expands into a broad aponeurosis, which is inserted in front of the gracilis and semitendinosus into the upper part of the medial surface of the body of the tibia, nearly as far forward as the anterior crest. The upper part of the aponeurosis is curved backward over the upper edge of the tendon of the gracilis to be inserted behind it. An offset from its upper margin blends with the capsule of the knee joint and another from its lower border with the fascia on the medial side of the leg. The sartorius is supplied by the femoral nerve. It flexes the leg on the thigh and, continuing to act, flexes the thigh on the pelvis; it next abducts and rotates the thigh outward. When the knee is bent, the sartorius assists the semitendinosus, semimembranosus and popliteus in rotating the tibia inward. Taking its fixed point from the leg, it flexes the pelvis on the thigh and assists in rotating the pelvis.

2.22

Answer: C   It crosses two joints

The biceps femoris is situated on the posterior and lateral aspect of the thigh. It has two heads of origin, a long head and a short head. The long head arises from the lower and inner impression on the back part of the tuberosity of the ischium by a tendon common to it and the semitendinosus and from the lower part of the sacrotuberous ligament. The fibres of the long head form a fusiform belly, which passes obliquely downward and lateralward across the sciatic nerve to end in an aponeurosis which covers the posterior surface of the muscle and receives the fibres of the short head. This aponeurosis becomes gradually contracted into a tendon, which is inserted into the lateral side of the head of the fibula and by a small slip into the lateral condyle of the tibia. At its insertion, the tendon divides into two portions, which embrace the fibular collateral ligament of the knee joint. From the posterior border of the tendon, a thin expansion is given off to the fascia of the leg. The tendon of insertion of this muscle forms the lateral hamstring; the common peroneal nerve descends along its medial border. At its origin, it crosses the hip joint and at its insertion it crosses the knee joint. It is supplied by the tibial nerve. Being a hamstring, it flexes the leg on the thigh. When

lower limb

the knee is semi-flexed, the biceps femoris (because of its oblique direction) rotates the leg slightly outward.

2.23

Answer: D   One of the posterior compartment leg muscles laterally rotates the femur

The muscles of the back of the leg are subdivided into two groups: superficial and deep. Those of the superficial group constitute a powerful muscular mass, forming the calf of the leg. Their large size is one of the most characteristic features of the muscular apparatus in man and bears a direct relation to his erect attitude and his mode of progression.

Superficial muscles include gastrocnemius, soleus and plantaris. Gastrocnemius and soleus are supplied by the first and second sacral nerves and plantaris by the fourth and fifth lumbar and first sacral nerves, through the tibial nerve. The muscles of the calf are the chief extensors of the foot at the ankle joint. They possess considerable power and are constantly called into use in standing, walking, dancing and leaping; hence the large size they usually present. In walking, these muscles raise the heel from the ground; the body being so supported on the raised foot, the opposite limb can be carried forward. In standing, the soleus, taking its fixed point from below, steadies the leg on the foot and prevents the body from falling forward. Gastrocnemius, acting from below, serves to flex the femur on the tibia, assisted by the popliteus. The plantaris is the rudiment of a large muscle which in some of the lower animals is continued over the calcaneus to be inserted into the plantar aponeurosis. In man, it is an accessory to gastrocnemius, extending the ankle if the foot is free, or bending the knee if the foot is fixed.

Deep muscles include tibialis posterior, flexor hallucis longus, flexor digitorum longus and popliteus. The popliteus is supplied by the fourth and fifth lumbar and first sacral nerves, the flexor digitorum longus and tibialis posterior by the fifth lumbar and first sacral, and the flexor hallucis longus by the fifth lumbar and the first and second sacral nerves, through the tibial nerve. Popliteus assists in flexing the leg on the thigh; when the leg is flexed, it will rotate the tibia inward. It is especially called into action at the beginning of the act of bending the knee, inasmuch as it produces the slight inward rotation of the tibia which is essential in the early stage of this movement. Tibialis posterior is a direct extensor of the foot at the ankle joint. Acting in conjunction with tibialis anterior, it turns the sole of the foot upward and medialward and inverts the foot, antagonizing the peronei, which turn it upward and lateralward (evert it). In the sole of the foot, the tendon of the tibialis posterior lies directly below the plantar calcaneonavicular ligament and is therefore an important factor in maintaining the arch of the foot. The flexor digitorum longus and flexor hallucis longus muscles are the direct flexors of the phalanges and, continuing their action, extend the foot on the leg. They assist gastrocnemius and soleus in extending the foot, as in the act of walking, or in standing on tiptoe. In consequence of the oblique direction of its tendons, the flexor digitorum longus would draw the toes medialward were it not for the quadratus plantae, which is inserted into the lateral side of the tendon and draws it to the middle line of the foot. Taking their fixed point from the foot, these muscles serve to maintain the upright posture by steadying the tibia and fibula perpendicularly on the talus.

2.24

Answer: D   Is supplied by the superior gluteal nerve

The gluteus medius is a broad, thick, radiating muscle, situated on the outer surface of the pelvis. Its posterior third is covered by the gluteus maximus, its anterior two-thirds by the gluteal aponeurosis, which separates it from the superficial fascia and integument. It arises from the outer surface of the ilium between the iliac crest and posterior gluteal line above and the anterior gluteal line below; it also arises from the gluteal aponeurosis covering its outer surface. The fibres converge to a strong flattened tendon, which is inserted into the oblique ridge which runs downward and forward on the lateral surface of the greater trochanter. A bursa separates the tendon of the muscle from the surface of the trochanter over which it glides. The gluteus medius is supplied by the fourth and fifth lumbar and first sacral nerves through the superior gluteal nerve. The gluteus medius (along with minimus) abducts the thigh when the limb is extended. It is principally called into action in supporting the body

lower limb

on one limb, in conjunction with the tensor fascia latae. Its anterior fibres, along with those of gluteus minimus, by drawing the greater trochanter forward, rotate the thigh inward, in which action they are also assisted by the tensor fascia latae.

2.25

Answer: E Would result from damage to the nerve that innervates the pectineus muscle

The pectineus is supplied by the second, third and fourth lumbar nerves through the femoral nerve and by the third lumbar through the accessory obturator when this exists. Occasionally it receives a branch from the obturator nerve. The anterior surface of the thigh receives its innervation from, the femoral nerve as well so that is the nerve most likely to be injured. In the thigh, the anterior division of the femoral nerve gives off anterior cutaneous branches. The anterior cutaneous branches comprise the intermediate and medial cutaneous nerves. The intermediate cutaneous nerve pierces the fascia lata (and generally the sartorius) about 7.5 cm below the inguinal ligament and divides into two branches that descend in immediate proximity along the forepart of the thigh to supply the skin as low as the front of the knee. Here they communicate with the medial cutaneous nerve and the infrapatellar branch of the saphenous, to form the patellar plexus. In the upper part of the thigh, the lateral branch of the intermediate cutaneous communicates with the lumboinguinal branch of the genitofemoral nerve.

2.26

Answer: E Could be damaged by a fracture of the neck of the fibula

The peroneus brevis is supplied by the fourth and fifth lumbar and first sacral nerves through the superficial peroneal nerve. The superficial peroneal nerve is one of the two terminal branches of the common peroneal nerve. The common peroneal nerve winds around the neck of the fibula and can be injured in cases of fracture neck of fibula. Such an injury can result in paralysis or paresis of peroneus brevis due to indirect involvement of the superficial peroneal nerve.

2.27

Answer: D   Serves as an attachment for adductors of the thigh

The linea aspera is a prominent longitudinal ridge or crest on the middle third of the femur. It has a medial and a lateral lip and a narrow, rough, intermediate line. Superiorly, the linea aspera is prolonged by three ridges. The lateral ridge is very rough, and runs almost vertically upward to the base of the greater trochanter. It is called the gluteal tuberosity and gives attachment to part of the gluteus maximus. Its upper part is often elongated into a roughened crest, on which a more or less well-marked, rounded tubercle, the third trochanter, is occasionally developed. The intermediate ridge or pectineal line is continued to the base of the lesser trochanter and gives attachment to the pectineus muscle. The medial ridge is lost in the intertrochanteric line, with a portion of the iliacus muscle inserted between the two. Inferiorly, the linea aspera is prolonged into two ridges which enclose between them a triangular area, the popliteal surface, on which the popliteal artery rests. Of these two ridges, the lateral is the more prominent, and descends to the summit of the lateral condyle. The medial is less marked, especially at its upper part, where it is crossed by the femoral artery. It ends below at the summit of the medial condyle, in a small tubercle, the adductor tubercle, which provides insertion to the tendon of the adductor magnus. The vastus medialis arises from the medial lip of the linea aspera and its superior and inferior prolongations. The vastus lateralis takes origin from the lateral lip and its upward prolongation. The adductor magnus is inserted into the linea aspera, and to its lateral prolongation above and its medial prolongation below. Two muscles are attached between the vastus lateralis and the adductor magnus: the gluteus maximus is inserted above and the short head of the biceps femoris arises below. Four muscles are inserted between the adductor magnus and the vastus medialis: the iliacus and pectineus superiorly, and the adductor brevis and adductor longus inferiorly. The linea aspera is perforated a little below its centre by the nutrient canal, which is directed obliquely upward.

lower limb

2.28

Answer: E   It is found in the medical compartment of the thigh

The obturator artery, a branch of the internal iliac artery, passes anteroinferiorly (forward and downward) on the lateral wall of the pelvis, to the upper part of the obturator foramen and, escaping from the pelvic cavity through the obturator canal, it divides into an anterior and a posterior branch. In the pelvic cavity this vessel is in relation laterally with the obturator fascia; medially, with the ureter, ductus deferens and peritoneum; while a little below it is the obturator nerve. Inside the pelvis, the obturator artery gives off iliac branches to the iliac fossa, which supply the bone and the iliacus and anastomose with the iliolumbar artery. A vesical branch, which runs backward to supply the bladder, and a pubic branch, which is given off from the vessel just before it; leaves the pelvic cavity. The pubic branch ascends on the back of the pubis, communicating with the corresponding vessel of the opposite side and with the inferior epigastric artery. Outside the pelvis, the obturator artery divides at the upper margin of the obturator foramen into an anterior and a posterior branch, which encircle the foramen under cover of the obturator externus. The anterior branch runs forward on the outer surface of the obturator membrane and then curves downward along the anterior margin of the foramen. It distributes branches to the obturator externus, pectineus, adductors and gracilis and anastomoses with the posterior branch and with the medial femoral circumflex artery. The posterior branch follows the posterior margin of the foramen and turns forward on the inferior ramus of the ischium, where it anastomoses with the anterior branch. It gives twigs to the muscles attached to the ischial tuberosity and anastomoses with the inferior gluteal. It also supplies an articular branch, which enters the hip joint through the acetabular notch, ramifies in the fat at the bottom of the acetabulum and sends a twig along the ligamentum teres to the head of the femur. It is the chief source of arterial supply to the medial compartment of the thigh.

2.29

Answer: D Anterior talofibular ligament

The anterior talofibular ligament, the shortest of the three lateral ankle ligaments, passes from the anterior margin of the fibular malleolus, forward and medially to the talus, in front of its lateral articular facet. It is the most commonly sprained ligament, as part of the lateral ligament of the ankle.

2.30

Answer: B Posterior tibial, flexor digitorum longus, flexor hallucis longus

The medial surface of the lower end of the tibia is prolonged downward to form a strong pyramidal process, flattened from without inward – the medial malleolus. The medial surface of this process is convex and subcutaneous. Its lateral or articular surface is smooth and slightly concave and articulates with the talus. Its anterior border is rough, for the attachment of the anterior fibres of the deltoid ligament of the ankle joint. Its posterior border presents a broad groove, the malleolar sulcus, directed obliquely downward and medialward and occasionally double. This sulcus lodges the tendons of the tibialis posterior and flexor digitorum longus. The summit of the medial malleolus is marked by a rough depression behind, for the attachment of the deltoid ligament. The flexor retinaculum is immediately posterior to the medial malleolus. The structures that pass under the flexor retinaculum are coming from the posterior compartment of the leg to enter the foot. These tendons, vessels and nerve are all organised behind the flexor retinaculum in a very characteristic way. From anterior to posterior, the structures are the tendon of Tibialis posterior, tendon of flexor Digitorum longus, posterior tibial Artery (and vein), tibial Nerve and tendon of flexor Hallucis longus – Tom, Dick an' Harry!

lower limb

2.31

Answer: A   Ischial tuberosities

Posteriorly, the superior ramus of the ischium of the hip bone (os coxae) forms a large swelling, the tuberosity of the ischium (or ischial tuberosity). It marks the lateral boundary of the pelvic inlet. When sitting, the weight is frequently placed upon the ischial tuberosity. It is divided into two portions: a lower, rough, triangular part and an upper, smooth, quadrilateral portion. The lower portion is subdivided by a prominent longitudinal ridge, passing from base to apex, into two parts: the outer gives attachment to the adductor magnus, the inner to the sacrotuberous ligament. The upper portion is subdivided into two areas by an oblique ridge, which runs downward and outward: from the upper and outer area the semimembranosus arises; from the lower and inner, the long head of the biceps femoris and the semitendinosus.

2.32

Answer: C   Extension of the hip and flexion of the knee

The semimembranosus, so called because of its membranous tendon of origin, is situated at the back and medial side of the thigh. It arises by a thick tendon from the upper and outer impression on the tuberosity of the ischium, above and lateral to the biceps femoris and semitendinosus. The tendon of origin expands into an aponeurosis, which covers the upper part of the anterior surface of the muscle; from this aponeurosis muscular fibres arise and converge to another aponeurosis, which covers the lower part of the posterior surface of the muscle and contracts into the tendon of insertion. It is inserted mainly into the horizontal groove on the posterior medial aspect of the medial condyle of the tibia. The tendon of insertion gives off certain fibrous expansions: one, of considerable size, passes upward and lateralward to be inserted into the back part of the lateral condyle of the femur, forming part of the oblique popliteal ligament of the knee joint; a second is continued downward to the fascia which covers the popliteus muscle; while a few fibres join the tibial collateral ligament of the joint and the fascia of the leg. The muscle overlaps the upper part of the popliteal vessels. It is supplied by the tibial nerve. Being a hamstring (the others being semitendinosus and biceps femoris), it flexes the leg on the thigh. When the knee is semiflexed, the biceps femoris (in consequence of its oblique direction) rotates the leg slightly outward; and the semitendinosus and to a slight extent the semimembranosus, rotate the leg inward, assisting the popliteus. Taking their fixed point from below, these muscles serve to support the pelvis on the head of the femur and to draw the trunk directly backward, as in raising it from the stooping position or in feats of strength, when the body is thrown backward in the form of an arch. Extension of the hip is mainly performed by the gluteus maximus, assisted by the hamstring muscles and the ischial head of the adductor magnus.

2.33

Answer: A   The muscles plantarflex the foot and are innervated by the tibial nerve

The muscles of the back of the leg are subdivided into two groups: superficial and deep. Superficial muscles include gastrocnemius, soleus and plantaris. The gastrocnemius and soleus muscles are supplied by the first and second sacral nerves and the plantaris by the fourth and fifth lumbar and first sacral nerves, through the tibial nerve. Deep muscles include tibialis posterior, flexor hallucis longus, flexor digitorum longus and popliteus. The popliteus is supplied by the fourth and fifth lumbar and first sacral nerves, the flexor digitorum longus and tibialis posterior by the fifth lumbar and first sacral, and the flexor hallucis longus by the fifth lumbar and the first and second sacral nerves, through the tibial nerve. The muscles of the calf are the chief extensors (plantarflexors) of the foot at the ankle joint. They possess considerable power and are constantly called into use in standing, walking, dancing and leaping; hence the large size they usually present (see also *Answer* to **2.23**).

lower limb

2.34

Answer: B   Vastus intermedius

The tuberosity of the tibia gives attachment to the ligamentum patellae (which is the single strong tendon of the quadriceps femoris, including rectus femoris, vasti medialis, intermedius and lateralis). A bursa intervenes between the deep surface of the ligament and the part of the bone immediately above the tuberosity.

2.35

Answer: C   There would still be cutaneous sensation over the anteromedial surface of the thigh

The sciatic nerve is a large nerve that runs down the lower limb. It is the longest single nerve in the body. The sciatic nerve supplies nearly the whole of the skin of the leg, the muscles of the back of the thigh and those of the leg and foot. A transection of the sciatic nerve at its exit from the pelvis will affect all the above-mentioned functions except cutaneous sensation over the anteromedial surface of the thigh, which comes from the femoral nerve.

2.36

Answer: B   Medical femoral circumflex

The medial femoral circumflex artery (internal circumflex artery, medial circumflex femoral artery) is an artery in the upper thigh that helps supply blood to the head and neck of the femur. It arises from the posteromedial aspect of the profunda femoris (the deep femoral artery), and winds around the medial side of the femur. It passes first between pectineus and psoas major, and then between obturator externus and adductor brevis. At the upper border of the adductor brevis it gives off two branches. One of these two branches is distributed to the adductors, gracilis and obturator externus, and anastomoses with the obturator artery. The other descends under adductor brevis, to supply it and adductor magnus. The continuation of the medial circumflex femoral artery passes backward and divides into superficial, deep, and acetabular branches. The superficial branch appears between quadratus femoris and the upper border of adductor magnus and participates in the cruciate anastomosis. In forming the cruciate anastomosis, the superficial branch of the medial circumflex femoral artery anastomoses with the inferior gluteal, lateral femoral circumflex, and first perforating arteries. The deep branch runs obliquely upward on the tendon of the obturator externus and anterior to the quadratus femoris toward the trochanteric fossa, where it anastomoses with branches from the gluteal arteries. The acetabular branch arises opposite the acetabular notch and enters the hip joint beneath the transverse ligament, accompanied by an articular branch from the obturator artery. It supplies the fat in the bottom of the acetabulum, and is continued along the round ligament to the head of the femur.

2.37

Answer: C   Perforating

The perforating arteries, usually three in number, are so named because they perforate the tendon of the adductor magnus to reach the back of the thigh. They pass backward close to the linea aspera of the femur under cover of small tendinous arches in the muscle. The first is given off above the adductor brevis, the second in front of that muscle and the third immediately below it.

The first perforating artery passes backward between the pectineus and adductor brevis (sometimes it perforates the latter). It then pierces the adductor magnus close to the linea aspera. It gives branches to the adductores brevis and magnus, biceps femoris and gluteus maximus and anastomoses with the inferior gluteal, medial and lateral femoral circumflex and second perforating arteries.

The second perforating artery, larger than the first, pierces the tendons of the adductores brevis and magnus and divides into ascending and descending branches, which supply the posterior femoral muscles, anastomosing with the first and third perforating vessels. The second artery frequently arises in common with the first. The nutrient artery of the femur is usually given off from the second perforating artery. When two nutrient arteries exist, they usually spring from the first and third perforating vessels.

The third perforating artery is given off below the adductor brevis. It pierces the adductor magnus and divides into branches, which

lower limb

supply the posterior femoral muscles, anastomosing above with the higher perforating arteries and below with the terminal branches of the profunda and the muscular branches of the popliteal. The nutrient artery of the femur may arise from this branch. The terminal part of the profunda is sometimes called the fourth perforating artery.

2.38

Answer: C   Posterior tibial artery

The posterior tibial artery begins at the lower border of the popliteus, opposite the interval between the tibia and the fibula. It extends obliquely downward and, as it descends, it approaches the tibial side of the leg, lying behind the tibia, and in the lower part of its course is situated midway between the medial malleolus and the medial process of the calcaneal tuberosity. Here it divides beneath the origin of the adductor hallucis into the medial and lateral plantar arteries. It is the main source of blood supply to the posterior compartment of the leg and plantar surface of the foot.

2.39

Answer: E   Anterior cruciate ligament

The drawer test is a test used by doctors to detect rupture of the cruciate ligaments in the knee. The patient should be supine with the hips flexed to 45°, the knees flexed to 90° and the feet flat on table. The examiner sits on the patient's feet and grasps the patient's tibia and pulls it forward (anterior drawer test) or pushes it backward (posterior drawer test). If the tibia moves forward or backward more than normal, the test is considered positive.

The anterior cruciate ligament (ACL) is one of the four major ligaments of the knee. It connects from a posterolateral (back and outside) part of the femur to an anteromedial (front and inside) part of the tibia. These attachments allow it to resist forces pushing the tibia forward relative to the femur. More specifically, it is attached to the depression in front of the intercondyloid eminence of the tibia, being blended with the anterior extremity of the lateral meniscus. It passes up, backward and laterally and is fixed into the medial and back part of the lateral condyle of the femur. Tearing of the ACL is a common injury in athletes. This often occurs when athletes decelerate rapidly, followed by a sharp or sudden change in direction (cutting). In jump sports, ACL failure has been linked to heavy or stiff landing as well as twisting or turning the knee while landing, especially when the knee is in the 'valgus' ('knock-knee') position.

2.40

Answer: A   Obturator artery

The posterior branch of the obturator artery also supplies an articular branch, which enters the hip joint through the acetabular notch, ramifies in the fat at the bottom of the acetabulum and sends a twig along the ligamentum teres (round ligament) to the head of the femur.

2.41

Answer: D   Biceps femoris

The popliteal fossa or space is a lozenge-shaped space at the back of the knee joint. Laterally it is bounded by the biceps femoris above and by the plantaris and the lateral head of the gastrocnemius below; medially it is limited by the semitendinosus and semimembranosus above and by the medial head of the gastrocnemius below. The floor is formed by the popliteal surface of the femur, the oblique popliteal ligament of the knee joint, the upper end of the tibia and the fascia covering the popliteus; the fossa is covered in by the fascia lata. The popliteal fossa contains the popliteal vessels, the tibial and common peroneal nerves, the termination of the small saphenous vein, the lower part of the posterior femoral cutaneous nerve, the articular branch from the obturator nerve, a few small lymph glands and a considerable quantity of fat.

lower limb

2.42

Answer: C   Superficial peroneal nerve

The superficial peroneal nerve supplies the peronei longus and brevis and the skin over the greater part of the dorsum of the foot. It passes forward between the peronei and the extensor digitorum longus, pierces the deep fascia at the lower third of the leg and divides into a medial and an intermediate dorsal cutaneous nerve. In its course between the muscles, the nerve gives off muscular branches to the peronei longus and brevis and cutaneous filaments to the skin of the lower part of the leg.

2.43

Answer: D   Posterior cruciate

The posterior cruciate ligament (PCL) is stronger, but shorter and less oblique in its direction, than the anterior. It is attached to the posterior intercondyloid fossa of the tibia and to the posterior extremity of the lateral meniscus, and passes upward, forward and medialward, to be fixed into the lateral and front part of the medial condyle of the femur. This configuration allows the PCL to resist forces pushing the tibia posteriorly relative to the femur.

2.44

Answer: A   Ampulla of the rectum

The inguinal lymph nodes, from 12 to 20 in number, are situated at the upper part of the femoral triangle. They can be divided into two groups by a horizontal line at the level of the termination of the great saphenous vein. Those lying above this line are called the superficial inguinal lymph nodes and those below it the subinguinal lymph nodes, the latter group consisting of a superficial and a deep set. The superficial inguinal lymph nodes form a chain immediately below the inguinal ligament. They receive as afferents lymphatic vessels from the skin of the penis, scrotum, perineum, buttock and abdominal wall below the level of the umbilicus. The superficial subinguinal lymph nodes are placed on either side of the upper part of the great saphenous vein. Their afferents consist chiefly of the superficial lymphatic vessels of the lower extremity, but they also receive some of the vessels which drain the skin of the penis, scrotum, perineum and buttock.

2.45

Answer: A   Vertical group of superficial inguinal lymph nodes

The lymph from the big toe will drain to the vertical group of superficial inguinal lymph nodes (see also *Answer* to **2.44**).

2.46

Answer: C   Nerve to vastus medialis

The adductor canal (Hunter's canal) is an aponeurotic tunnel in the middle third of the thigh, extending from the apex of the femoral triangle to the opening in adductor magnus. It is bounded in front and laterally by the vastus medialis; behind by the adductors longus and magnus; and is covered in by a strong aponeurosis which extends from the vastus medialis, across the femoral vessels to the adductors longus and magnus. Lying on the aponeurosis is the sartorius muscle. The canal contains the femoral artery and vein, the saphenous nerve and the nerve to vastus medialis.

2.47

Answer: C   It has the femoral nerve lying lateral to it

The femoral artery, a direct continuation of the external iliac artery, begins immediately behind the inguinal ligament, midway between the anterior superior spine of the ilium and the symphysis pubis, and passes down the front and medial side of the thigh. It ends at the junction of the middle with the lower third of the thigh, where it passes through an opening in the adductor magnus to become the popliteal artery. At the upper part of the thigh, the vessel lies in front of the hip joint. In the lower part of its course it lies to the medial side of the body of the femur and between these two parts, where it crosses the angle between the head and body, the vessel is some distance from the bone. The first 4 cm of the vessel is enclosed,

lower limb

247

together with the femoral vein, in a fibrous sheath – the femoral sheath. In the upper third of the thigh the femoral artery is contained in the femoral triangle (Scarpa's triangle) and in the middle third of the thigh, in the adductor canal (Hunter's canal). The course of the femoral artery on the surface is represented by the upper two-thirds of a line from a point midway between the anterior superior iliac spine and the symphysis pubis to the adductor tubercle, with the thigh abducted and rotated outward.

2.48

Answer: D Superficial external pudental artery

The saphenous opening is an oval opening in the fascia lata. The centre of the opening is 4 cm lateral and 4 cm below the pubic tubercle. It is about 2.5 cm long and 2 cm broad with its long axis directed downwards and laterally. The opening has a sharp crescentic lateral margin or falciform margin, which lies in front of the femoral sheath. The medial margin of the opening lies at a deeper level. It is formed by the fascia overlying the pectineus. The fascia passes behind the femoral sheath. The saphenous opening is covered by the cribriform fascia, so called because it is perforated by the great saphenous vein and by numerous blood and lymphatic vessels. Exposure of the great saphenous vein at the saphenous opening will also reveal the superficial external pudendal artery piercing the cribriform fascia. The superficial external pudendal vein, superficial epigastric vein and superficial iliac circumflex vein all join the great saphenous vein before it enters the saphenous opening.

2.49

Answer: A Tibial nerve

The flexor retinaculum is immediately posterior to the medial malleolus. The structures that pass under the flexor retinaculum are coming from the posterior compartment of the leg to enter the foot. These tendons, vessels and nerve are all organised behind the flexor retinaculum in a very characteristic way. From anterior to posterior, the structures are: tendon of Tibialis posterior, tendon of flexor Digitorum longus, posterior tibial Artery (and vein), tibial Nerve and

lower limb

tendon of flexor Hallucis longus – Tom, Dick an' Harry! Out of all the answer choices, the tibial nerve is the only one which lies behind the flexor retinaculum, so that's your answer. Tibialis anterior is in the anterior compartment of the leg – its tendon just crosses under the extensor retinaculum to enter the dorsum of the foot. The anterior tibial artery is also in the anterior compartment of the leg. It crosses the ankle under the extensor retinaculum and enters the dorsum of the foot as dorsalis pedis. Quadratus plantae is a deep muscle of the plantar surface of the foot – it insures that the tendons from flexor digitorum longus flex the toes properly. The plantar arterial arch is a structure that supplies blood to the deep foot. None of these other structures are associated with the flexor retinaculum.

2.50

Answer: B   Just lateral to the tendon of extensor hallucis longus

The dorsalis pedis artery is the continuation of the anterior tibial artery, which continues on to the dorsum of the foot. The name change from anterior tibial to dorsalis pedis occurs at the level of the ankle. As the artery crosses into the foot, it lies just lateral to the tendon of extensor hallucis longus, so that is where you would feel a pulse. The pulse of the posterior tibial artery, which comes from the posterior compartment of the leg, might be felt behind the medial malleolus. The pulse of the fibular artery might be felt behind the lateral malleolus, but that pulse would be very weak. There are no special pulses associated with the tendon of fibularis tertius or the second dorsal metatarsal space.

2.51

Answer: B   Dorsalis pedis artery

The deep plantar artery is a branch of the dorsalis pedis artery. It descends into the sole of the foot, between the two heads of the first dorsal interosseous muscle, and anastomoses with the termination of the lateral plantar artery, to complete the plantar arch. It supplies a branch to the medial side of the great toe and continues forward along the first interosseous space as the first plantar metatarsal artery. The first plantar metatarsal artery bifurcates to supply the adjacent sides of the great and second toes.

2.52

Answer: B   Dorsalis pedis artery

The lateral tarsal artery arises from the dorsalis pedis, as that vessel crosses the navicular bone. It passes in an arched direction lateralward, lying on the tarsal bones and covered by the extensor digitorum brevis. It supplies this muscle and the articulations of the tarsus and anastomoses with branches of the arcuate, anterior lateral malleolar and lateral plantar arteries and with the perforating branch of the peroneal artery.

2.53

Answer: C   Peroneal

The peroneal artery is deeply seated on the back of the fibular side of the leg. It arises from the posterior tibial, about 2.5 cm below the lower border of the popliteus, passes obliquely toward the fibula and then descends along the medial side of that bone, contained in a fibrous canal between the tibialis posterior and the flexor hallucis longus, or in the substance of the latter muscle. It then runs behind the tibiofibular syndesmosis and divides into lateral calcaneal branches, which ramify on the lateral and posterior surfaces of the calcaneus. It is covered in the upper part of its course by the soleus and deep transverse fascia of the leg; below, by the flexor hallucis longus. Its branches are:

- Muscular
- Nutrient
- Perforating
- Lateral calcaneal
- Communicating.

2.54

Answer: E   Tibialis posterior

The navicular bone is situated at the medial side of the tarsus, between the talus behind and the cuneiform bones in front. Its anterior surface is convex from side to side and subdivided by two ridges into three facets for articulation with the three cuneiform bones. The posterior surface is oval, concave, broader laterally than medially and articulates with the rounded head of the talus. The dorsal surface is convex from side to side and rough, for the attachment of ligaments. The plantar surface is irregular and also rough for the attachment of ligaments. The medial surface presents a rounded tuberosity, the lower part of which gives attachment to part of the tendon of the tibialis posterior. Hence, the injury in this vignette will affect the action of tibialis posterior. The lateral surface is rough and irregular for the attachment of ligaments and occasionally presents a small facet for articulation with the cuboid bone. The navicular articulates with four bones, the talus and the three cuneiforms; and occasionally with a fifth, the cuboid.

2.55

Answer: C   First cuneiform

The first cuneiform bone is the largest of the three cuneiforms. It is situated at the medial side of the foot, between the navicular behind and the base of the first metatarsal in front. Its medial surface is subcutaneous, broad and quadrilateral; at its anterior plantar angle is a smooth oval impression into which part of the tendon of the tibialis anterior is inserted. For the rest of its extent it is rough for the attachment of ligaments. The lateral surface is concave, presenting, along its superior and posterior borders a narrow L-shaped surface, the vertical limb and posterior part of the horizontal limb of which articulate with the second cuneiform, while the anterior part of the horizontal limb articulates with the second metatarsal bone; the rest of this surface is rough for the attachment of ligaments and part of the tendon of the peroneus longus. The anterior surface, kidney-shaped and much larger than the posterior, articulates with the first metatarsal bone. The posterior surface is triangular, concave and articulates with the medial and largest of the three facets on the anterior surface of the navicular. The plantar surface is rough and forms the base of the wedge. At its back part is a tuberosity for the insertion of part of the tendon of tibialis posterior. It also gives insertion in front to part of the tendon of tibialis anterior. The dorsal surface is the narrow end of the wedge and is directed upward and lateralward; it is rough, for the attachment of ligaments.

SECTION 3:
THORAX – ANSWERS

3.1

Answer: B   varies in length from 38 to 45 cm

The thoracic duct conveys the greater part of the lymph and chyle into the blood. It is the common trunk of all the lymphatic vessels of the body, excepting those on the right side of the head, neck and thorax, right upper extremity, right lung, right side of the heart and the convex surface of the liver. In the adult, it varies in length from 38 to 45 cm and extends from the second lumbar vertebra to the root of the neck. It begins in the abdomen by a triangular dilatation, the cisterna chyli, which is situated on the front of the body of the second lumbar vertebra, to the right side of and behind the aorta, by the side of the right crus of the diaphragm. It enters the thorax through the aortic hiatus of the diaphragm and ascends through the posterior mediastinal cavity between the aorta and azygos vein. The thoracic duct has several valves; at its termination it is provided with a pair, the free borders of which are turned toward the vein, so as to prevent the passage of venous blood into the duct.

3.2

Answer: C   Sternal angle

The sternal angle is the point where the costal cartilage attaches the second rib to the sternum. This is an important anatomical landmark to remember – it is used to find the valves when auscultating the heart. The costal margins are formed by the medial borders of the seventh to tenth costal cartilages. They are easily palpable and extend inferolaterally from the xiphisternal joint. The sternal notch/jugular notch is the notch located at the superior border of the manubrium, between the sternal ends of the clavicles. The sternoclavicular joints are simply the joints connecting the sternum with the clavicles. Finally, the xiphoid process is the bone that forms the inferior part of the sternum.

thorax

3.3

Answer: A   Costodiaphragmatic recess

The costodiaphragmatic recess is the lowest extent of the pleural cavity or sac. It is the part of the pleural sac where the costal pleura changes into the diaphragmatic pleura. Because this is the inferior part of the pleural sac, fluid in the pleural sac will fall to this region when a patient adopts the erect posture. The costodiaphragmatic recess is also the area into which a needle is inserted for thoracocentesis and it is found at different levels in different areas of the thorax. At the midclavicular line, the costodiaphragmatic recess is between ribs 6 and 8; at the midaxillary line it is between ribs 8 and 10; and at the paravertebral line it is between ribs 10 and 12.

The costomediastinal recess is found where the costal pleura becomes the mediastinal pleura. The cupola is the part of the pleural cavity, which extends above the level of the first rib into the root of the neck. The hilar reflection is the point at the root of the lung where the mediastinal pleura is reflected and becomes continuous with the visceral pleura. Finally, the middle mediastinum is the space in the mediastinum which contains the heart, pericardium, great vessels and bronchi (at the roots of the lung).

3.4

Answer: D   External intercostals – internal intercostals – innermost intercostals – parietal pleura

A needle inserted for aspiration of fluid from the pleural space will pass through the skin, subcutaneous tissue, external intercostals, internal intercostals, innermost intercostals and parietal pleura in that order from superficial to deep.

3.5

Answer: E   Latissimus dorsi

Latissimus dorsi is a triangular, flat muscle that covers the lumbar region and the lower half of the thoracic region. It has an extensive origin from the spinous processes of the lower six thoracic vertebrae, from the posterior layer of the lumbodorsal fascia, from the external lip of the crest of the ilium lateral to the margin of the sacrospinalis, and from the three or four lower ribs by fleshy digitations, which are interposed between similar processes of the external oblique. Through the posterior layer of the lumbodorsal fascia it is attached to the spines of the lumbar and sacral vertebrae, to the supraspinal ligament, and to the posterior part of the crest of the ilium. From this extensive origin the fibres converge and form a thick, narrow tendon which crosses the inferior angle of the scapula (usually receiving a few fibres from it). The muscle curves around the lower border of the teres major muscle, and is twisted on itself, so that the superior fibres become at first posterior and then inferior, and the vertical fibres become at first anterior and then superior. It is inserted into the bottom of the intertubercular groove of the humerus above the tendon of the pectoralis major through a quadrilateral tendon that is about 7 cm. long. The lower border of its tendon is united with that of teres major, the surfaces of the two being separated near their insertions by a bursa; another bursa is sometimes interposed between the muscle and the inferior angle of the scapula. The tendon of the muscle gives off an expansion to the deep fascia of the arm.

Latissimus dorsi is supplied by the sixth, seventh and eighth cervical nerves through the thoracodorsal (long subscapular) nerve. When the latissimus dorsi muscle acts on the humerus, it depresses and draws it backward, and at the same time rotates it inward. It is the muscle that is principally employed in giving a downward blow, as in felling a tree. With the arm fixed, the muscle can act in various ways on the trunk; it can raise the lower ribs and assist in forcible inspiration; or, if both arms are fixed, the two muscles can assist the abdominal muscles and pectorals in suspending and drawing the trunk forward, as in climbing.

thorax

3.6

Answer: D   Inferior vena cava – right atrium – tricuspid valve
– right ventricle – pulmonary trunk – left pulmonary
artery – left superior lobar artery – left apical
segmental artery

Pulmonary embolism is a blockage of an artery in the lungs by a
blood clot, fat, air or clumped tumour cells. By far the most common
form of pulmonary embolism is a thromboembolism, which occurs
when a blood clot, generally a venous thrombus, becomes dislodged
from its site of formation and embolises to the arterial blood supply
of one of the lungs. Symptoms may include dyspnoea, pain during
breathing and, more rarely, circulatory instability and death. A clot
originating in the leg vein will travel up the inferior vena cava, into
the right atrium, through the tricuspid valve, into the right ventricle,
through the pulmonary trunk, into the left pulmonary artery, into the
left superior lobar artery, to finally reach the left apical segmental
artery and block it.

3.7

Answer: C   The great cardiac vein is the largest tributary of the
coronary sinus and this vein starts at the apex of
the heart and ascends with the anterior ventricular
branch of the left coronary artery

Most of the veins of the heart open into the coronary sinus. This
is a wide venous channel, about 2.25 cm in length, situated in the
posterior part of the coronary sulcus and covered by muscular fibres
from the left atrium. It ends in the right atrium between the opening
of the inferior vena cava and the atrioventricular aperture, its orifice
being guarded by a semilunar valve, the valve of the coronary sinus
(valve of Thebesius). Its tributaries are the great, small and middle
cardiac veins, the posterior vein of the left ventricle and the oblique
vein of the left atrium, all of which, except the last, are provided
with valves at their orifices.

The great cardiac vein begins at the apex of the heart and ascends
along the anterior longitudinal sulcus to the base of the ventricles. It
then curves to the left in the coronary sulcus and, reaching the back
of the heart, opens into the left extremity of the coronary sinus. It

thorax

is the largest tributary of the coronary sinus. It receives tributaries from the left atrium and from both ventricles: one, the left marginal vein, is of considerable size and ascends along the left margin of the heart. The small cardiac vein runs in the coronary sulcus between the right atrium and ventricle and opens into the right extremity of the coronary sinus. It receives blood from the back of the right atrium and ventricle; the right marginal vein ascends along the right margin of the heart and joins it in the coronary sulcus, or opens directly into the right atrium. The middle cardiac vein commences at the apex of the heart, ascends in the posterior longitudinal sulcus and ends in the coronary sinus near its right extremity. The posterior vein of the left ventricle runs on the diaphragmatic surface of the left ventricle to the coronary sinus, but may end in the great cardiac vein.

The oblique vein of the left atrium (oblique vein of Marshall) is a small vessel that descends obliquely on the back of the left atrium and ends in the coronary sinus near its left extremity; it is continuous above with the ligament of the left vena cava and the two structures form the remnant of the left Cuvierian duct.

The following two groups of cardiac veins do not end in the coronary sinus: the anterior cardiac veins, comprising three or four small vessels which collect blood from the front of the right ventricle and open into the right atrium (the right marginal vein frequently opens into the right atrium and is therefore sometimes regarded as belonging to this group) the smallest cardiac veins (veins of Thebesius), consisting of a number of minute veins which arise in the muscular wall of the heart (the majority open into the atria, but a few end in the ventricles).

thorax

3.8

Answer: A   Foramen ovale

Atrial septal defect is a congenital heart defect that results in a communication between the atria of the heart and may involve the interatrial septum. The interatrial septum is the tissue that separates the right and left atria from each other. Without this septum, or if there is a defect in this septum, it is possible for blood to travel from the left side of the heart to the right side of the heart, or the other way around, resulting in mixing of arterial and venous blood.

During development of the fetus, the interatrial septum develops to eventually separate the left and right atria. The foramen ovale remains open during fetal development to allow blood from the venous system to bypass the lungs and go to the systemic circulation. This is because, before birth, the oxygenation of the blood is via the placenta and not the lungs. A layer of tissue begins to cover the foramen ovale during fetal development and will close it completely soon after birth. After birth, the pressure in the pulmonary circulation drops and the foramen ovale closes. In approximately 25% of adults the foramen ovale does not seal over. In this case, elevation of pressure in the pulmonary circulation (in pulmonary hypertension due to various causes, or transiently during a cough) can cause opening of the foramen ovale. This is known as a patent foramen ovale.

3.9

Answer: C   Moderator band (septomarginal trobecula)

A muscular band, well marked in sheep and some other animals, frequently extends from the base of the anterior papillary muscle to the ventricular septum. From its attachments it was thought to prevent overdistension of the ventricle and was named the 'moderator band'. However, more recent research has indicated that it is more properly considered part of the electrical conduction system of the heart and in that capacity it is now called the septomarginal trabecula.

3.10

Answer: B   Sternal angle

The sternal angle is the point where the costal cartilage attaches the second rib to the sternum. This is an important anatomical landmark to remember − it is used to find the valves when auscultating the heart. The costal margins are formed by the medial borders of the seventh to tenth costal cartilages. They are easily palpable and extend inferolaterally from the xiphisternal joint. The sternal notch/jugular notch is the notch located at the superior border of the manubrium, between the sternal ends of the clavicles. The sternoclavicular joints are simply the joints connecting the sternum with the clavicles. Finally, the xiphoid process is the bone that forms the inferior part of the sternum.

3.11

Answer: B   Intercostal nerves

Intercostal nerves are the ventral primary rami of spinal nerves T1–T11. They provide motor innervation to intercostal muscles, abdominal wall muscles (via T7–T11) and muscles of the forearm and hand (via T1). They provide sensory innervation to the skin of the chest and abdomen on the anterior and lateral sides. The other nerves listed do not innervate the chest wall. Dorsal primary rami provide motor innervation to true back muscles and sensory innervation to the skin on the back. The lateral pectoral nerve provides motor innervation to pectoralis major only, while the medial pectoral nerve provides motor innervation to pectoralis major and minor. The thoracodorsal nerve provides motor innervation to latissimus dorsi.

3.12

Answer: A   Costodiaphragmatic recess

The costodiaphragmatic recess is the lowest extent of the pleural cavity or sac. It is the part of the pleural sac where the costal pleura changes into the diaphragmatic pleura. Because this is the inferior part of the pleural sac, fluid in the pleural sac will fall to this region when a patient sits up. The costodiaphragmatic recess is also the area into which a needle is inserted for thoracocentesis and it is found at different levels at different areas of the thorax. At the midclavicular line, the costodiaphragmatic recess is between ribs 6 and 8; at the midaxillary line it is between ribs 8 and 10; and at the paravertebral line it is between ribs 10 and 12. The costomediastinal recess is found where the costal pleura becomes the mediastinal pleura. The cupola is the part of the pleural cavity that extends above the level of the first rib into the root of the neck. The hilar reflection is the point at the root of the lung where the mediastinal pleura is reflected and becomes continuous with the visceral pleura. Finally, the middle mediastinum is the space in the mediastinum that contains the heart, pericardium, great vessels and bronchi (at the roots of the lung).

thorax

3.13

Answer: D   Oblique pericardial sinus

The oblique pericardial sinus is an area of the pericardial cavity located behind the left atrium of the heart where the serous pericardium reflects onto the inferior vena cava and pulmonary veins. If you slide your fingers under the heart, they will be in the oblique sinus. The other pericardial sinus that you should be familiar with is the transverse sinus. The transverse sinus is an area of the pericardial cavity located behind the aorta and pulmonary trunk and anterior to the superior vena cava. It separates the outflow vessels from the inflow vessels. The coronary sinus is a large vein on the heart that drains into the right atrium. The coronary sulcus is a groove on the heart that separates the atria from the ventricles. The costomediastinal recess is an area in the pleural sac where the costal pleura changes to the mediastinal pleura.

3.14

Answer: D   Sternoclavicular joint

The first rib articulates with the sternum directly below the sternoclavicular joint. The nipple is found in the fourth intercostal space, between the fourth and fifth ribs. The sternal angle is connected to the costal cartilage of rib 2. Finally, the xiphoid process is located just below the point where the costal cartilage of rib 7 articulates with the sternum. The root of the lung consists of the main bronchus, pulmonary and bronchial vessels, lymphatic vessels and nerves entering and leaving the lung.

3.15

Answer: D   Oblique pericardial sinus

The oblique pericardial sinus is an area of the pericardial cavity located behind the left atrium of heart where the serous pericardium reflects onto the inferior vena cava and pulmonary veins. If you slide your fingers under the heart, they will be in this space. The other pericardial sinus that you should be familiar with is the transverse sinus. The transverse sinus is an area of the pericardial cavity located behind the aorta and pulmonary trunk and anterior to the superior vena cava. It separates the outflow vessels from the inflow vessels. The cardiac notch is an indentation in the superior lobe of the left lung, which creates the lingula. The costomediastinal recess is an area in the pleural sac where the costal pleura changes to the mediastinal pleura. Finally, the hilar reflection is the reflection of pleura on the root of the lung, where visceral pleura on the lung becomes continuous with the mediastinal pleura.

3.16

Answer: D   Cupola

The cupola is the cervical parietal pleura which extends slightly above the level of the first rib into the root of the neck. The costodiaphragmatic recess is the part of the pleural sac where the costal pleura changes into the diaphragmatic pleura. It is the lowest extent of the pleural sac. The costomediastinal recess is found where the costal pleura becomes the mediastinal pleura. The endothoracic fascia is connective tissue between the inner chest wall and the costal parietal pleura. The costocervical recess is a made-up term.

3.17

Answer: C   Left vagus

The left vagus nerve lies against the lateral surface of the arch of the aorta. The left recurrent laryngeal nerve is an especially important nerve arising from the vagus, which loops around the aortic arch. This nerve innervates the muscles of the left larynx. If it is damaged, a patient may experience hoarseness after surgery. Care must be taken to preserve this nerve, especially during thyroid surgery. The left and right phrenic nerves, which innervate the diaphragm, are lateral to the vagus nerves and are not looping near the aortic arch. The left and right sympathetic trunks lie on the posterior chest wall and are not involved with the aortic arch.

thorax

3.18

Answer: E   Transverse pericardial sinus

The transverse pericardial sinus is an area of the pericardial cavity located behind the aorta and pulmonary trunk and anterior to the superior vena cava. When entering the transverse pericardial sinus, a surgeon will insert an index finger between the aorta and pulmonary trunk on the ventral side and the superior vena cava on the dorsal side. The oblique pericardial sinus is an area of the pericardial cavity located behind the left atrium of the heart. If a surgeon places fingers under the apex of the heart, then moves the fingers until they are stopped by a pericardial reflection, then the fingers are in the oblique sinus. The cardiac notch is a structure on the left lung that separates the lingula below from the upper portion of the superior lobe of the left lung. The coronary sinus is a venous sinus on the posterior surface of the heart which receives blood from the smaller veins that drain the heart. The coronary sulcus is a groove on the heart between the atria and ventricles. The coronary sinus, circumflex artery and right coronary artery lie in the coronary sulcus.

3.19

Answer: B   Pulmonary trunk and aorta

The transverse pericardial sinus is an area of the pericardial cavity located behind the aorta and pulmonary trunk and anterior to the superior vena cava. Therefore, the two large vessels lying ventral to his finger are the pulmonary trunk and aorta; the large vessel lying dorsal to his finger is the superior vena cava (see also *Answer* to **3.18**).

3.20

Answer: B   Costodiaphragmatic recess

The costodiaphragmatic recess is the lowest extent of the pleural cavity or sac. It is the part of the pleural sac where the costal pleura changes into the diaphragmatic pleura. It is also the area into which a needle is inserted for thoracocentesis and it is found at different levels in different areas of the thorax. At the midclavicular line, the costodiaphragmatic recess is between ribs 6 and 8; at the midaxillary line it is between ribs 8 and 10; and at the paravertebral line it is between ribs 10 and 12. Therefore, inserting the needle just above the ninth rib at the midaxillary line should put you in the costodiaphragmatic recess.

The cardiac notch is a structure on the left lung which separates the lingula below from the upper portion of the superior lobe of the left lung. The costomediastinal recess is found where the costal pleura becomes the mediastinal pleura. The cupola is the part of the pleural cavity which extends above the level of the first rib into the root of the neck. The oblique pericardial sinus is an area of the pericardial cavity located behind the left atrium of the heart.

3.21

Answer: A   Costodiaphragmatic recess

The costodiaphragmatic recess is the lowest extent of the pleural cavity or sac. It is the part of the pleural sac where the costal pleura changes into the diaphragmatic pleura. It is also the area into which a needle is inserted for thoracocentesis and it is found at different levels in different areas of the thorax. At the midclavicular line, the costodiaphragmatic recess is between ribs 6 and 8; at the mid-axillary line it is between ribs 8 and 10; and at the paravertebral line it is between ribs 10 and 12. Therefore, inserting the needle just above the ninth rib at the midaxillary line should put the surgeons's needle in the costodiaphragmatic recess.

The costomediastinal recess is found where the costal pleura becomes the mediastinal pleura. The cupola is the part of the pleural cavity that extends above the level of the first rib into the root of the neck. The hilar reflection is the point at the root of the lung where the mediastinal pleura is reflected and becomes continuous with the visceral pleura. The pulmonary ligament is a fold of pleura located below the root of the lung where the visceral pleura and the mediastinal parietal pleura are continuous with each other.

thorax

3.22

Answer: B   Costomediastinal recess

The costomediastinal recess is an area right next to the cardiac notch, which is an indentation in the superior lobe of the left lung. If you take a very deep breath, the lingula of the left lung, which is formed by the cardiac notch, will tend to expand into the costomediastinal recess. The costodiaphragmatic recess is the lowest extent of the pleural cavity or sac. It is the part of the pleural sac where the costal pleura changes into the diaphragmatic pleura. The cupola is the part of the pleural cavity that extends above the level of the first rib into the root of the neck. The hilum is found on the medial surface of the lung – it is the point at which the structures forming the root enter and leave the lung. The pulmonary ligament is a fold of pleura located below the root of the lung where the visceral pleura and the mediastinal parietal pleura are continuous with each other.

3.23

Answer: E   Transverse process of the vertebra T7

The tubercle of a rib is a projection located posteroinferior and lateral to the neck of the rib. It articulates with the transverse process of the vertebra of the same number. So, the tubercle of rib 7 should articulate with the transverse process of the T7 vertebra. The head of the rib is the part of the rib that articulates with the demifacets of two adjacent vertebral bodies. So, the head of rib 7 should articulate with the sixth vertebra superiorly and the seventh vertebra inferiorly.

3.24

Answer: B   Cupola

The cupola is the part of the plural cavity that extends above the level of the first rib into the root of the neck. Therefore, if a patient was stabbed above the clavicle, it would be very likely that the cupola was damaged. The costal pleura is the layer of parietal pleura that covers the costal surface. The hilar reflection is the point where the visceral pleura of the lung reflects to become continuous with the parietal pleura. The mediastinal pleura is the parietal pleura on the mediastinal surface, found medial to the lung. Finally, the pulmonary ligament is a double layer of pleura extending from the inferior end of the hilar reflection downward to the diaphragm below.

3.25

Answer: D Left recurrent laryngeal nerve

The left recurrent laryngeal nerve is a branch of the vagus that wraps around the aorta, posterior to the ductus arteriosus or ligamentum arteriosum. It then travels superiorly to innervate muscles of the larynx. It is important to protect this nerve during surgery. If the left recurrent laryngeal nerve becomes paralysed, a patient might experience a hoarse voice or even have difficulty breathing due to a laryngeal spasm. You should make sure that you understand what this nerve does, what types of procedures might injure this nerve and the effects of a damaged left recurrent laryngeal. The accessory hemiazygos vein is a vein on the left side of the body. It drains the posterolateral chest wall and empties blood into the azygos vein. The left internal thoracic artery is a branch of the left subclavian artery that supplies blood to the anterior thoracic wall. The left phrenic nerve runs laterally to the vagus nerve and its branches in the thorax; it is not close enough to be damaged by the surgery. The thoracic duct is deep in the chest — it travels between the azygos vein and the aorta, posterior to the oesophagus.

3.26

Answer: E Pulmonary ligament

The pulmonary ligament is a double layer of pleura extending from the inferior end of the hilar reflection downward to the diaphragm. Therefore, it is a structure that would block you from moving your finger posteriorly at the root of a lung. The costodiaphragmatic recess is the space at the inferior border of the lung where the costal pleura touches the diaphragmatic pleura. The cupola is the part of the pleura that extends superiorly above the first rib — it is not associated with the root of the lung in any way. The inferior vena cava is found in the mediastinum and would not be near the root of

thorax

the lung. The left pulmonary veins are part of the root of the lung and would not block someone from reaching behind the lung.

3.27

Answer: B   Endothoracic fascia

The endothoracic fascia is the connective tissue between the inner aspect of the chest wall and the costal parietal pleura. By clearing the endothoracic fascia, it is easy to separate the costal pleura from the thoracic wall. Deep fascia is a fascial layer that invests a muscle or muscle group – it is not present around the lungs. The parietal pleura comprises the cupola or cervical pleura, costal pleura, diaphragmatic pleura and mediastinal pleura. It lines the inner surfaces of the walls of the pleural cavity. The visceral pleura is the serous membrane that covers the lungs. Finally, the transversus thoracis muscle fascia is only associated with the transversus thoracis – it would not provide a natural cleavage plane for separating the costal pleura from the thoracic wall.

3.28

Answer: A   Costodiaphragmatic recess

The costodiaphragmatic recess is the area inferior to the lung where the costal and diaphragmatic pleura are continuous. This is the lowest extent of the pleural cavity. The costomediastinal recess is a small anterior recess where the costal and mediastinal pleura are continuous. The cupola is the pleural space that extends above the first rib. The inferior mediastinum is a term sometimes used to refer to the anterior, middle and posterior subdivisions of the mediastinum all together. The pulmonary ligament is a fold of pleura located beneath the root of the lung.

thorax

3.29

Answer: C   Second costal cartilage

The sternal angle is a very important anatomical landmark which is used when placing the stethoscope and listening for heart sounds. The sternal angle is the location of the attachment of the costal cartilage of the second rib to the sternum. Therefore, once you locate the sternal angle on a patient, you know the location of the second rib and you can use that landmark to find the right spots to auscultate each valve of the heart. Also remember that a horizontal plane through the sternal angle passes through the T4/T5 intervertebral disc and marks the inferior boundary of the superior mediastinum.

3.30

Answer: D   The bottom of interspace 9 in the midaxillary line

For a thoracocentesis, the needle needs to be inserted below the level of the lungs, in the costodiaphragmatic recess. At the midclavicular line, the recess is between intercostal spaces 6 and 8; at the midaxillary line it is between 8 and 10 and at the paravertebral line between 10 and 12. Additionally, the needle needs to be inserted at the top of the rib (or the bottom of the intercostal space). This is essential for avoiding damage to the neurovascular bundle that is found below the rib, running in the costal groove. Taken together, these two pieces of information point to the conditions listed in option D as the only appropriate ones for a thoracocentesis.

3.31

Answer: C   Costomediastinal recess

The costomediastinal recess is an area right next to the cardiac notch, which is an indentation in the superior lobe of the left lung. This is where the medial area of the superior lobe of the left lung would tend to expand if it became very inflated. The lung would not enter the anterior mediastinum, which is an area between the two pleural sacs, bounded anteriorly by the sternum and posteriorly by the pericardium. The anterior mediastinum contains areolar tissue,

thorax

sternopericardial ligaments, lymph vessels and nodes, but no lung tissue. The costodiaphragmatic recess is the recess at the inferior border of a lung. This is the space into which the inferior lobe of the lung would expand following deep inhalation. The cupola is the serous membrane lining the pleural cavity, which extends above the level of the first rib into the root of the neck. The most superior portion of the superior lobe might expand into this space. The pulmonary ligament is the fold of pleura located below the root of the lung where the visceral pleura and the mediastinal parietal pleura are continuous with each other.

3.32

Answer: A   Cardiac notch

The cardiac notch is only found on the left lung, which makes sense because the heart is located on the left side of the mediastinum. The horizontal fissure is a deep groove that separates the middle lobe from the upper lobe of the right lung. The left lung does not have a horizontal fissure. The oblique fissure is found in both lungs. It separates the upper lobe from the lower lobe in both lungs and the middle lobe from the lower lobe in the right lung. Both lungs also have a superior lobar bronchus leading to their superior lobes. Finally, the right lung has three lobes while the left lung has two lobes.

3.33

Answer: D   Left recurrent laryngeal

The tracheobronchial nodes are at the tracheal bifurcation. There are three groups of these nodes: right superior, left superior and inferior. The aorta loops over the left bronchus, near the tracheal bifurcation. Therefore, it is reasonable to assume that any nerve that is closely associated with the aorta might be irritated if the tracheobronchial lymph nodes became inflamed. This means that the correct answer is the left recurrent laryngeal nerve, which loops under the aorta to ascend to the larynx. The right and left phrenic nerves are lateral and would not be irritated by the inflammation. The right recurrent laryngeal nerve loops around the right subclavian

thorax

artery and is not close enough to this area. Finally, the right vagus is not closely associated with the aorta.

3.34

Answer: D   Lingula

When inspiring fully, the lingula of the left lung might partially fill the costomediastinal recess. The lingula, a tongue-like projection of the left lung below the cardiac notch, is right next to the costomediastinal recess. If the apex of the lung was highly inflated, it might expand to fill the cupola. The hilum is the part of the lung where the structures forming the root of the lung – the main bronchus, pulmonary vessels, bronchial vessels, lymphatics and nerve – enter and leave the lung. It does not expand on inspiration. The middle lobe of the lung can expand to fill the costomediastinal recess, but remember that the question is specifically asking about a left lung structure and the middle lobe is only found in the right lung!

3.35

Answer: C   Lower lode from both upper and middle lobes

The oblique fissure cuts across the right lung in such a way as to separate the lower lobe from both the middle and upper lobes. So what does the horizontal fissure do? It separates the middle lobe from the upper lobe. Remember: the lingula is only on the left lung and is part of the superior lobe.

3.36

Answer: B   Inferior lobe

Because of the sharp angle of the oblique fissure, the posterior surface of the left lung is almost entirely composed of the inferior lobe. Therefore, a stab wound halfway between the apex and the diaphragmatic surface of the lung would result in injury to the inferior lobe. The hilum is the point at which the structures forming the root of the lung enter the lung. The lingula is part of the superior lobe, which forms the anterior and superior sides of the lung. In addition,

thorax

remember that the middle lobe is not relevant here because it is on the right lung. (Besides, it does not even contribute to the posterior surface of the right lung.)

3.37

Answer: D   Right main bronchus

There are several reasons why inhaled objects will be more likely to enter the right lung instead of the left lung. First, the carina, a ridge-like structure at the bifurcation of the trachea, is set a little toward the left. Therefore, there is a more direct path for objects to fall to the right. In addition, the right bronchus is shorter, wider and more vertical than the left bronchus. All of these factors mean that an inhaled object will enter the right main bronchus. It would be almost impossible for a bead to be lodged in the terminal bronchiole of the right lung – that is a very small space!

3.38

Answer: D   Its upper lobar bronchus lies behind and above the right pulmonary artery

The structures at the root of the lung have different relationships in the right and left lungs. On both sides the pulmonary veins are anterior and inferior while the bronchus is posterior. The difference between the two sides involves the pulmonary arteries. On the right side, the arteries are anterior to the bronchus, while on the left side the arteries are superior to the bronchus. The right lung is slightly larger than the left lung and the lingula is found in the left lung only. Neither lung is in the mediastinum – the mediastinum is the space between the two pleural sacs. Finally, the phrenic nerve passes anterior to the root of the lung – on both the left and right sides.

3.39

Answer: D   Right bronchus

The right bronchus receives blood from a single right bronchial artery. This artery may branch from one of the left bronchial arteries or it

thorax

may branch from the right third posterior intercostal artery, the first intercostal artery that arises from the descending aorta. Damaging this artery might stop the blood supply to the main bronchus. The intercostal arteries to the first and second intercostal spaces are derived from the highest intercostal artery, so the blood supply to either of these spaces would not be disrupted. The left bronchus is supplied by two left bronchial arteries, which branch directly from the descending aorta. The fibrous pericardium is a fibrous sac that contains the pericardial cavity and the heart. Its blood supply is not a major concern.

3.40

Answer: C   Superior segmental bronchus of the right inferior lobe

Remember: inhaled material tends to go into the right bronchus because it is bigger and more vertically orientated than the left! The superior segmental bronchus branches posteriorly off the intermediate bronchus or the inferior lobe bronchus, so it is the segmental bronchus most likely to receive the foreign bodies that enter the right main bronchus (see also *Answer* to **3.37**).

3.41

Answer: A   Carina

The carina is a keel-shaped cartilage lying at the tracheal bifurcation – it separates the right main stem bronchus from the left main stem bronchus. The carina is a little to the left of the tracheal bifurcation, so if there is an inhaled body the carina will tend to divert foreign objects to the right main bronchus. The cricoid cartilage is the inferior and posterior cartilage of the larynx. The costal cartilages prolong the ribs anteriorly and contribute to the elasticity of the thoracic wall. They increase in length through the first seven and then gradually decrease. The pulmonary ligament is a fold of pleura located below the root of the lung. Tracheal rings are the cartilaginous structures that support the trachea and keep it patent.

thorax

3.42

Answer: E   The middle lobe from the upper lobe

The horizontal fissure cuts across the right lung in such a way as to separate the middle lobe from the upper lobe. The oblique fissure separates the lower lobe from both the middle and upper lobes. Remember: the lingula is only on the left lung and it is part of the superior lobe.

3.43

Answer: E   Superior segment of the lower lobe

The superior segmental bronchus to the lower lobe of the right lung branches posteriorly off the intermediate bronchus or the inferior lobe bronchus. Therefore, it is the segmental bronchus most likely to receive the fluid or foreign bodies that enter the right main bronchus. This segment of the lung is even more likely to accumulate fluid when the patient is supine.

3.44

Answer: C   Left brachiocephalic vein

The left brachiocephalic vein joins with the right brachiocephalic vein to form the superior vena cava on the right side of the body. Therefore, the left brachiocephalic vein must course across the mediastinum to reach its destination. The left subclavian artery and vein are lateral to the mediastinum, while the left jugular and common carotid travel vertically.

3.45

Answer: C   Left brachiocephalic

Remember: the ascending aorta is the short part of the aorta emerging from the heart before the aortic arch. The left brachiocephalic vein is the only vein listed which is anterosuperior to that part of the aorta. It crosses horizontally through the mediastinum to join with the right brachiocephalic vein and form the superior vena cava. The right brachiocephalic vein stays on the right side of the chest and would not be affected by the aortic aneurysm. The azygos vein is also on the right side of the chest and it lies deep in the thoracic cavity. The internal thoracic vein lies on the interior surface of the anterior wall of the chest. Although it drains into the brachiocephalic vein, it would not be affected by the aneurysm. The left superior intercostal vein crosses the aortic arch laterally, but its blockage would only affect drainage of intercostal spaces 2–4 on the left side.

3.46

Answer: A   Azygos vein

The azygos vein begins opposite the first or second lumbar vertebra by a branch known as the ascending lumbar vein. It can also originate by a branch from the right renal vein, or from the inferior vena cava. It enters the thorax through the aortic hiatus in the diaphragm and passes in the posterior mediastinum along the right side of the vertebral column to the fourth thoracic vertebra. At this level it arches forward over the root of the right lung, and ends in the superior vena cava, just before the superior vena cava pierces the pericardium. In the aortic hiatus it lies with the thoracic duct on the right side of the aorta. In the thorax it lies on the intercostal arteries, on the right side of the aorta and thoracic duct, and is partly covered by pleura.

It receives the right subcostal and intercostal veins. The upper three or four intercostal veins open by a common stem called the highest superior intercostal vein. It receives the hemiazygos veins, several oesophageal, mediastinal, and pericardial veins and, near its termination, the right bronchial vein. A few imperfect valves are found in the azygos vein, but its tributaries are provided with complete valves.

3.47

Answer: A   Left brachiocephalic vein

The thymus is a very superficial structure found in the anterior mediastinum. The left brachiocephalic vein courses through the

thorax

mediastinum to join the right brachiocephalic vein and form the superior vena cava on the right side of the thorax. Because the left brachiocephalic vein is fairly superficial, it travels just deep to the thymus. So it might be compressed by the tumor. The left pulmonary vein, left bronchial vein and right pulmonary arteries are deep structures that enter and exit the lung at its root – they are not near the thymus. The right superior intercostal vein drains intercostal spaces 2–4. It drains into the arch of the azygos vein and is not associated with the thymus.

3.48

Answer: C   Oesophagus

In the mid-thorax, the aorta, thoracic duct and azygos vein are all posterior to the oesophagus. (They are in that order, from left to right.) The superior vena cava and the trachea are not located in the mid-thorax – the superior vena cava terminates as it feeds into the right atrium and the trachea ends as it splits into the two main stem bronchi, which enter the lungs.

3.49

Answer: B   Voluntary muscle activity

The posterior mediastinum is bounded superiorly by the plane through the sternal angle and T4/5, inferiorly by the diaphragm, anteriorly by the middle mediastinum and posteriorly by the spinal cord. This area contains the descending thoracic aorta, the azygos system, the oesophagus, the thoracic duct and lymph nodes. Of the answer choices, the oesophagus is the only one in the posterior mediastinum. The great vessels and bronchi at the roots of the lung are in the middle mediastinum.

3.50

Answer: E

The sympathetic nervous system is not responsible for voluntary muscle activity. The neurones that supply voluntary muscles originate

thorax

from the ventral horn of the spinal cord. One of the main functions of sympathetic nerves is maintaining the tone of blood vessels – if these nerves were damaged, it would be difficult to regulate vascular tone. The sympathetic nervous system also regulates the arrector pili muscles, sweat production and visceral reflexes.

3.51

Answer: B   Ascending aorta

The mediastinum lies between the right and left pleurae in and near the median sagittal plane of the chest. It extends from the sternum in front to the vertebral column behind and contains all the thoracic viscera except the lungs. It can be divided for purposes of description into two parts: an upper portion, above the upper level of the pericardium, which is called the superior mediastinum; and a lower portion, below the upper level of the pericardium. This lower portion is again subdivided into three parts: that in front of the pericardium, the anterior mediastinum; that containing the pericardium and its contents, the middle mediastinum; and that behind the pericardium, the posterior mediastinum.

The middle mediastinum is the broadest part of the interpleural space. It contains the heart enclosed in the pericardium, the ascending aorta, the lower half of the superior vena cava with the azygos vein opening into it, the bifurcation of the trachea and the two bronchi, the pulmonary artery dividing into its two branches, the right and left pulmonary veins, the phrenic nerves and some bronchial lymph glands. Of all the options, this patient is most likely to have an aneurysm of the ascending aorta.

3.52

Answer: D   Superior vena cava

The posterior mediastinum is an irregular triangular space running parallel with the vertebral column; it is bounded in front by the pericardium above and by the posterior surface of the diaphragm below, behind by the vertebral column from the lower border of the fourth to the twelfth thoracic vertebra and on either side by the

thorax

mediastinal pleura. It contains the thoracic part of the descending aorta, the azygos and the two hemiazygos veins, the vagus and splanchnic nerves, the oesophagus, the thoracic duct and some lymph glands. In this clinical vignette, the lymph glands are the correct choice.

3.53

Answer: B   Fourth thoratic

The superior mediastinum is that portion of the interpleural space that lies between the manubrium sterni in front and the upper thoracic vertebrae behind. It is bounded below by a slightly oblique plane passing backward from the junction of the manubrium and body of the sternum to the lower part of the body of the fourth thoracic vertebra and laterally by the pleurae. It contains the origins of the sternohyoid muscles and sternothyroid muscles and the lower ends of the longi colli; the aortic arch; the innominate artery and the thoracic portions of the left common carotid and the left subclavian arteries; the innominate veins and the upper half of the superior vena cava; the left highest intercostal vein; the vagus, cardiac, phrenic and left recurrent nerves; the trachea and oesophagus; the thoracic duct; the remains of the thymus; and some lymph glands.

3.54

Answer: E   Thoracic duct

The cervical portion of the oesophagus is in relation, in front, with the trachea; and at the lower part of the neck, where it projects to the left side, with the thyroid gland. Behind, it rests on the vertebral column and longus colli muscles; on either side it is in relation with the common carotid artery (especially the left, as it inclines to that side) and parts of the lobes of the thyroid gland; the recurrent nerves ascend between it and the trachea; to its left side is the thoracic duct. Of all the options given in the vignette, the thoracic duct is the most likely structure to be at risk of injury.

thorax

3.55

Answer: A   Aortic arch

The mediastinal surface of each lung is in contact with the mediastinal pleura. It presents a deep concavity, the cardiac impression, which accommodates the pericardium. The cardiac impression is larger and deeper on the left than on the right lung, mainly because the heart projects further to the left than to the right side of the median plane. Above and behind this concavity is a triangular depression called the hilum. The structures which form the root of the lung enter and leave the lung at the hilum. These structures are invested by pleura that forms the pulmonary ligament below the hilum and behind the pericardial impression. On the right lung, immediately above the hilum, is an arched depression which accommodates the azygos vein. Superior to this there is a wide groove for the superior vena cava and right brachiocephalic vein, some little distance below the apex. There is a depression for the innominate artery behind the groove for the superior vena cava and right brachiocephalic vein, nearer the apex. Behind the hilum and the attachment of the pulmonary ligament is a vertical groove for the oesophagus. The oesophageal groove becomes less distinct below, due to the inclination of the lower part of the oesophagus to the left of the midline. In front and to the right of the lower part of the oesophageal groove is a deep concavity for the extrapericardiac portion of the thoracic part of the inferior vena cava. On the left lung, immediately above the hilum, is a well-marked curved depression produced by the aortic arch (one of the options given in this question), and running upward from this toward the apex is a groove which accommodates the left subclavian artery. The left brachiocephalic vein lies in a slight impression in front of the groove for the left subclavian artery, close to the margin of the lung. Behind the hilum and pulmonary ligament is a vertical depression produced by the descending aorta and in front of this, near the base of the lung, the lower part of the oesophagus causes a shallow impression.

thorax

SECTION 4: ABDOMEN – ANSWERS

4.1

Answer: C   Short gastric

The short gastric arteries branch from the splenic artery near the hilum of the spleen. They travel back in the gastrosplenic ligament to supply the fundus of the stomach. So, these arteries might be damaged if the gastrosplenic ligament was disrupted. The left gastric artery is a branch of the coeliac trunk that supplies the left half of the lesser curvature. The splenic artery travels deep to the stomach to reach the hilum of the spleen. Although its branches travel in the gastrosplenic ligament, the splenic artery does not travel in this structure and it would not be damaged in this particular case. The middle colic artery is a branch of the superior mesenteric artery that supplies the transverse colon. The left gastroepiploic artery is the largest branch of the splenic artery and runs from left to right about a finger's breadth or more from the greater curvature of the stomach, between the layers of the greater omentum, and anastomoses with the right gastroepiploic. In its course, it distributes several ascending branches to both surfaces of the stomach; others descend to supply the greater omentum and anastomose with branches of the middle colic.

4.2

Answer: E   It has sparse aggregated lymph nodules

The jejunum is wider, its diameter being about 4 cm, and is thicker, more vascular and of a deeper colour than the ileum, so that a given length weighs more. The circular folds (valvulae conniventes) of its mucous membrane are large and thickly set and its villi are larger than those in the ileum. The aggregated lymph nodules are almost absent in the upper part of the jejunum and in the lower part are less frequently found than those in the ileum, are smaller and tend to assume a circular form. By grasping the jejunum between the finger and thumb, the circular folds can be felt through the walls of the gut; these are absent in the lower part of the ileum and it is possible in this way to distinguish the upper from the lower part of the small intestine. Finally, the jejunum for the most part occupies the umbilical and left iliac regions, while the ileum occupies chiefly the umbilical, hypogastric, right iliac and pelvic regions.

4.3

Answer: D   Obturator

The obturator nerve arises from the ventral divisions of the second, third and fourth lumbar nerves. The branch from the third is the largest, while that from the second is often very small. It descends through the fibres of psoas major and emerges from its medial border near the brim of the pelvis. The iliohypogastric nerve arises from the first lumbar nerve. It emerges from the upper part of the lateral border of the psoas major. The ilioinguinal nerve, smaller than the iliohypogastric nerve, arises with it from the first lumbar nerve. It emerges from the lateral border of the psoas major just below the iliohypogastric nerve. The lateral femoral cutaneous nerve arises from the dorsal divisions of the second and third lumbar nerves. It emerges from the lateral border of the psoas major, about its middle. The femoral nerve, the largest branch of the lumbar plexus, arises from the dorsal divisions of the second, third and fourth lumbar nerves. It descends through the fibres of the psoas major, emerging from the muscle at the lower part of its lateral border.

4.4

Answer: C   The left ovarian vein drains into the left renal vein

The testicular (spermatic) veins emerge from the back of the testis and receive tributaries from the epididymis. They unite and form a convoluted plexus, called the pampiniform plexus, which constitutes the greater mass of the spermatic cord. The vessels composing this plexus are very numerous and ascend along the cord, in front of the ductus deferens. Below the superficial inguinal ring they unite to form three or four veins, which pass along the inguinal canal and, entering the abdomen through the deep inguinal ring,

abdomen

coalesce to form two veins, which ascend on psoas major, behind the peritoneum, lying one on either side of the testicular artery. These unite to form a single vein, which opens on the right side into the inferior vena cava, at an acute angle and on the left side into the left renal vein, at a right angle. The testicular veins are provided with valves. The left testicular vein passes behind the iliac colon and is so exposed to pressure from the contents of that part of the bowel. The ovarian veins correspond with the testicular in the man. They form a plexus in the broad ligament near the ovary and uterine tube and communicate with the uterine plexus. They end in the same way as the testicular veins in the man. Valves are occasionally found in these veins. Like the uterine veins, they become much enlarged during pregnancy.

4.5

Answer: C   Descending part of the duodenum

The major duodenal papilla is situated at the medial side of the descending portion of the duodenum, a little below its middle and about 7 to 10 cm from the pylorus. The common bile and pancreatic ducts unite and open by a common orifice on the summit of the duodenal papilla.

4.6

Answer: D   Obliterated umbilical arteries

The medial umbilical ligament is a paired structure found in humans. It is on the deep surface of the anterior abdominal wall and is covered by the medial umbilical folds. It represents the remnant of the fetal umbilical artery, which serves no purpose in humans after birth. In an adult it will be shrivelled. It can be used as a landmark for surgeons exploring the medial inguinal fossa during laparoscopic inguinal hernia repair. Other than this, it has no purpose in an adult and it may be cut or damaged with impunity.

abdomen

4.7

Answer: C   Gastroduodenal

The gastroduodenal artery is a short but large-calibre branch of the hepatic artery, which descends, near the pylorus, between the superior (first) part of the duodenum and the neck of the pancreas and divides at the lower border of the duodenum into two branches, the right gastroepiploic and the superior pancreaticoduodenal. Previous to its division, it gives off two or three small branches to the pyloric end of the stomach and to the pancreas. In this clinical vignette, it is the artery most likely to be the source of bleeding, as it lies posterior to the first part of the duodenum.

4.8

Answer: A   Coeliac artery

The branches of the abdominal aorta can be divided into three sets: visceral, parietal and terminal.

Visceral branches:

- Coeliac artery
- Superior mesenteric artery
- Inferior mesenteric artery
- Middle suprarenal arteries
- Renal arteries
- Gonadal (testicular/ovarian) arteries.

Parietal branches:

- Inferior phrenic arteries
- Lumbar arteries
- Middle sacral artery.

Terminal branches:

- Common iliac arteries.

Of the visceral branches, the coeliac artery and the superior and inferior mesenteric arteries are unpaired, while the suprarenal, renal, testicular and ovarian arteries are paired. Of the parietal branches the inferior phrenic and lumbar arteries are paired; the middle sacral artery is unpaired. The terminal branches are paired.

4.9

Answer: D Give rise to the splenic, left gastric and common hepatic arteries

The coeliac trunk is a short thick trunk, about 1.25 cm in length, which arises from the front of the aorta, just below the aortic hiatus of the diaphragm and, passing nearly horizontally forward, divides into three large branches, the left gastric, the hepatic and the splenic. It occasionally gives off one of the inferior phrenic arteries. It is covered by the lesser omentum. On the right side it is in relation to the right coeliac ganglion and the caudate process of the liver; on the left side, to the left coeliac ganglion and the cardiac end of the stomach. Below, it is in relation to the upper border of the pancreas and the splenic vein.

4.10

Answer: B Suspensory ligament (of Treitz)

The suspensory muscle of the duodenum is the official name of what is commonly known as the ligament of Treitz, and it refers to tissue that connects the duodenum to the diaphragm. It is also known as the suspensory ligament of the duodenum. It arises from the connective tissue around the stems of the coeliac trunk and superior mesenteric artery and inserts into the third and fourth portions of the duodenum and frequently into the duodenojejunal flexure (between the duodenum and the jejunum) as well. It is composed of a slip of skeletal muscle from the right crus of the diaphragm and a fibromuscular band of smooth muscle from the third and fourth parts of the duodenum. Its contraction leads to opening of the duodenojejunal flexure, which results in the flow of chyme. While commonly referred to as a ligament, it is officially both a suspensory muscle and a suspensory ligament because of its composition and function. This muscle/ligament is an important anatomical landmark

abdomen

because it is used to divide the gastrointestinal tract into an upper portion and a lower portion. It is an especially important landmark to look for when examining the bowel for the presence of malrotation of the gut, a syndrome often suspected in young children when they have episodes of recurrent vomiting. Visualising a normal location of the ligament of Treitz in radiological images is critical in ruling out malrotation of the gut in a child; it is located abnormally when malrotation is present.

4.11

Answer: E   Pancreas

Mobility of abdominal contents depends on the presence of mesentery. Structures such as the stomach, transverse colon and appendix all have mesenteries and therefore are relatively mobile. In addition, the greater omentum is a large mobile fold of peritoneum that hangs down from the stomach and extends from the stomach to the transverse colon. In contrast, the pancreas is a retroperitoneal structure and therefore it is fixed.

4.12

Answer: A   Pancreas

The retroperitoneum is the anatomical space behind the abdominal cavity. It has no specific delineating anatomical structures. Organs that were once suspended within the abdominal cavity by mesentery but which migrated posterior to the peritoneum during the course of embryogenesis to become retroperitoneal are considered to be secondarily retroperitoneal organs. Structures that lie behind the peritoneum are termed 'retroperitoneal'. These include:

- Primarily retroperitoneal:
  - kidneys
  - suprarenal glands
  - bladder
  - ureter
  - inferior vena cava

- rectum

- oesophagus (part)

- Secondary retroperitoneal:

  - part of the pancreas

  - the second, third and fourth portions of the duodenum (but not the first portion)

  - ascending and descending portions of the colon.

4.13

Answer: A Oesophageal hiatus

The oesophageal hiatus is situated in the muscular part of the diaphragm at the level of the tenth thoracic vertebra and is elliptical in shape. It is placed above, in front and a little to the left of the aortic hiatus and transmits the oesophagus, the vagus nerves and some small oesophageal arteries.

4.14

Answer: B It is an important anastomatic site for the portal and caval (systematic) venous systems

The rectum is continuous above with the sigmoid colon, while below it ends in the anal canal. From its origin at the level of the third sacral vertebra it passes downward, lying in the sacrococcygeal curve, and extends for about 2.5 cm in front of and a little below the tip of the coccyx, as far as the apex of the prostate. It then bends sharply backward into the anal canal. It therefore presents two anteroposterior curves: an upper, with its convexity backward; and a lower, with its convexity forward. Two lateral curves are also described: one to the right, opposite the junction of the third and fourth sacral vertebrae, and the other to the left, opposite the left sacrococcygeal articulation (though these are of little importance). The rectum is about 12 cm long and at its commencement its calibre is similar to that of the sigmoid colon, but near its termination it is dilated to form the rectal ampulla. The rectum has no sacculations

abdomen

285

comparable to those of the colon, but when the lower part of the rectum is contracted, its mucous membrane is thrown into a number of folds, which are longitudinal in direction and are effaced by the distension of the gut. Besides these, there are certain permanent transverse folds, of a semilunar shape, known as Houston's valves. They are usually three in number; sometimes a fourth is found; and occasionally only two are present. One is situated near the commencement of the rectum, on the right side; a second extends inward from the left side of the tube, opposite the middle of the sacrum; a third, the largest and most constant, projects backward from the forepart of the rectum, opposite the fundus of the urinary bladder. When a fourth is present, it is situated nearly 2.5 cm above the anus on the left and posterior wall of the tube. These folds are about 12 mm in width and contain some of the circular fibres of the gut. In the empty state of the intestine, they overlap each other so effectually as to require considerable manoeuvring to insert a bougie or the finger along the canal. These folds support the weight of faecal matter and prevent it from migrating toward the anus, where its presence always stimulates the urge to defecate.

The peritoneum is related to the upper two-thirds of the rectum, covering at first its front and sides, but lower down its front only. From the latter it is reflected onto the seminal vesicles in men and the posterior vaginal wall in women. The level at which the peritoneum leaves the anterior wall of the rectum to be reflected onto the viscus in front of it is of considerable importance from a surgical point of view, in connection with the removal of the lower part of the rectum. It is higher in men than in women. In men, the height of the rectovesical excavation is about 7.5 cm, the height to which an ordinary index finger can reach from the anus. In women the height of the rectouterine excavation is about 5.5 cm from the anal orifice. The rectum is surrounded by a dense tube of fascia derived from the fascia endopelvina, but fused behind with the fascia covering the sacrum and coccyx. The fascial tube is loosely attached to the rectal wall by areolar tissue to allow for distension of the viscus.

The upper part of the rectum is in relation, behind, to the superior haemorrhoidal vessels, the left piriformis and the left sacral plexus of nerves, which separate it from the pelvic surfaces of the sacral vertebrae. In its lower part it lies directly on the sacrum, coccyx and levatores ani, a dense fascia alone intervening. In front, it is separated above, in the man from the fundus of the bladder, and in the woman from the intestinal surface of the uterus and its appendages, by some convolutions of the small intestine and frequently by the sigmoid colon. Below, it is in relation in the man with the triangular portion of the fundus of the bladder, the vesiculae seminales and ductus deferentes and more anteriorly with the posterior surface of the prostate; in the woman, with the posterior wall of the vagina.

The rectum is supplied by the superior rectal (haemorrhoidal) branch of the inferior mesenteric artery. The veins of the rectum commence in a plexus of vessels that surrounds the anal canal. In the vessels forming this plexus are smaller saccular dilatations just within the margin of the anus; from the plexus, about six vessels of considerable size are given off. These ascend between the muscular and mucous coats for about 12.5 cm, running parallel to each other; they then pierce the muscular coat and, by their union, form a single trunk, the superior haemorrhoidal vein. This arrangement is called the haemorrhoidal plexus. It communicates with the tributaries of the middle and inferior haemorrhoidal veins at its commencement and so a communication is established between the systemic and portal circulations.

4.15

Answer: B   Prostatic urethra

The ejaculatory ducts are two in number, one on either side of the middle line. Each is formed by the union of the duct from the seminal vesicles with the ductus deferens and is about 2 cm long. They commence at the base of the prostate and run forward and downward between its middle and lateral lobes and along the sides of the prostatic utricle, to end by separate slit-like orifices close to or just within the margins of the utricle in the prostatic urethra. The ducts diminish in size and also converge, toward their terminations.

4.16

Answer: E   External abdominal oblique aponeurosis

The inguinal ligament is the lower border of the aponeurosis of the external oblique and extends from the anterior superior iliac spine to the pubic tubercle, from which point it is reflected backward

abdomen

and lateralward to be attached to the pectineal line for about 1.25 cm, forming the lacunar ligament. Its general direction is convex downward toward the thigh, where it is continuous with the fascia lata. Its lateral half is rounded and oblique in direction; its medial half gradually widens at its attachment to the pubis, is more horizontal in direction and lies beneath the spermatic cord.

4.17

Answer: C   Internal abdominal oblique muscle

The cremaster is a thin muscular layer that is composed of a number of fasciculi which take origin from the middle of the inguinal ligament. At its origin its fibres are continuous with those of the internal oblique and also occasionally with the transversus abdominis. It passes along the lateral side of the spermatic cord and descends with it through the superficial inguinal ring on the front and sides of the cord. It forms a series of loops which differ in thickness and length in different people. At the upper part of the cord the loops are short, but they become successively longer and longer, the longest reaching down as low as the testis, where a few are inserted into the tunica vaginalis. These loops are united together by areolar tissue and form a thin covering over the cord and testis called the cremasteric fascia. The fibres ascend along the medial side of the cord and are inserted by a small pointed tendon into the pubic tubercle and crest, as well as into the front of the sheath of the rectus abdominis.

4.18

Answer: C   T10

The umbilicus is an important landmark on the abdomen, because its position is relatively consistent among humans. The skin around the waist at the level of the umbilicus is supported by the tenth thoracic spinal nerve (T10 dermatome). The umbilicus is at the level of the fibrocartilage between the third and fourth lumbar vertebrae.

4.19

Answer: B   Liver, duodenum and gallbladder

Referred pain is an unpleasant sensation localised to an area separate from the site of the causative injury or other painful stimulation. Often, referred pain arises when a nerve is compressed or damaged at or near its origin. In this circumstance, the sensation of pain will generally be felt in the territory that the nerve serves, even though the damage originates elsewhere. A common example is spinal disc herniation, in which a nerve root arising from the spinal cord is compressed by adjacent disc material. Although pain may arise from the damaged disc itself, pain and/or other symptoms will also be felt in the region served by the compressed nerve (for example, the thigh, knee, or foot). Relieving the pressure on the nerve root may ameliorate the referred pain, provided that permanent nerve damage has not occurred. A similar mechanism may be responsible for some instances of the phantom limb syndrome in amputees.

In another classic example of referred pain, patients who are suffering a myocardial infarction feel pain in their left arm. Other examples of referred pain are the common 'ice cream headache' or 'brain freeze' which happens when you accidentally chill the vagus nerve when you eat ice-cold food too quickly, as well as pain from an inflamed gallbladder which may refer pain to the right shoulder and pain from a herniated cervical disc refers pain down one or both arms into the hands. In addition, tooth pain may refer pain that should be localised to the affected tooth to the opposite side of the mouth as opposed to actually feeling pain in the tooth with the cavity or abscess.

In cases of damage to viscera, referred pain may be due to convergence of visceral nerves that innervate the damaged organs with somatic nerves that innervate sections of skin. Because a neurone from the organ and one from the skin can form a synapse with the same projection neurone in the dorsal horn, input from either neurone will be interpreted the same way by it and all neurones further up the pathway. Because the brain is more 'accustomed' to receiving sensation from the peripheral structure than from the viscus, it may interpret the pain as originating from the former. So, there is an array of diseases that cause damage to organs and which produce characteristic patterns of pain in unrelated places in the body's periphery.

abdomen

4.20

Answer: C   Distal jejunum, caecum, vermiform appendix

For convenience of description of the viscera and for reference to morbid conditions of the contained parts, the abdomen is divided into nine regions by imaginary planes, two horizontal and two sagittal, the edges of the planes being indicated by lines drawn on the surface of the body. In the older method the upper, or subcostal, horizontal line encircles the body at the level of the lowest points of the tenth costal cartilages. The lower, or intertubercular, is a line carried through the highest points of the iliac crests seen from the front, that is through the tubercles on the iliac crests about 5 cm behind the anterior superior spines. An alternative method is that of Addison, who adopts the following lines:

- An upper transverse, the transpyloric, halfway between the jugular notch and the upper border of the symphysis pubis. This indicates the margin of the transpyloric plane, which in most cases cuts through the pylorus, the tips of the ninth costal cartilages and the lower border of the first lumbar vertebra.

- A lower transverse line midway between the upper transverse line and the upper border of the symphysis pubis; this is known as the transtubercular, line because it practically corresponds to that passing through the iliac tubercles; behind, its plane cuts the body of the fifth lumbar vertebra.

By means of these horizontal planes, the abdomen is divided into three zones named, from above, the subcostal, umbilical and hypogastric zones. Each of these is further subdivided into three regions by the two sagittal planes, which are indicated on the surface by a right and a left lateral line drawn vertically through points halfway between the anterior superior iliac spines and the middle line. The middle region of the upper zone is called the epigastric and the two lateral regions the right and left hypochondrium. The central region of the middle zone is the umbilical and the two lateral regions the right and left lumbar. The middle region of the lower zone is the hypogastric or pubic and the lateral regions are the right and left iliac or inguinal. The middle regions, viz. epigastric, umbilical and pubic, can each be divided into right and left portions by the middle line.

abdomen

4.21

Answer: A   The superior meseriteric artery courses between the body and uncinate process of the pancreas before the artery supplies the jejunum and ileum

The small intestine is a convoluted tube, extending from the pylorus to the ileocaecal valve, where it ends in the large intestine. It is contained in the central and lower part of the abdominal cavity and is surrounded above and at the sides by the large intestine. A portion of the small intestine extends below the superior inlet of the pelvis and lies anterior to the rectum. It is about 7 metres long, and gradually diminishes in size from its commencement to its termination. It is related anteriorly to the greater omentum and abdominal wall. It is connected to the vertebral column by a fold of peritoneum called the mesentery. The small intestine is divisible into three portions: the duodenum, the jejunum and the ileum. The jejunum and ileum are supplied by the superior mesenteric artery, which courses between the body and uncinate process of the pancreas, before it gives rise to the intestinal branches. These intestinal branches, having reached the attached border of the bowel, run between the serous and muscular coats, with frequent branches given off to the free border, where they also anastomose with other branches running around the opposite surface of the gut. Numerous branches are given off from these vessels and these pierce the muscular coat, supplying it and forming an intricate plexus in the submucous tissue. From this plexus, minute vessels pass to the glands and villi of the mucous membrane.

4.22

Answer: D   Arcuate line

The rectus sheath is a tough, tendinous sheath over the rectus abdominis muscle. It covers the entire anterior surface of the rectus abdominis. However, on the posterior side of the muscle the sheath is incomplete – it ends inferiorly at the arcuate line. Below the arcuate line the rectus abdominis is covered by transversalis fascia, not the rectus sheath! The rectus sheath is formed by the aponeuroses of the external oblique, internal oblique and transversus abdominis, which are arranged in the following manner. At the lateral margin

abdomen

of the rectus, the aponeurosis of the internal oblique divides into two lamellae, one of which passes in front of the rectus, blending with the aponeurosis of the external oblique, the other, behind it, blending with the aponeurosus of the transversus and these, joining again at the medial border of the rectus, are inserted into the linea alba. This arrangement of the aponeuroses exists from the costal margin to midway between the umbilicus and symphysis pubis, where the posterior wall of the sheath ends in a thin curved margin, the linea semicircularis or arcuate line, the concavity of which is directed downward; below this level the aponeuroses of all three muscles pass in front of the rectus. The rectus, in the situation where its sheath is deficient below, is separated from the peritoneum by the transversalis fascia. Because the tendons of the internal oblique and transversus abdominis only reach as high as the costal margin, it follows that above this level the sheath of the rectus is deficient behind, the muscle resting directly on the cartilages of the ribs and being covered merely by the tendon of the external oblique.

The linea alba is an aponeurotic band on the midline of the anterior abdominal wall, which extends from the xiphoid process to the pubic symphysis. It is formed by the combined abdominal muscle aponeuroses. Because there are no major arteries or nerves running in the linea alba, it provides a useful site for a midline incision in the abdomen. All of the other answer choices are related to the inguinal canal. The falx inguinalis (sometimes called the inguinal falx or conjoint tendon), is the inferomedial attachment of transversus abdominis with some fibres of the internal abdominal oblique – it contributes to the posterior wall of the inguinal canal. The inguinal ligament is the ligament that connects the anterior superior iliac spine with the pubic tubercle – it makes the floor of the inguinal canal. The internal (deep) inguinal ring is the entrance to the inguinal canal, where the transversalis fascia pouches out and creates an opening through which structures can leave the abdominal cavity.

4.23

Answer: C   Pubic tubercle

The pubic tubercle is a bony process that would be felt lateral to the edge of the spermatic cord at the superficial inguinal ring. (This is really the only answer choice that could feel like a bony prominence when palpated.) The pubic tubercle serves as the point of attachment for the inguinal ligament, which makes up the floor of the inguinal canal. The pubic pecten is the ridge on the superior surface of the superior pubic ramus. This is the place where you find the pectineal ligament, a thickening of fascia on the pecten of the pubis. The pectineal ligament is a good place to put sutures when performing surgery. The pubic symphysis is the joint between the two pubic bones. The iliopubic eminence is a bony process on the pubis found near its articulation with the ilium. The iliopectineal line is a line formed by the arcuate line of the ilium and the pectineal line of the pubis. This line forms a plane that marks the transition between the abdominal and pelvic cavity.

4.24

Answer: A   Epigastric region

The abdomen is divided into nine regions for descriptive purposes by two vertical lines that pass through the midpoint between the anterior superior iliac spine and the symphysis pubis and two horizontal lines – the subcostal plane and the intertubercular plane. The regions so formed are: from top to bottom (left side), left hypochondrium, left lumbar region, left iliac fossa; from top to bottom (centre), epigastrium, umbilical area, hypogastrium or suprapubic area; from top to bottom (right side), right hypochondrium, right lumbar region, right iliac fossa. The epigastric region contains the first part of the duodenum, part of the stomach, part of the liver and the pancreas. This is the region that the surgeon would need to enter to reach an ulcer in the first part of the duodenum. The left inguinal region contains the sigmoid colon. The left lumbar region contains the descending colon and kidney. The right hypochondrial region contains part of the liver and the gallbladder. Finally, the hypogastric region contains the bladder and rectum (see also *Answer* to **4.20**).

abdomen

4.25

Answer: B   Iliohypogastric

The iliohypogastric nerve arises from the first lumbar nerve. It emerges from the upper part of the lateral border of psoas major and crosses obliquely in front of quadratus lumborum to the iliac crest. It then perforates the posterior part of the transversus abdominis, near the crest of the ilium, and divides between that muscle and the internal oblique into a lateral and an anterior cutaneous branch. It provides sensory innervation to the skin of the lower abdominal wall, upper hip and upper thigh. This is the region where the patient is experiencing paraesthesia, so this nerve must be injured. The genitofemoral nerve is another nerve from the lumbar plexus. It provides sensory innervation to the skin of the anterior scrotum or labia majora and upper medial thigh. The subcostal nerve is the ventral primary ramus of T12 − it is the equivalent of an intercostal nerve at a higher thoracic level. It provides sensory innervation to the anterolateral abdominal wall, but in an area superior to the pubic region. A spinal nerve would not have been injured in the operation. Remember: the spinal nerve is just that small segment of nerve that exists once the dorsal and ventral rootlets come together, before the dorsal and ventral primary rami branch off. In any case, the T9 and T10 dermatomes are superior to the area where the patient is experiencing paraesthesia.

4.26

Answer: B   Posterior rectus sheath

Remember: the transverse suprapubic incision (also called the Pfannenstiel incision) is made below the arcuate line. Therefore, there is no longer a posterior layer of the rectus sheath and the inner surface of the rectus abdominis is lined only with transversalis fascia. When making this incision, the abdominal wall layers are incised as follows: skin, superficial fascia (fatty and membranous), deep fascia, anterior rectus sheath, rectus abdominis muscle, transversalis fascia, extraperitoneal connective tissue and peritoneum.

4.27

Answer: B   Inferior epigastric

The inferior epigastric artery arises from the external iliac artery immediately above the inguinal ligament. It curves forward in the subperitoneal tissue and then ascends obliquely along the medial margin of the deep inguinal ring. It continues to ascend between the rectus abdominis and the posterior lamella of its sheath after piercing the fascia transversalis and passing anterior to the linea semicircularis. It finally divides into numerous branches, which anastomose above the umbilicus with the superior epigastric branch of the internal mammary artery and with the lower intercostal arteries. As the inferior epigastric artery passes obliquely upward from its origin it lies along the lower and medial margins of the deep inguinal ring and posterior to the commencement of the spermatic cord. The ductus deferens, as it leaves the spermatic cord in the male and the round ligament of the uterus in the female, winds around the lateral and posterior aspects of the artery. The inferior epigastric vessels are found in the preperitoneal fat of the abdomen. They lie just superficial to the peritoneum and form the lateral umbilical fold. Hernias can pass either lateral or medial to these vessels. If the hernia is lateral to the vessels (which is what happened in this case), it is an indirect inguinal hernia. If the hernia is medial to these vessels, it is a direct inguinal hernia.

The deep circumflex artery courses along the iliac crest on the inner surface of the abdominal wall. This artery lies very laterally on the abdominal wall, and hernias would pass medial to this vessel. The superficial circumflex iliac, superficial epigastric, and superficial external pudendal arteries are all superficial arteries that arise from the femoral artery. They are all found in the superficial fascia, not in the preperitoneal fat.

4.28

Answer: E   Linea alba

The linea alba is a tendinous raphé in the middle line of the abdomen, stretching between the xiphoid process and the symphysis pubis. It is placed between the medial borders of the recti and is formed by the blending of the aponeuroses of the external and internal obliques and transversi. It is narrow below, corresponding to the

abdomen

linear interval existing between the recti; but broader above, where these muscles diverge from one another. At its lower end the linea alba has a double attachment – its superficial fibres passing in front of the medial heads of the recti to the symphysis pubis, while its deeper fibres form a triangular lamella, attached behind the recti to the posterior lip of the crest of the pubis and called the adminiculum lineae albae. It presents apertures for the passage of vessels and nerves. The umbilicus, which in the fetus exists as an aperture and transmits the umbilical vessels, is closed in the adult. It is a good place to make a vertical incision.

The linea aspera is a vertical ridge on the posterior surface of the femur. The arcuate line is the point at which the posterior lamina of the rectus sheath ends and transversalis fascia lines the inner surface of rectus abdominis. The semilunar line is the lateral margin of the rectus abdominis, formed by the fused aponeuroses of the abdominal wall muscles. The iliopectineal line is a line on the pelvic bones, formed by the arcuate line of the ilium and the pectineal line of the pubis. (Note: the arcuate line of the ilium is very different from the arcuate line of the rectus sheath!) This line is important because it marks the boundary between the abdominal cavity and the pelvic cavity.

4.29

Answer: B   Inferior epigastric artery

If the internal thoracic artery was ligated or divided, blood would no longer flow to the superior epigastric artery, which is the branch of the internal thoracic that supplies blood to rectus abdominis. However, the superior epigastric artery communicates with the inferior epigastric artery, a branch of the external iliac artery. This means that blood could flow from the external iliac, to the inferior epigastric, to the superior epigastric and the rectus abdominis. The superficial epigastric and superficial circumflex iliac arteries are two superficial branches of the femoral artery. They do not supply deep structures in the abdomen. The distal portions of the umbilical arteries are obliterated in adults – they are the medial umbilical ligaments that form the medial umbilical folds. The deep circumflex iliac artery courses along the iliac crest on the inner surface of the abdominal wall. It is too lateral to supply blood to rectus abdominis.

4.30

Answer: E   Level of the umbilicus

The umbilicus is an important landmark for venous and lymphatic drainage of the abdominal wall. Above the umbilicus, lymphatics drain into the axillary lymph nodes and the venous blood drains into the superior epigastric vein, which drains to the internal thoracic vein. Below the umbilicus, lymphatics drain into the superficial inguinal lymph nodes, while venous blood drains into the inferior epigastric vein and the external iliac vein (see also *Answer* to **4.18**).

4.31

Answer: D   Medical umbilical ligament and inferior epigastric artery

Remember: the medial umbilical fold is made by the medial umbilical ligament (the obliterated portion of the umbilical artery), while the lateral umbilical fold is a fold of peritoneum over the inferior epigastric vessels. The median umbilical fold is a midline structure made by the median umbilical ligament (obliterated urachus). The medial inguinal fossa is the space on the inner abdominal wall between the medial umbilical fold and the lateral umbilical fold. This is the place in the abdominal wall where there is an area of weak fascia called the inguinal triangle – direct inguinal hernias can break through this space. The lateral inguinal fossa is a space lateral to the lateral umbilical fold – indirect inguinal hernias push through the deep inguinal ring in this space.

4.32

Answer: E   Transversus abdominis muscle and peritoneum

The inferior epigastric vessels lie on the inner surface of the transversus abdominis and are covered by parietal peritoneum. Remember: the peritoneum lies over the inferior epigastric vessels to make the lateral umbilical fold. Camper's fascia and Scarpa's fascia are two layers of the superficial fascia – Camper's is the fatty layer and Scarpa's is the membranous layer (see also *Answer* to **4.27**).

abdomen

4.33

Answer: E   An indirect inguinal hernia

An indirect inguinal hernia leaves the abdominal cavity lateral to the inferior epigastric vessels and enters the inguinal canal through the deep inguinal ring. Commonly, these hernias traverse the entire inguinal canal, leave the canal through the superficial inguinal ring and enter the scrotum. The indirect inguinal hernias are the most common type of hernia and are often caused by heavy lifting. Direct inguinal hernias leave the abdominal cavity medial to the inferior epigastric vessels, through the weak fascia. These usually do not traverse the entire inguinal canal and they rarely enter the scrotum. Direct inguinal hernias can be caused by a weakness of abdominal musculature.

Congenital inguinal hernias are indirect hernias that occur due to the persistence of the processus vaginalis, an embryonic structure that is a diverticulum of the peritoneal cavity extending into the labial or scrotal folds. A femoral hernia is caused by abdominal viscera pushing through the femoral ring into the femoral canal. An incisional hernia occurs after surgery, when omentum or an organ protrudes through a surgical incision due to poor healing.

4.34

Answer: E   Round ligament of the uterus

The deep inguinal ring is situated in the transversalis fascia, midway between the anterior superior iliac spine and the symphysis pubis and about 1.25 cm above the inguinal ligament. It is of an oval form, the long axis of the oval being vertical; it varies in size in different subjects and is much larger in the man than in the woman. It is bounded, above and laterally, by the arched lower margin of the transversus abdominis; below and medially, by the inferior epigastric vessels. It transmits the spermatic cord in the man and the round ligament of the uterus in the woman. From its circumference a thin funnel-shaped membrane, the infundibuliform fascia, is continued around the cord and testis, enclosing them in a distinct covering. The round ligament of the uterus is a derivative of the gubernaculum, a structure that pulled the gonads into place during embryonic development. In men, the scrotal ligament is what remains from the gubernaculum. Of the other answer choices, the ilioinguinal nerve is the only other one that courses through the inguinal canal. Remember: it leaves through the superficial ring and gives off the anterior labial or scrotal branch as a cutaneous continuation. However, the ilioinguinal nerve does not pass through the deep ring – it enters the inguinal canal on the side.

The iliohypogastric nerves run between the internal oblique and transversus abdominis in the abdominal wall, piercing the internal oblique at the anterior superior iliac spine to travel just deep to the external oblique. The inferior epigastric artery runs between the transversus abdominis and the peritoneum, forming the lateral umbilical fold. The medial umbilical ligament is the obliterated umbilical artery – it lies within the medial umbilical fold of peritoneum.

4.35

Answer: C   Medical inguinal fossa

A direct inguinal hernia passes through the weak fascia in the medial inguinal fossa. This is the area between the medial and lateral umbilical folds (made of the obliterated umbilical artery and inferior epigastric vessels, respectively). A direct inguinal hernia does not pass through the deep inguinal ring or the lateral inguinal fossa – that is what an indirect hernia does. Although it is much more common for an indirect hernia to pass through the superficial inguinal ring, direct hernias can go through this ring too. However, the question is asking you to identify which region the hernia enters on the abdominal side, so superficial inguinal ring is not the correct answer. The supravesicular fossa is between the median and medial umbilical folds – it is formed where the peritoneum reflects from the anterior abdominal wall onto the bladder. Potentially, a very rare external supravesicular hernia could form here.

4.36

Answer: E   Round ligament of the uterus

In women, the round ligament of the uterus is the main structure traversing the inguinal canal. In men, the most important structure

abdomen

in the inguinal canal is the spermatic cord. The iliohypogastric nerve innervates the abdominal wall. It runs between the transversus abdominis and internal oblique muscles, then pierces the internal oblique at the anterior superior iliac spine to run between the internal and external obliques. The inferior epigastric artery lies between the peritoneum and the transversus abdominis, creating the lateral umbilical fold. The ovarian artery and vein are branches from the descending aorta and inferior vena cava, which supply the ovary in the pelvis. The pectineal ligament is a thick layer of fascia over the pectineal line of the pubis. Although the pectineal ligament helps define the boundaries of the inguinal canal, you cannot really say that the pectineal ligament traverses the canal. That is why the round ligament is the best answer.

4.37

Answer: B   Anterior labial

The anterior labial nerve (anterior scrotal in men) is the terminal branch of the ilioinguinal nerve. It innervates the skin of the mons pubis in women and the skin of the anterior scrotum in men. The femoral branch of the genitofemoral nerve provides sensory innervation to the upper medial thigh. The iliohypogastric nerve innervates muscles of the abdominal wall. The subcostal nerve is the ventral primary ramus of the twelfth thoracic nerve. It innervates muscles of the abdominal wall and skin of the lower abdominal wall.

4.38

Answer: E   Either a direct or an indirect inguinal hernia

You cannot tell if an inguinal hernia is direct or indirect just by palpating it! Although indirect hernias are the ones that usually come out of the superficial inguinal ring and enter the scrotum, direct inguinal hernias might do this too! As for the other answers, a femoral hernia goes through the femoral ring into the femoral canal – it has nothing to do with the superficial inguinal ring. A superficial inguinal lymph node lies in the superficial fascia, parallel to the inguinal ligament. It would feel more superficial and should not be mistaken for a hernia protruding through the inguinal ring (see also *Answers* to **4.33, 4.35**).

4.39

Answer: B   Above the midpoint of the inguinal ligamnet

The deep inguinal ring is found near the midpoint of the inguinal ligament, below the anterior superior iliac spine. This ring is lateral to the inferior epigastric artery. The superficial inguinal ring is found above the pubic tubercle. Remember: the supravesical fossa is the space between the median and medial umbilical folds (see also *Answer* to **4.34**).

4.40

Answer: D   Ilioinguinal nerve

The ilioinguinal nerve arises with the iliohypogastric nerve from the first lumbar nerve. It emerges from the lateral border of psoas major just below the iliohypogastric and, passing obliquely across the quadratus lumborum and iliacus muscles, perforates the transversus abdominis, near the anterior part of the iliac crest and communicates with the iliohypogastric nerve between the transversus and the internal oblique. The nerve then pierces the internal oblique, distributing filaments to it and, accompanying the spermatic cord through the subcutaneous inguinal ring, is distributed to the skin of the upper and medial part of the thigh, to the skin over the root of the penis and upper part of the scrotum in the man and to the skin covering the mons pubis and labium majus in the woman. The size of this nerve is in inverse proportion to that of the iliohypogastric. Occasionally it is very small and ends by joining the iliohypogastric; in such cases, a branch from the iliohypogastric takes the place of the ilioinguinal, or the latter nerve may be altogether absent. As the ilioinguinal nerve runs in the inguinal canal, so this nerve could easily be compressed by an inguinal hernia. The ilioinguinal nerve also gives off the anterior scrotal nerve, which is the nerve responsible for sensory innervation to the anterior scrotum. The location of this hernia and the scrotal pain both fit with an injury to the ilioinguinal nerve.

abdomen

The femoral branch of the genitofemoral provides sensory innervation to the upper medial thigh. The femoral nerve innervates the anterior compartment of the thigh and has some cutaneous sensory branches to the thigh. The iliohypogastric nerve innervates the skin of the lower abdominal wall, upper hip and upper thigh. Finally, the subcostal nerve is the ventral primary ramus of T12, which innervates the skin of the anterolateral abdominal wall.

4.41

Answer: D   Perineum

To understand this question, you need to understand the descent of the testes. The testes begin as retroperitoneal structures in the posterior abdominal wall. They are attached to the anterolateral abdominal wall by the gubernaculum. The gubernaculum 'pulls' the testes through the deep inguinal ring, inguinal canal and superficial inguinal ring and over the pelvic brim. The gubernaculum is preceded by the processus vaginalis, which is derived from the peritoneum anterior to the testes. The processus vaginalis 'pushes' the muscle and fascia layers, which will eventually make up the canal and spermatic cord, into the scrotum. After the testes are in position in the scrotum, the gubernaculum persists as the scrotal ligament, while part of the processus vaginalis remains as a bursa-like sac called the tunica vaginalis testis. Therefore, the testes could be caught in the deep inguinal ring, the inguinal canal, at the superficial inguinal ring, or at the pelvic brim. The testes are never in the perineum and they would not be stuck there.

4.42

Answer: E   Sigmoid colon

The sigmoid colon is the most likely intestinal segment to be involved in a left-sided indirect inguinal hernia, as it is mobile due to the presence of sigmoid mesocolon. Although the descending colon is also on the left side of the abdomen, it is a bit superior to be herniating through the deep inguinal ring and is also retroperitoneal. The ascending colon and caecum are on the right side of the abdomen, so they would not be involved in a left-sided hernia.

Finally, the rectum is a structure in the pelvis; it is too inferior to enter the deep inguinal ring and cause an indirect inguinal hernia.

4.43

Answer: C Ilioinguinal

A direct inguinal hernia is caused by a weakness in the abdominal muscles which prevents a patient from contracting these muscles strongly. If this patient cannot contract his muscles, he cannot pull the falx inguinalis down to cover the thin area of weak fascia on the posterior wall of the inguinal canal. The ilioinguinal nerve is important for innervating the muscles of the lower abdominal wall. Therefore, if this nerve was damaged during the appendicectomy, the man might not be able to contract his abdominal muscles and pull the falx inguinalis over the weak fascia. This could have led him to develop the direct inguinal hernia.

The genitofemoral nerve innervates the cremaster muscle. An injury to this muscle would lead to an inability to elevate the testes, but it would not compromise the strength of the abdominal wall. The subcostal nerve and the ventral primary ramus of T10 innervate muscles, skin and fascia of the upper abdominal wall. These nerves are too superior to affect the inguinal region (see also *Answer* to **4.41**).

4.44

Answer: A External abdominal oblique aponeurosis

The superficial inguinal ring is an opening in the aponeurosis of the external oblique just above and lateral to the pubic crest. This opening is oblique in direction, somewhat triangular in form, and corresponds to the course of the fibres of the aponeurosis. It usually measures about 2.5 cm from base to apex and about 1.25 cm transversely. It is bounded inferiorly by the crest of the pubis, on either side by the margins of the opening in the aponeurosis (called the crura of the ring), and superiorly by a series of curved intercrural fibres. The inferior crus (or external pillar) is the stronger and is formed by the portion of the inguinal ligament that is inserted into

abdomen

the pubic tubercle. The inferior crus is curved to form a kind of groove, which the spermatic cord rests on in the male. The superior crus (or internal pillar) is a broad, thin, flat band, attached to the front of the symphysis pubis and interlacing with its fellow from the opposite side. The superficial inguinal ring gives passage to the spermatic cord and the ilioinguinal nerve in the male, and to the round ligament of the uterus and the ilioinguinal nerve in the female. It is much larger in men than in women because of the large size of the spermatic cord.

The falx inguinalis is composed of arching fibres of the transversalis fascia and the internal abdominal oblique. It forms the posterior wall of the inguinal canal. The internal abdominal oblique forms the roof of the inguinal canal and contributes fibres to the falx inguinalis. Scarpa's fascia is the membranous layer of subcutaneous fascia. Finally, transversalis fascia is found on the posterior wall of the inguinal canal, forming an area of weak fascia in that wall.

4.45

Answer: B   Ilioinguinal

The ilioinguinal nerve enters the inguinal canal from the side (instead of passing through the deep inguinal ring). It leaves the inguinal canal by passing through the superficial inguinal ring to exit the canal, so it might be injured during inguinal hernia repair. The femoral branch of the genitofemoral nerve travels lateral to the superficial inguinal ring. The iliohypogastric nerve and the subcostal nerve travel superior to the inguinal canal and superficial inguinal ring. Finally, the obturator nerve is a branch of the lumbar plexus, which innervates muscles in the thigh. To reach the thigh, this nerve travels deep to the inguinal canal and it is not involved with this region (see also *Answers* to **4.41**, **4.43**).

4.46

Answer: B   Direct inguinal hernia

The boundaries listed in this question are the boundaries of the inguinal triangle, which is the site for direct inguinal hernias. Remember: direct inguinal hernias protrude through the weak fascia of the abdominal wall, medial to the inferior epigastric vessels. Indirect inguinal hernias (which can also be called congenital inguinal hernias) occur lateral to the inferior epigastric vessels – they protrude through the deep inguinal ring. Femoral hernias protrude through the femoral ring, into the femoral canal. They can be felt in the femoral triangle, inferior to the pubic tubercle. Finally, an umbilical hernia is an abnormal protrusion of abdominal contents into a defect in the umbilical area. These are common in the newborn, but they usually resolve by the age of 2 years.

4.47

Answer: C   Inferior mesenteric

The inferior mesenteric vein and inferior mesenteric artery do not run in tandem. The inferior mesenteric vein is part of the portal venous system – it drains into the splenic vein, which drains into the hepatic portal vein. The inferior mesenteric artery is a branch off the descending aorta at the level of the L3 vertebral body. However, the inferior mesenteric artery and vein supply/drain the same region: the descending and sigmoid colon and the rectum.

The superior epigastric vessels run together and are the continuation of the internal thoracic artery and vein. The superficial circumflex iliac vessels run together in the superficial fat of the abdominal wall. The superior rectal vessels are the terminal ends of the inferior mesenteric vessels, found on the superior surface of the rectum. The ileocolic artery and vein are branches off the superior mesenteric vessels. They both run in the mesentery, supplying/draining the caecum, appendix and terminal portion of the ileum.

4.48

Answer: A   Circular folds of the mucosa

The small intestine features circular folds of tissue that are covered with villi – these folds are very obvious on an X-ray with barium contrast. The colon does not have similar folds in the mucosa. Some other things that distinguish the small intestine from the large intestine are: (i) the large intestine has three strips of longitudinal muscle, called taenia coli, instead of a continuous surrounding

abdomen

longitudinal muscle layer; (ii) the taenia coli are shorter than the colon, so the colon forms bulges, called haustra; (iii) the surface of the colon is covered with fatty omental appendages. The colon and small intestine share similar circular smooth muscle layers and a serosa. Although the gland structure is different in the colon from that in the small intestine, this would not be visible on n X-ray. The same goes for the longitudinal muscle layer – there are differences between the two organs, but not ones that you would see on barium contrast radiography.

4.49

Answer: C   Middle colic artery

The middle colic artery is the branch from the superior mesenteric artery (SMA) that supplies the transverse colon. This is the most distal part of the colon that receives blood from the SMA. Branches from the middle colic go to the marginal artery, which would be able to supply the descending colon, sigmoid colon and rectum if the inferior mesenteric artery was occluded. The ileocolic and right colic arteries are also branches of the SMA that supply the colon (and contribute to the marginal artery), but the middle colic, which serves a more distal part of the colon, is a better answer. The gastroduodenal artery is a branch off the common hepatic artery, which supplies parts of the duodenum, pancreas and stomach. The splenic artery is one of the three branches of the coeliac trunk. It supplies the spleen, pancreas and curvature of the stomach.

4.50

Answer: A   Looking at the confluence of the taenia coli

The vermiform appendix is a long, narrow, worm-shaped tube that arises from the apex of the caecum. Although its base is constant it can pass in one of several directions, such as upward behind the caecum, to the left behind the ileum and mesentery, or downward into the lesser pelvis. Its average length is about 8.3 cm, varying from 2 cm to 20 cm. It is retained in position by a fold of peritoneum (mesenteriole), derived from the left leaf of the mesentery. This fold, in the majority of cases, is more or less triangular in shape, and as a rule extends along the entire length of the tube. Between its two layers and close to its free margin lies the appendicular artery. The lumen of the vermiform appendix, although small, extends throughout the whole length of the tube and communicates with the caecum by an orifice which is placed below and behind the ileocaecal opening. It is sometimes guarded by a semilunar valve formed from a fold of mucous membrane.

The taenia coli are three bands of longitudinal muscle on the surface of the large intestine. (Remember, the large intestine does not have a continuous layer of longitudinal muscle, it has these three taenia coli.) These three bands meet at the appendix, which is the terminal portion of the caecum. The appendix is below the ileocaecal valve, not above it. It is not near the right colic artery, which supplies the ascending colon. The appendix would not be found by removing a layer of the mesentery of the jejuno-ileum – in fact, the appendix has its own mesentery, the mesoappendix. Finally, the appendix is not on the pelvic brim.

4.51

Answer: B   Is a site of ectopic pancreatic tissue

Meckel's diverticulum is an outpouching of the small bowel that is present in 2% of the people and usually occurs about 0.6 m (2 ft) before the junction with the caecum. It can be lined by the mucosa of the stomach and ulcerate. Alternatively, it can be lined with ectopic pancreatic tissue. Its calibre is generally similar to that of the ileum and its blind extremity may be free or may be connected with the abdominal wall or with some other portion of the intestine by a fibrous band. It represents the remains of the proximal part of the vitelline duct, the duct of communication between the yolk sac and the primitive digestive tube in early fetal life. An abnormal persistence of the urachus is called an urachal fistula. Because the urachus is attached to the bladder, this can be detected if yellow fluid (urine) is seen coming from the umbilicus of a newborn. A failure of the midgut loop to return to the abdominal cavity is called an omphalocele. In this instance, the midgut remains in the body stalk, where it had left the gut to rotate. Polyhydramnios is an excess production of amniotic fluid, often caused by anencephaly or an oesophageal fistula.

abdomen

4.52

Answer: A   Left colic flexure

The left colic flexure, also called the splenic flexure, is the point where the colon takes a sharp downward turn. This flexure is the point where the transverse colon ends and the descending colon begins. It is located immediately inferior to the spleen, so an enlarged spleen must move medially to avoid this colic flexure. The left suprarenal gland is a retroperitoneal structure, which sits superior to the kidney. The suspensory muscle of the duodenum or ligament of Treitz is a thin sheet of muscle derived from the right crus of the diaphragm — it suspends the fourth part of the duodenum from the posterior abdominal wall. Both the pancreas and stomach lie medial to the spleen. These organs would not prevent the spleen from descending inferiorly.

4.53

Answer: E   Sigmoid colon

The vagus nerve supplies parasympathetic fibres to all of the abdominal organs which receive blood from the coeliac trunk or superior mesenteric artery. This means that the vagus supplies parasympathetics to the entire gastrointestinal tract, up to the last part of the transverse colon. The end of the transverse colon and all gastrointestinal structures distal to that point receive parasympathetic innervation from the pelvic splanchnic nerves and blood from the inferior mesenteric artery. So, the ascending colon, caecum, jejunum and ileum would all be affected by damage to the vagus nerve. The sigmoid colon, which receives parasympathetic innervation from the pelvic splanchnics, would not be affected.

4.54

Answer: D   Epiploic appendages

There are three features that distinguish the large intestine from the small intestines. The large intestine does not have a continuous longitudinal muscle layer — instead, it has three strips of longitudinal muscle known as taeniae coli. The large intestine is covered with omental appendages (appendices epiploicae), which are fat-filled pendants of peritoneum the surface of the large intestine. Finally, the large intestine is folded into sacculations known as haustra, which form where the longitudinal muscle layer of the wall of the large intestine is deficient.

Serosa is a general term for the outermost coat or serous layer of a visceral structure that lies in the body cavities of the abdomen or thorax. Complete circular folds are only found in the small intestine. In the large intestine, there are mostly semicircular folds which do not continue around the entire intestine. Valvulae conniventes or valves of Kerckring is another name for the circular folds which are large valvular flaps projecting into the lumen of the small bowel. They are composed of reduplications of the mucous membrane, the two layers of the fold being bound together by submucous tissue. Unlike the folds in the stomach, they are permanent and are not obliterated when the intestine is distended. The majority extend transversely around the cylinder of the intestine for about a half or two-thirds of its circumference, but some form complete circles and others have a spiral direction. The latter usually extend a little more than once around the bowel, but occasionally two or three times. The larger folds are about 8 mm in depth at their broadest part; but the greater number are of smaller size. The larger and smaller folds alternate with each other. They are not found at the commencement of the duodenum, but begin to appear about 2.5 to 5 cm beyond the pylorus. In the lower part of the descending portion, below the point where the bile and pancreatic ducts enter the intestine, they are very large and closely approximated. In the horizontal and ascending portions of the duodenum and upper half of the jejunum they are large and numerous, but from this point, down to the middle of the ileum, they diminish considerably in size. In the lower part of the ileum they almost entirely disappear; hence the comparative thinness of this portion of the intestine, as compared with the duodenum and jejunum. The circular folds retard the passage of the food along the intestines and afford an increased surface for absorption.

abdomen

4.55

Answer: A   Caecum

The inferior mesenteric artery supplies blood to the end of the transverse colon and all distal structures in the gastrointestinal tract. This means that the splenic flexure, descending colon, sigmoid colon and rectum would all be deprived of blood if the inferior mesenteric artery was occluded. The caecum receives blood from the superior mesenteric artery, so it would not be affected by the obstruction.

4.56

Answer: E   Marginal

The marginal artery is an important anastomosis for the large intestine. It runs around the border of the large intestine and it is formed by the anastomosis of branches of the ileocolic artery, right colic artery, middle colic artery, left colic artery and sigmoid artery. If a small artery becomes occluded, these branches allow blood to reach all segments of the colon. In addition, it is another reason that in abdominal aortic aneurysm repair sometimes the inferior mesenteric artery does not have to be re-implanted into the repaired abdominal aorta. Arcades are anastomotic loops between arteries that provide alternative pathways for blood flow. These arcades are more prominent in the small intestine than the large intestine. Arteriae rectae (straight arteries) are the small branches that run from the marginal artery to reach the colon. The ileocolic artery is the branch of the superior mesenteric artery that supplies the caecum, appendix and terminal portion of the ileum. The coronary arteries supply blood to the heart.

4.57

Answer: B   Left and middle colic

To answer this question, you need to identify which branches represent an anastomosis between the superior mesenteric artery (SMA) and the inferior mesenteric artery (IMA). Therefore, you want to find the answer choice listing the most distal branch of the SMA and the most proximal branch of the IMA. Those branches are the

abdomen

middle colic (from the SMA) and the left colic (from the IMA). The ileocolic, right colic and middle colic arteries are branches of the SMA; the left colic, sigmoid and superior rectal arteries are branches of the inferior mesenteric artery.

4.58

Answer: E   Superior mesenteric

The superior mesenteric artery is the artery of the midgut. It is a large vessel and supplies the whole length of the small intestine, except for the superior part of the duodenum. It also supplies the caecum and the ascending colon and about half of the transverse part of the colon. It arises from the front of the aorta, about 1.25 cm below the coeliac trunk, and is crossed at its origin by the lineal (splenic) vein and the neck of the pancreas. It passes downward and forward, anterior to the uncinate process of the head of the pancreas and the inferior part of the duodenum, and descends between the layers of the mesentery to the right iliac fossa. At this level it is considerably diminished in size and anastomoses with one of its own branches, namely the ileocolic. In its course it crosses in front of the inferior vena cava, the right ureter and psoas major. It forms an arch, the convexity of which is directed forward and downward to the left side, the concavity backward and upward to the right. It is accompanied by the superior mesenteric vein, which lies to its right side, and it is surrounded by the superior mesenteric plexus of nerves. Its branches include the inferior pancreaticoduodenal, intestinal, ileocolic, right colic and middle colic arteries.

The coeliac trunk is the artery of the foregut, and the inferior mesenteric artery is the artery of the hindgut. The splenic artery is a branch of the coeliac artery, and the proper hepatic artery is a branch of the common hepatic artery, which in turn is a branch of the coeliac artery.

4.59

Answer: B   Left gastric

The left gastric artery is the artery that supplies the lesser curvature of the stomach (along with the right gastric artery).

abdomen

These two arteries would be most likely to cause bleeding at the lesser curvature of the stomach. The left gastric is one of the three arteries that comes off the coeliac trunk. The other two branches are the hepatic artery and the splenic artery. It is the smallest of the three branches of the coeliac artery. It passes upward and to the left, posterior to the omental bursa, to the cardiac orifice of the stomach. Here it distributes branches to the oesophagus, which anastomose with the aortic oesophageal arteries; others supply the cardiac part of the stomach, anastomosing with branches of the splenic (lineal) artery. It then runs from left to right, along the lesser curvature of the stomach to the pylorus, between the layers of the lesser omentum; it gives branches to both surfaces of the stomach and anastomoses with the right gastric artery. The left and right gastroepiploic arteries are the two arteries that supply the greater curvature of the stomach. The gastroduodenal artery is a branch off the common hepatic artery that supplies the duodenum, head of the pancreas and the greater curvature of the stomach. The short gastric arteries are four or five small arteries from the splenic artery that supply the fundus of the stomach.

4.60

Answer: D   Greater omentum

During the development of the gut, there are two mesogastria attaching to the developing stomach: the dorsal mesogastrium and the ventral mesogastrium. Different organs begin to develop in each mesogastrium – the spleen and pancreas develop in the dorsal mesogastrium and the liver develops in the ventral mesogastrium. Therefore, the structures involving the spleen and the posterior part of the developing stomach (which becomes the greater curvature) are derived from the dorsal mesogastrium. These include the greater omentum (gastrophrenic ligament, gastrosplenic ligament, gastrocolic ligament) and splenorenal ligament. The structures involved with the liver and its attachment to the stomach wall form from the ventral mesogastrium. These include the lesser omentum (hepatogastric ligament, hepatoduodenal ligament) and the ligaments of the liver (falciform ligament, coronary ligaments, right and left triangular ligaments). Of the answer choices, only the greater omentum is part of the dorsal mesogastrium.

abdomen

4.61

Answer: A   It develops in the dorsal mesogastrium

The spleen and pancreas develop behind the stomach in the dorsal mesogastrium; the liver develops in the ventral mesogastrium. The spleen is not a retroperitoneal organ – it is covered by visceral peritoneum on all its surfaces. The spleen appears about the fifth week as a localised thickening of the mesoderm in the dorsal mesogastrium above the tail of the pancreas. With the change in position of the stomach, the spleen is carried to the left and comes to lie behind the stomach and in contact with the left kidney. The part of the dorsal mesogastrium that intervened between the spleen and the greater curvature of the stomach forms the gastrosplenic ligament.

4.62

Answer: D   Splenorenal ligament

The splenorenal ligament is the peritoneal structure that connects the spleen to the posterior abdominal wall over the left kidney. It also contains the tail of the pancreas. To avoid postoperative pancreatic fistula it is extremely important to identify the tail of the pancreas at the time of splenectomy. The gastrocolic ligament connects the greater curvature of the stomach with the transverse colon. The gastrosplenic ligament connects the greater curvature of the stomach with the hilum of the spleen. The phrenicocolic ligament connects the splenic flexure of the colon to the diaphragm. Finally, the transverse mesocolon connects the transverse colon to the posterior abdominal wall.

4.63

Answer: D   Spleen

The spleen is the only organ listed which is covered entirely by visceral peritoneum. About the other organs: the kidney and suprarenal glands are retroperitoneal organs. This is different from the secondarily retroperitoneal organs that started out in a mesentery and then got pushed against the posterior wall. The kidneys and the suprarenal

abdomen

glands began developing in the retroperitoneum and stayed there. The duodenum and pancreas are partially peritonealised and partially retroperitoneal. The first two centimetres of the superior duodenum is peritonealised, but the rest of the duodenum, to the duodenojejunal junction, is retroperitoneal. For the most part, the pancreas is secondarily retroperitoneal, although the tail of the pancreas is peritonealised, lying within the splenorenal ligament (see also *Answer* to **4.12**).

4.64

Answer: B   Gastroduodenal

The gastroduodenal artery is a branch of the common hepatic artery; it descends behind the first part of the duodenum. Therefore, if an ulcer destroyed the posterior wall of the duodenum, gastric juices could escape and destroy the gastroduodenal artery. The common hepatic artery is a branch of the coeliac trunk found superior to the duodenum. The left gastric artery is a branch of the coeliac trunk which supplies the left side of the lesser curvature of the stomach. The proper hepatic artery is a branch of the common hepatic artery; it travels superiorly from the common hepatic artery to give off the right, middle and left hepatic arteries. Finally, the superior mesenteric artery originates from the aorta at the bottom of the L1 level, posterior to the pancreas. It travels over the third part of the duodenum and supplies the intestines, up to the last third of the transverse colon.

4.65

Answer: D   Spleen

The spleen is usually well protected by the ninth to the twelfth ribs on the left side. Nevertheless, if one or more of these ribs is fractured, the spleen is the first organ to be ruptured. The spleen can also be damaged if there is blunt trauma to the abdomen or a sudden increase in intra-abdominal pressure. This patient has several symptoms of a ruptured spleen – he has tenderness on the left mid- and posterior axillary lines and hypotension. (Because of its spongy parenchyma and thin capsule, a ruptured spleen will bleed profusely

abdomen

and a patient may become hypotensive.) The stomach, splenic flexure of the colon, tail of the pancreas, left kidney and suprarenal gland are in the same quadrant of the abdomen and they are also at risk of injury. Nevertheless, you should remember that the spleen is at greatest risk because of its close relationship with the ninth to the twelfth ribs.

4.66

Answer: D   Spleen

The spleen is a peritonealised organ that is attached to the left colic flexure. It could tear if there was too much traction while pulling the descending colon away from the body wall. Another clue in this scenario that points to a ruptured spleen is the large amount of blood that fills the operative field. The spleen is covered by a very thin capsule and it has a soft and pulpy parenchyma. Therefore, when it is ruptured, the spleen bleeds profusely. The duodenum and liver are not associated with the left colic flexure. The kidney and suprarenal glands are retroperitoneal organs that are not associated with any mesenteric attachment (see also *Answer* to **4.65**).

4.67

Answer: D   Splenic

The splenic artery is a branch of the coeliac trunk. It passes deep to the stomach and sends branches to the pancreas before reaching the spleen. If the posterior wall of the stomach eroded, gastric juices could damage the splenic artery. The gastroduodenal artery lies behind the first portion of the duodenum. An ulcer in this portion of the duodenum might jeopardise the gastroduodenal artery. The common hepatic artery is a branch of the coeliac trunk, which runs superior to the lesser curvature of the stomach. The left gastroepiploic artery runs on the left side of the greater curvature of the stomach. Finally, the superior mesenteric artery arises from the aorta at the L1 level, posterior to the pancreas. It crosses over the third portion of the duodenum.

abdomen

4.68

Answer: E Splenic

As it enters the hilum of the spleen, the splenic artery gives off short gastric arteries, which supply blood to the fundus of the stomach. These short gastric arteries travel in the gastrosplenic ligament to reach the fundus. The common hepatic artery does not directly supply the stomach – it gives off the gastroduodenal artery, which supplies the right portion of the greater curvature of the stomach with the right gastroepiploic artery. The inferior phrenic artery is a branch of the aorta, and supplies blood to the diaphragm. The left gastroepiploic artery is a branch of the splenic artery, and supplies the left half of the greater curvature. The right gastric artery is a branch of the proper hepatic artery, and supplies the right half of the lesser curvature (see also *Answer* to **4.1**).

4.69

Answer: C Short gastric

The short gastric arteries branch from the splenic artery near the hilum of the spleen. They travel back in the gastrosplenic ligament to supply the fundus of the stomach. So, these arteries might be damaged if the gastrosplenic ligament was disrupted. The left gastric artery is a branch of the coeliac trunk, and supplies the left half of the lesser curvature. The splenic artery travels deep to the stomach to reach the hilum of the spleen. Although its branches travel in the gastrosplenic ligament, the splenic artery does not travel in this structure and it would not be damaged by the surgery. The middle colic artery is a branch of the superior mesenteric artery which supplies the transverse colon. The caudal pancreatic artery is a branch of the splenic artery which supplies the tail of the pancreas.

4.70

Answer: B Right gastroepiploic

If the gastroduodenal artery and its branches were ligated, blood would flow in a retrograde direction from the left gastroepiploic artery, which is a branch of the splenic artery, to the right

abdomen

gastroepiploic artery, a ligated branch of the gastroduodenal artery. This flow from the left to right gastroepiploic artery would allow blood to reach the entire greater curvature of the stomach. Remember: there are many anastomoses around the stomach that will allow this organ to receive blood even if one branch is ligated. The left hepatic artery is a branch of the proper hepatic artery; it supplies blood to the left and quadrate lobes of the liver, as well as part of the caudate lobe. The short gastric arteries are branches of the splenic artery which supply the fundus of the stomach. The left gastric artery is a branch of the coeliac trunk, and supplies the left portion of the lesser curvature. Omental branches are branches of the left and right gastro-omental (gastroepiploic) arteries which supply the greater omentum.

4.71

Answer: B   Gastroduodenal artery

The gastroduodenal artery lies behind the superior part of the duodenum. It has three branches: the posterior superior pancreaticoduodenal artery, the anterior superior pancreaticoduodenal artery and the right gastro-omental artery. The other vessels are not near the superior duodenum. The coronary vein is formed from the right and left gastric veins and is located in the lesser curvature of the stomach. The inferior pancreaticoduodenal arcade is found in the inferior part of the head of the pancreas. It supplies the pancreas and duodenum. It is near the horizontal (third) part of the duodenum, not the superior part. The proper hepatic artery is a branch of the common hepatic artery, which delivers oxygenated blood to the liver. Finally, the splenic vein comes from the spleen – it joins the superior mesenteric vein to form the portal vein (see also *Answer* to **4.7**).

4.72

Answer: B   Inferior vena cava

The epiploic foramen, also called the omental foramen, is the passageway between the greater and lesser peritoneal sacs. The inferior vena cava lies immediately posterior to this foramen, so this

abdomen

is the vessel that was probably cut. The aorta lies next to the inferior vena cava, but it is a little more to the left and a little deeper – it does not lie immediately posterior to the epiploic foramen. The hepatic portal vein is anterior to the epiploic foramen. The right renal artery is a branch off the aorta. Like the aorta, it is too deep to be a vessel immediately behind the foramen. Finally, the superior mesenteric vein is anterior to the foramen. Remember: this is one of the two vessels that make up the hepatic portal vein, so if the hepatic portal vein is anterior to the foramen, the superior mesenteric vein should be too.

4.73

Answer: C   Gallbladder fossa and the inferior vena cava

This question is asking you to identify the structures that make the line that separates the true/functional lobes of the liver. The concept of functional lobes contrasts with traditional anatomical terminology, which separated the liver into the left, right, quadrate and caudate lobes. These traditional lobes were based on the anatomical appearance, while the functional lobes are based on the distribution of the portal vein, hepatic arteries and hepatic bile ducts. The functional lobes of the liver are separated into a right and left lobe by the gallbladder fossa and the inferior vena cava. Therefore, the old 'right lobe' corresponds to the functional right lobe, while the caudate, quadrate and left lobes according to anatomical terminology are lumped together as one big left lobe.

4.74

Answer: A   Duodenum

The duodenum receives blood from the gastroduodenal artery, a branch of the common hepatic artery. It also receives blood from the inferior pancreaticoduodenal artery, which is a branch of the superior mesenteric artery. Therefore, the duodenum is receiving blood from the common hepatic artery and the superior mesenteric artery, but it is not receiving any blood from the splenic artery. The splenic artery supplies blood to the body of the pancreas with the dorsal and superior pancreatic arteries; it supplies blood to the tail of the pancreas with the caudal pancreatic artery. The splenic artery supplies the fundus of the stomach with short gastric arteries and the left portion of the greater curvature with the left gastro-omental artery. The left gastro-omental artery also supplies blood to the greater omentum through omental branches. All of these structures would be affected if the splenic artery was ligated.

4.75

Answer: A   Head

Tumours in the head of the pancreas often obstruct the common bile duct, blocking the normal bile recycling circuit. This blockade prevents excretion of bilirubin, a yellow-coloured pigment that is a red blood cell breakdown product. The accumulation of bilirubin in various tissues, including the skin, causes jaundice. Tumours in other areas of the pancreas are not as likely to block the common bile duct and cause jaundice.

4.76

Answer: A   Duodenum

The superior mesenteric artery crosses over the third part of the duodenum and the aorta is posterior to the third part of the duodenum. If something causes these vessels to become enlarged, they can crush the duodenum and food will not be able to pass through the duodenum. This is often called the 'nutcracker effect', and it is only seen in the third part of the duodenum.

4.77

Answer: A   Common hepatic duct, liver and cystic duct

The triangle of Calot is formed by the cystic duct laterally, the liver superiorly and the common hepatic duct medially. It is an important landmark in this region because the cystic artery can be found in the triangle of Calot. During a cholecystectomy, the cystic artery needs to be ligated. Although the cystic artery usually branches from the

abdomen

right hepatic artery, there is some variation. However, if you locate the triangle of Calot, you can find the cystic artery in that triangle, trace it back to its origin and then ligate it there.

4.78

Answer: D   Splenic vein to left renal vein

The splenic vein is a major vein of the portal system, while the left renal vein is a major vein of the caval system. These veins are large, so a bypass between them could be useful for relieving the portal hypertension. The coronary vein, right gastroepiploic vein, left colic vein, sigmoid vein, inferior mesenteric vein and splenic vein are all part of the portal system. Any bypasses among these veins will not relieve the portal hypertension. The superior and inferior rectal veins already form a portal–caval anastomosis; surgery would not be needed to connect these two venous channels. However, if too much blood tries to flow through this anastomosis, haemorrhoids will develop. These veins are not large enough to help relieve severe portal hypertension.

4.79

Answer: B   Superior mesenteric artery

The superior mesenteric artery crosses over the third part of the duodenum and the aorta is posterior to the third part of the duodenum. If something causes these vessels to become enlarged, they can crush the duodenum and food will not be able to pass through the duodenum. This is often called the 'nutcracker effect', and it is only seen in the third part of the duodenum. You should know what structures are involved in the 'nutcracker effect' and how they are causing an upper bowel obstruction!

4.80

Answer: B   Right crus

The right crus is the part of the diaphragm that takes origin from L1–L3. It splits to enclose the oesophagus. So, in the case of an

abdomen

oesophageal hernia, the herniating stomach would be entirely surrounded by the fibres of the right crus. The left crus is the part of the diaphragm that takes origin from L1 and L2. It is smaller and shorter than the right crus and it intermingles with the right crus around the aortic hiatus. It does not contribute to the oesophageal hiatus. The central tendon is the tendon in the middle of the diaphragm where all the fibres of the diaphragm attach. It provides an opening for the inferior vena cava. Finally, sternal and costal fibres refer to muscle fibres in the diaphragm that take origin from the xiphoid process or the ribcage. This could not refer to the right crus, because it originates on the lumbar vertebrae.

4.81

Answer: B   Inferior vena cava

Remember: the inferior vena cava (IVC) is a little off-centre, on the right side of the abdomen. This means that structures on the right might be closely associated with this vessel, while structures on the left will need to have longer venous channels to connect with the IVC and drain into it. In the case of the suprarenal glands, you can see that the IVC is lying over the right suprarenal gland and is very far from the left gland. (This means that the right gland is draining directly into the inferior vena cava, while the left gland is draining into the renal vein.) As far as the other structures in the question go, the aorta lies fairly evenly between the suprarenal glands – it is not overlying either gland. The left hepatic vein, which drains blood from the liver to the inferior vena cava, is superior to the kidneys and not really involved with this area. The right crus of the diaphragm is a set of fibres that splits to make the oesophageal hiatus, and the right renal artery is a branch off the aorta to the kidney which enters the kidney below the level of the suprarenal gland.

4.82

Answer: C   Left renal vein

The suprarenal vein returns the blood from the medullary venous plexus and receives several branches from the cortical substance; it emerges from the hilum of the gland and on the right side opens into

abdomen

the inferior vena cava, on the left into the renal vein. So, a tumour in the left suprarenal vein will next involve the left renal vein.

4.83

Answer: E   Pancreas

The left suprarenal, slightly larger than the right, is crescentic in shape, its concavity being adapted to the medial border of the upper part of the left kidney. It presents a medial border, which is convex, and a lateral, which is concave; its upper end is narrow and its lower rounded. Its anterior surface has two areas: an upper one, covered by the peritoneum of the omental bursa, which separates it from the cardiac end of the stomach and sometimes from the superior extremity of the spleen; and a lower one, which is in contact with the pancreas and splenic artery and is therefore not covered by the peritoneum. The structure most likely to be injured in this vignette is the pancreas. On the anterior surface, near its lower end, is a furrow or hilum, directed downward and forward, from which the suprarenal vein emerges. Its posterior surface presents a vertical ridge, which divides it into two areas. The lateral area rests on the kidney, the medial and smaller resting on the left crus of the diaphragm. The Inferior vena cava, duodenum and liver are all relations of the right suprarenal gland.

4.84

Answer: B   Inferior vena cava

The clue in this question is the location of the vascular structure. Of all the structures mentioned, the inferior vena cava is the most likely correct option because it is formed by the junction of the two common iliac veins, on the right side of the fifth lumbar vertebra. It ascends along the front of the vertebral column on the right side of the aorta up to the liver, where it is lodged in a groove on the posterior surface. It then perforates the diaphragm between the median and right portions of its central tendon. It subsequently inclines forward and medially for about 2.5 cm, and opens into the posteroinferior part of the right atrium after piercing the fibrous pericardium and passing behind the serous pericardium. There is a semilunar valve, the valve of the inferior vena cava, guarding the atrial opening of the inferior vena cava. This valve is rudimentary in the adult, but is large and performs an important function in the fetus.

4.85

Answer: B Left gastroepiploic

The arteries supplying the stomach are the left gastric, the right gastric and right gastroepiploic branches of the hepatic and the left gastroepiploic and short gastric branches of the splenic. The superior mesenteric artery supplies the whole length of the small intestine, except the superior part of the duodenum; it also supplies the caecum and the ascending part of the colon and about half of the transverse part of the colon. Its ligation will therefore affect these organs and not the stomach.

4.86

Answer: B Hepatic

The hepatic artery is the largest of the three branches of the coeliac artery in the fetus. In the adult, it is intermediate in size between the left gastric and splenic. It is first directed forward and to the right, to the upper margin of the superior part of the duodenum, forming the lower boundary of the epiploic foramen (foramen of Winslow). It then crosses the portal vein anteriorly and ascends between the layers of the lesser omentum and in front of the epiploic foramen, to the porta hepatis, where it divides into two branches, right and left, which supply the corresponding lobes of the liver, accompanying the ramifications of the portal vein and hepatic ducts. The hepatic artery, in its course along the right border of the lesser omentum, is in relation with the common bile duct and portal vein, the duct lying to the right of the artery and the vein behind. Its branches are:

- Right gastric artery
- Cystic artery
- Gastroduodenal artery, which divides into:

- right gastroepiploic artery
- superior pancreaticoduodenal artery.

4.87

Answer: C   Gastroduodenal artery

The gastroduodenal artery divides at the lower border of the duodenum into two branches, the right gastroepiploic and the superior pancreaticoduodenal. The superior pancreaticoduodenal artery descends between the contiguous margins of the duodenum and pancreas. It supplies both these organs and anastomoses with the inferior pancreaticoduodenal branch of the superior mesenteric artery and with the pancreatic branches of the splenic artery.

4.88

Answer: E   Superior mesenteric artery

The inferior pancreaticoduodenal artery is given off from the superior mesenteric artery or from its first intestinal branch, opposite the upper border of the inferior part of the duodenum. It courses to the right between the head of the pancreas and the duodenum and then ascends to anastomose with the superior pancreaticoduodenal artery. It distributes branches to the head of the pancreas and to the descending and inferior parts of the duodenum.

4.89

Answer: A   Common bile duct

The head of the pancreas is flattened anteroposteriorly and is lodged within the curve of the duodenum. Its upper border is overlapped by the superior part of the duodenum and its lower border overlies the horizontal part of the duodenum. Its right and left borders overlap in front of, and insinuate themselves behind the descending and ascending parts of the duodenum respectively. The angle of junction of the lower and left lateral borders forms a prolongation that is called the uncinate process. The superior and inferior pancreaticoduodenal arteries anastomose anteriorly in the groove

abdomen

between the duodenum and the right lateral and lower borders of the head of pancreas. The common bile duct descends posteriorly, close to the right border, to its termination in the descending part of the duodenum. The posterior surface of the head of pancreas is in relation with the inferior vena cava, the common bile duct, the renal veins, the right crus of the diaphragm, and the aorta.

4.90

Answer: D   Superior mesenteric artery

The neck of pancreas starts from the right upper portion of the front of the head. It is about 2.5 cm long, and is directed at first upward and forward, and then upward and to the left, to join the body. It is somewhat flattened from above downward and backward. Its anterosuperior surface supports the pylorus. Its posteroinferior surface is related to the commencement of the portal vein. It is grooved by the gastroduodenal artery on the right side.

4.91

Answer: E   Superior mesenteric

The arteries of the pancreas are derived from the splenic and the pancreaticoduodenal branches of the hepatic and superior mesenteric arteries.

4.92

Answer: B   Left inferior phrenic

The arteries supplying the oesophagus are derived from the inferior thyroid branch of the thyrocervical trunk, from the descending thoracic aorta, from the left gastric branch of the coeliac artery and from the left inferior phrenic of the abdominal aorta. They have for the most part a longitudinal direction.

abdomen

4.93

Answer: C   Left gastroepiploic

Ligation of the splenic artery at its origin in theory will reduce flow in its direct branches. The branches of the splenic artery are:

- Pancreatic branches
- Short gastric arteries
- Left gastroepiploic artery.

Of the options given in the vignette, the left gastroepiploic is the correct option. The left gastroepiploic artery, the largest branch of the splenic, runs from left to right about a finger's breadth or more from the greater curvature of the stomach, between the layers of the greater omentum, and anastomoses with the right gastroepiploic. In its course, it distributes several ascending branches to both surfaces of the stomach; others descend to supply the greater omentum and anastomose with branches of the middle colic.

4.94

Answer: E   Superior mesenteric artery

The ileocolic artery is the lowest branch arising from the concavity of the superior mesenteric artery. It passes downward and to the right behind the peritoneum toward the right iliac fossa, where it divides into a superior and an inferior branch; the inferior anastomoses with the end of the superior mesenteric artery, the superior with the right colic artery. The inferior branch of the ileocolic runs toward the upper border of the ileocolic junction and supplies the following branches:

- Colic, which pass upward on the ascending colon
- Anterior and posterior caecal, which are distributed to the front and back of the caecum
- Appendicular artery, which descends behind the termination of the ileum and enters the mesentary of the vermiform process; it runs near the free margin of this mesentary and ends in branches, which supply the vermiform process

- Ileal, which run upward and to the left on the lower part of the ileum and anastomose with the termination of the superior mesenteric.

4.95

Answer: D   Splenic artery

The short gastric arteries consist of from five to seven small branches which arise from the end of the splenic artery and from its terminal divisions. They pass from left to right, between the layers of the gastrosplenic ligament and are distributed to the greater curvature of the stomach, anastomosing with branches of the left gastric and left gastroepiploic arteries.

4.96

Answer: B   Inferior mesenteric artery

The sigmoid arteries, branches of the inferior mesenteric artery, two or three in number, run obliquely downward and to the left behind the peritoneum and in front of psoas major, the ureter and the testicular vessels. Their branches supply the lower part of the descending colon, the iliac colon and the sigmoid or pelvic colon; anastomosing above with the left colic and below with the superior haemorrhoidal (rectal) artery.

4.97

Answer: A   Abdominal aorta

The middle suprarenal arteries are two small vessels that arise one from either side of the abdominal aorta, opposite the superior mesenteric artery. They pass lateralward and slightly upward, over the crura of the diaphragm, to the suprarenal glands, where they anastomose with suprarenal branches of the inferior phrenic and renal arteries. In the fetus, these arteries are of large size.

abdomen

4.98

Answer: C   Left inferior phrenic artery

The superior suprarenal artery arises from the inferior phrenic artery. Each inferior phrenic artery gives off superior suprarenal branches to the suprarenal gland of its own side.

4.99

Answer: A   Abdominal aorta

The middle sacral artery is a small vessel which arises from the back of the aorta, a little above its bifurcation. It descends in the midline in front of the fourth and fifth lumbar vertebrae, the sacrum and coccyx and ends in the glomus coccygeum. From it, minute branches are said to pass to the posterior surface of the rectum. On the last lumbar vertebra it anastomoses with the lumbar branch of the iliolumbar artery. In front of the sacrum, it anastomoses with the lateral sacral arteries and sends offsets into the anterior sacral foramina. It is crossed by the left common iliac vein and is accompanied by a pair of venae comitantes; these unite to form a single vessel which opens into the left common iliac vein.

4.100

Answer: A   Inferior mesenteric artery

The superior haemorrhoidal (rectal) artery is the continuation of the inferior mesenteric artery. It descends into the pelvis between the layers of the mesentery of the sigmoid colon. It crosses the left common iliac vessels. It divides into two branches opposite the third sacral vertebra, which descend on either side of the rectum, and about 10–12 cm from the anus these break up into several small branches. These pierce the muscular coat of the bowel and run downward, as straight vessels, placed at regular intervals from each other in the wall of the bowel, between its muscular and mucous coats, to the level of the internal anal sphincter. At this level these straight vessels form a series of loops around the lower end of the rectum, and anastomose with the middle haemorrhoidal branches of the internal iliac artery and with the inferior haemorrhoidal branches of the internal pudendal artery.

abdomen

SECTION 5:
PELVIS – ANSWERS

5.1

Answer: A   External anal sphincter

An episiotomy is an incision made in the perineum to enlarge the distal end of the birth canal and to prevent serious damage to the perineal structures. This procedure is often performed when there is a risk of tearing the birth canal during a breech or forceps delivery. When performing a median episiotomy, a cut is made immediately posterior to the vagina, through the perineal body. If this cut went too far, the physician might cut through the external anal sphincter or the rectum. It is important to remember that episiotomies are usually made in the posterolateral direction, not on the midline. If the incision tears further during the delivery, a median incision is more likely than a posterolateral incision to extend posteriorly through the external anal sphincter and the rectum. A posterolateral incision is much safer! The bulbospongiosus muscle, ischiocavernosus muscle and sphincter urethrae are anterior to the area that is cut during an episiotomy. The sacrospinous ligament extends from the sacrum to the ischial tuberosity – it is deep to the perineum and should not be involved in this procedure.

5.2

Answer: B   Pelvic splanchnics

Erection is mediated by parasympathetic nerves and the pelvic splanchnic nerves are the parasympathetic nerves that innervate the smooth muscle and glands of all pelvic viscera. Therefore, the pelvic splanchnic nerves are the nerves contributing the fibres to the prostatic plexus that innervate penile/clitoral erectile tissue to cause erection. None of the other listed nerves carry parasympathetic fibres which could innervate the penis and cause erection. Additionally, none of these other nerves contribute to the prostatic plexus, which is an extension of the inferior hypogastric plexus. The deep perineal nerve is a branch of the perineal nerve that innervates all the muscles of the urogenital triangle. The pudendal nerve is the major nerve of the perineal region. Its branches include the inferior rectal nerve, perineal nerve and the dorsal nerve of the penis/clitoris. The genitofemoral nerve provides motor innervation to the cremaster muscle and sensory innervation to the skin of the anterior scrotum/labium majus and the upper medial thigh. Finally, the dorsal nerve of the penis/clitoris is a branch of the pudendal nerve that provides sensory innervation to the skin of the shaft of the penis/clitoris.

5.3

Answer: C   Superficial inguinal nodes

The perineum and the external genitalia, including the scrotum and labia majora, drain to the superficial inguinal lymph nodes. However, in the man, remember that the testes do not drain to the superficial inguinal lymph nodes! The lymphatic vessels for the testes travel in the spermatic cord and drain the testes into the lumbar nodes (ovaries also drain to lumbar nodes). The internal iliac nodes drain the pelvis and gluteal region. The lumbar nodes drain the internal pelvic organs. The sacral nodes drain the prostate gland, uterus, vagina, rectum and posterior pelvic wall; the external iliac nodes drain the lower limb.

5.4

Answer: C   Levator ani and coccygeus muscles

Levator ani and coccygeus form the pelvic diaphragm. Levator ani is a broad, thin muscle, situated on the side of the pelvis. It is attached to the inner surface of the side of the lesser pelvis, and unites with its fellow from the opposite side to form the greater part of the floor of the pelvic cavity. It supports the viscera in the pelvic cavity, and surrounds the various structures which pass through it. It takes origin anteriorly from the posterior surface of the superior ramus of the pubis, lateral to the symphysis, and posteriorly from the inner surface of the spine of the ischium. It also arises from the obturator fascia between these two points. Posteriorly, this fascial origin corresponds, more or less closely, with the tendinous arch of the pelvic fascia, but anteriorly the muscle arises from the fascia at a varying distance above the arch, in some cases reaching nearly as high as the canal for the obturator vessels and nerve. The fibres pass downward and backward to the midline of the floor of the pelvis. The most posterior are inserted into the side of the last two segments of the coccyx. Those placed more anteriorly unite with the muscle of the opposite side in a median fibrous raphé (the anococcygeal raphé). The anococcygeal raphé extends between the coccyx and the margin of the anus. The middle fibres are inserted into the side of the rectum, blending with the fibres of the sphincter muscles. Finally, the anterior fibres descend on the side of the prostate to unite beneath it with the muscle of the opposite side, joining with the fibres of the external anal sphincter and transversus perinei at the central tendinous point of the perineum. The anterior portion is occasionally separated from the rest of the muscle by connective tissue and is known as the levator prostatae because it supports the prostate like a sling. In the female the anterior fibres of the levator ani descend on the side of the vagina. The levator ani is supplied by a branch from the fourth sacral nerve and by a branch that is sometimes derived from the perineal nerve and sometimes from the inferior haemorrhoidal division of the pudendal nerve.

The coccygeus is situated behind the levator ani. It is a triangular plane of muscular and tendinous fibres. It takes origin by its apex from the spine of the ischium and sacrospinous ligament and is inserted by its base into the margin of the coccyx and into the side of the lowest piece of the sacrum. It assists the levator ani and piriformis in closing in the back part of the outlet of the pelvis. The coccygeus is supplied by a branch from the fourth and fifth sacral nerves. The two levatores ani constrict the lower end of the rectum and vagina. They elevate and invert the lower end of the rectum after it has been protruded and everted during the expulsion of the faeces. They are also muscles of forced expiration. The coccygei pull forward and support the coccyx after it has been pressed backward during defecation or parturition. The levatores ani and coccygei together form a muscular diaphragm which supports the pelvic viscera.

pelvis

5.5

Answer: B   Pudendal

The pudendal nerve arises from the anterior branches of the second, third and fourth sacral nerves. It passes between the piriformis and coccygeus muscles and leaves the pelvis through the lower part of the greater sciatic foramen. It then crosses the spine of the ischium, and re-enters the pelvis through the lesser sciatic foramen. It accompanies the internal pudendal vessels, upward and forward along the lateral wall of the ischiorectal fossa, being contained in a sheath of the obturator fascia that is known as Alcock's (pudendal) canal, and divides into two terminal branches, the perineal nerve and the dorsal nerve of the penis or clitoris. Before its division it gives off the inferior haemorrhoidal nerve. It is the principal motor and sensory nerve of the perineum.

5.6

Answer: B   Fallopian tube

The portion of the broad ligament that stretches from the fallopian tube to the level of the ovary is known by the name of the mesosalpinx. The uterine tube lies between the layers of the mesosalpinx.

5.7

Answer: E   Urinary bladder, uterus/cervix/vagina, rectum

The location of the pain is indicative of pathology involving the pelvic viscera, including urinary bladder, uterus/cervix/vagina or rectum.

5.8

Answer: A   S2, S3, S4

The pudendal nerve derives its fibres from the ventral branches of the second, third and fourth sacral nerves and therefore its root value is S2,3,4.

5.9

Answer: E   Ischial tuberosities

The perineum corresponds to the outlet of the pelvis. Its deep boundaries are: in front, the pubic arch and the arcuate ligament of the pubis; behind, the tip of the coccyx; and on either side, the inferior rami of the pubis and ischium and the sacrotuberous ligament. The space is somewhat lozenge-shaped and is limited on the surface of the body by the scrotum in front, by the buttocks behind and laterally by the medial side of the thigh. A line drawn transversely across, in front of the ischial tuberosities divides the space into two portions. The posterior contains the termination of the anal canal and is known as the anal region; the anterior, which contains the external urogenital organs, is called the urogenital region.

5.10

Answer: D   Perineal membrane

The deep fascia of the urogenital region forms an investment for the deep transversus perinei and the sphincter urethrae membranaceae, but within it lie also the deep vessels and nerves of this part, the whole forming a transverse septum which is known as the urogenital diaphragm. Because of its shape, it is usually known as the triangular ligament and is stretched almost horizontally across the pubic arch, so as to close in the front part of the outlet of the pelvis. It consists of two dense membranous laminae, which are united along their posterior borders but are separated in front by intervening structures. The superficial of these two layers, the inferior fascia of the urogenital diaphragm or perineal membrane, is triangular in shape and about 4 cm in depth. Its apex is directed forward and is separated from the arcuate pubic ligament by an oval opening for the transmission of the deep dorsal vein of the penis. Its lateral margins are attached on either side to the inferior rami of the pubis and ischium, above the crus penis. Its base is directed toward the rectum and connected to the central tendinous point of the perineum. It is continuous with the deep layer of the superficial fascia behind the superficial transversus perinei and with the inferior layer of the diaphragmatic part of the pelvic fascia. It is perforated about

pelvis

2.5 cm below the symphysis pubis by the urethra, the aperture for which is circular and about 6 mm in diameter; by the arteries to the bulb and the ducts of the bulbourethral glands close to the urethral orifice; by the deep arteries of the penis, one on either side, close to the pubic arch and about halfway along the attached margin of the fascia; by the dorsal arteries and nerves of the penis, near the apex of the fascia. Its base is also perforated by the perineal vessels and nerves, while between its apex and the arcuate pubic ligament the deep dorsal vein of the penis passes upward into the pelvis.

If the inferior fascia of the urogenital diaphragm was detached on either side, the following structures will be seen between it and the superior fascia: the deep dorsal vein of the penis; the membranous portion of the urethra; the deep transversus perinei and sphincter urethrae membranaceae muscles; the bulbourethral glands and their ducts; the pudendal vessels and dorsal nerves of the penis; the arteries and nerves of the urethral bulb; and a plexus of veins.

5.11

Answer: B   coccygeus, iliococcygeus, pubococcygeus and puborectalis muscles

The levator ani and the coccygeus form the pelvic diaphragm. The levator ani may be divided into iliococcygeal and pubococcygeal parts. The iliococcygeus arises from the ischial spine and from the posterior part of the tendinous arch of the pelvic fascia and is attached to the coccyx and anococcygeal raphé; it is usually thin and may fail entirely, or is largely replaced by fibrous tissue. An accessory slip at its posterior part is sometimes called the iliosacralis. The pubococcygeus arises from the back of the pubis and from the anterior part of the obturator fascia and is directed backward almost horizontally along the side of the anal canal toward the coccyx and sacrum, to which it finds attachment. Between the termination of the vertebral column and the anus, the two pubococcygei muscles come together and form a thick, fibromuscular layer lying on the raphé formed by the iliococcygei. The greater part of this muscle is inserted into the coccyx and into the last one or two pieces of the sacrum. This insertion into the vertebral column is, however, not recognised by all observers. The fibres that form a sling for the rectum are called the puborectalis or sphincter recti. They arise from

pelvis

the lower part of the symphysis pubis and from the superior fascia of the urogenital diaphragm. They meet with the corresponding fibres of the opposite side around the lower part of the rectum and form a strong sling for it (see also *Answer* to **5.4**).

5.12

Answer: A   Obturator internus

The levator ani is a broad, thin muscle, situated on the side of the pelvis. It is attached to the inner surface of the side of the lesser pelvis and unites with its fellow of the opposite side to form the greater part of the floor of the pelvic cavity. It supports the viscera in this cavity and surrounds the various structures that pass through it. It arises, in front, from the posterior surface of the superior ramus of the pubis lateral to the symphysis; behind, from the inner surface of the spine of the ischium; and between these two points, from the obturator internus fascia (see also *Answer* to **5.4**).

5.13

Answer: C   uterine arteries

In the female, as it lies in relation to the wall of the pelvis, the ureter forms the posterior boundary of a shallow depression called the ovarian fossa, which lodges the ovary. It then runs medially and forward on the lateral aspect of the uterine cervix and upper part of the vagina to reach the fundus of the bladder. In this part of its course it is accompanied for about 2.5 cm by the uterine artery, which then crosses the ureter anteriorly and ascends between the two layers of the broad ligament. The ureter is situated about 2 cm from the side of the cervix of the uterus. The relationship of the ureters and uterine arteries is of clinical significance because the ureters are at risk of iatrogenic injury during hysterectomy.

pelvis

5.14

Answer: B   The origin of the ovarian arteries

The lymphatics of the ovary ascend with the ovarian artery to the lateral and preaortic glands.

5.15

Answer: C   Ischial spine

When performing a transvaginal pudendal nerve block, the ischial spine is palpated through the wall of the vagina and the needle is then passed through the vaginal mucous membrane toward the ischial spine. Eventually, the needle pierces the sacrospinous ligament, at which point the pudendal nerve is bathed with anaesthetic. Remember: the pudendal nerve is within the pudendal canal and it wraps around the ischial spine before it delivers its branches. Therefore, administering the nerve block at the ischial spine allows an anaesthetist to anaesthetise all the branches of the pudendal nerve. This is a very important landmark, which you want to remember!

Also remember: the pudendal nerve block does not need to be administered transvaginally. In a perineal pudendal nerve block, the ischial tuberosity is palpated through the buttock and the needle is inserted into the pudendal canal about 2.4 cm deep medial to the ischial tuberosity. The anaesthetic can then be injected to bathe the pudendal nerve. In this case, a different anatomical landmark, the ischial tuberosity, is used to deliver the nerve block.

Arcus tendineus levator ani is the origin for levator ani. It is a specialisation of the fascia of obturator internus, which runs from the spine of the ischium to the superior pubic ramus. The coccyx is the inferior portion of the vertebral column – it is found on the posterior wall of the pelvis. The lateral fornix of the vagina is the space found lateral to the cervix as it protrudes into the vagina. The obturator foramen is a large foramen on the anterior side of the pelvis, formed by the pubic and ischial rami. It is a site of attachment for obturator externus and internus. None of these structures are appropriate landmarks to use when performing a pudendal nerve block.

5.16

Answer: B External anal sphincter muscle

An episiotomy is an incision made in the perineum to enlarge the distal end of the birth canal and to prevent serious damage to the perineal structures. This procedure is often performed when there is a risk of tearing the birth canal during a breech or forceps delivery. When performing a medial episiotomy, a cut is made immediately posterior to the vagina, through the perineal body. If this cut went too far, the obstetrician might cut through the external anal sphincter or the rectum. Therefore, external anal sphincter is the correct answer.

It is important to remember that episiotomies are usually made in the posterolateral direction, not on the midline. If the incision tears further during the delivery, a median incision is more likely than a posterolateral incision to extend posteriorly through the external anal sphincter and the rectum. A posterolateral incision is much safer! The bulbospongiosus muscle, ischiocavernosus muscle and sphincter urethrae are anterior to the area that is cut during an episiotomy. The sacrospinous ligament extends from the sacrum to the ischial tuberosity – it is deep to the perineum and should not be involved in this procedure.

5.17

Answer: D Pelvic splanchnics

Erection is mediated by parasympathetic nerves and the pelvic splanchnic nerves are the parasympathetic nerves that innervate the smooth muscle and glands of all pelvic viscera. Therefore, the pelvic splanchnic nerves are the nerves contributing the fibres to the prostatic plexus which innervate penile/clitoral erectile tissue to cause erection. None of the other listed nerves carry parasympathetic fibres which could innervate the penis and cause erection. Additionally, none of these other nerves contribute to the prostatic plexus, which is an extension of the inferior hypogastric plexus. The deep perineal nerve is a branch of the perineal nerve that innervates all the muscles of the urogenital triangle. The dorsal nerve of the penis/clitoris is a branch of the pudendal nerve that provides sensory innervation to the skin of the shaft of the penis/

pelvis

clitoris. The genitofemoral nerve provides motor innervation to the cremaster muscle and sensory innervation to the skin of the anterior scrotum/labium majus and the upper medial thigh. Finally, the pudendal nerve is the major nerve of the perineal region. Its branches include the inferior rectal nerve, perineal nerve and the dorsal nerve of the penis/clitoris.

5.18

Answer: D　Superficial inguinal

The perineum and the external genitalia, including the labia majora and scrotum, drain to the superficial inguinal lymph nodes. However, in the man, remember that the testes do not drain to the superficial inguinal lymph nodes! The lymphatic vessels for testes travel in the spermatic cord and drain the testes into the lumbar nodes (ovaries also drain to lumbar nodes). The lumbar nodes drain the internal pelvic organs; the sacral nodes drain the prostate gland, uterus, vagina, rectum and posterior pelvic wall; the external iliac nodes drain the lower limb; the internal iliac nodes drain the pelvis and gluteal region.

5.19

Answer: E　Internal pudendal vein

The rectal venous plexus is one of the four portal/systemic anastomoses. Blood from the portal system can flow into the venous system at this junction. This means that portal blood, from the superior rectal vein, could flow through the rectal venous plexus, into the inferior rectal vein and into the systemic venous drainage. Now, you just need to figure out which vessel the inferior rectal vein drains into. It drains into the internal pudendal vein, so that is the answer. The external iliac vein is one of the two branches of the common iliac vein (along with the internal iliac vein). However, the internal iliac vein and its tributaries (including the pudendal vein) are much more important in draining the pelvic structures. The inferior gluteal vein is a branch of the anterior division of the internal iliac vein – it drains gluteus maximus. The inferior mesenteric vein is

pelvis

part of the portal venous system – it gives rise to the superior rectal veins, but not the inferior rectal veins.

5.20

Answer: D   Internal iliac artery

The uterine artery arises from the anterior division of the internal iliac artery and runs medially on the levator ani toward the uterine cervix. It crosses above and in front of the ureter, to which it supplies a small branch, about 2 cm from the cervix. Reaching the side of the uterus, it ascends in a tortuous manner between the two layers of the broad ligament to the junction of the Fallopian tube and uterus. It then runs laterally toward the hilum of the ovary, and ends by joining with the ovarian artery. It supplies branches to the uterine cervix and others which descend on the vagina. The branches descending on the vagina anastomose with branches of the vaginal arteries and form with them two median longitudinal vessels, the azygos arteries of the vagina, one of which runs down in front of and the other behind the vagina. It supplies numerous branches to the body of the uterus, and from its terminal portion branches are distributed to the Fallopian tube and the round ligament of the uterus.

5.21

Answer: D   Ureter

The ovaries are homologous with the testes in the male. They are two nodular structures, situated one on either side of the uterus in relation to the lateral wall of the pelvis, and attached to the back of the broad ligament of the uterus, posteroinferior to the Fallopian tubes. The ovaries are of a greyish-pink colour, and present either a smooth or a puckered, uneven surface. They are both about 4 cm in length, 2 cm in width, and about 8 mm in thickness, and weigh 2–3.5 g. Each ovary has a lateral and a medial surface, an upper or tubal and a lower or uterine extremity, and an anterior or mesovarian and a posterior free border. It lies in a shallow depression called the ovarian fossa on the lateral wall of the pelvis. This fossa is bounded superiorly by the external iliac vessels, anteriorly by the obliterated umbilical artery and posteriorly by the ureter. The ureter is at risk

pelvis

of iatrogenic injury in this location. The ovary becomes displaced during the first pregnancy, and probably never again returns to its original position. In the erect posture the long axis of the ovary is vertical. The tubal end is near the external iliac vein and provides attachment to the ovarian fimbria of the Fallopian tube and a fold of peritoneum, the suspensory ligament of the ovary, which is directed upward over the iliac vessels and contains the ovarian vessels. The uterine end is directed downward toward the pelvic floor. It is usually narrower than the tubal end and is attached to the lateral angle of the uterus, immediately behind the Fallopian tube, by a rounded cord called the ligament of the ovary. This ligament lies within the broad ligament and contains some non-striped, muscular fibres. The lateral surface of the ovary is in contact with the parietal peritoneum that lines the ovarian fossa while the medial surface is to a large extent covered by the fimbriated extremity of the Fallopian tube. The mesovarian border is straight and is directed toward the obliterated umbilical artery. It is attached to the back of the broad ligament by a short fold called the mesovarium. The blood vessels and nerves pass between the two layers of this fold to reach the hilum of the ovary. The free border is convex, and is directed toward the ureter. The Fallopian tube arches over the ovary, running upward in relation to its mesovarian border, then curves over its tubal pole, and finally passes downward on its free border and medial surface.

5.22

Answer: E   Urinary bladder

The prostate is a firm body, partly glandular and partly muscular, which is located immediately below the internal urethral orifice and around the commencement of the urethra. It is situated in the pelvic cavity, related superiorly to the lower part of the symphysis pubis, inferiorly to the superior fascia of the urogenital diaphragm, and posteriorly to the rectum, through which it can be distinctly felt, especially when it is enlarged. It is about the size of a chestnut and somewhat conical in shape. It has a base, an apex, an anterior, a posterior and two lateral surfaces. The prostate measures about 4 cm transversely at the base, 2 cm in its anteroposterior diameter, and 3 cm in its vertical diameter. It weighs about 8 g. It is held in its position by the puboprostatic ligaments, the superior fascia of the urogenital diaphragm and the anterior portions of the levatores ani, which pass backward from the pubis and embrace the sides of the prostate. These portions of the levatores ani are known as the levatores prostatae because they support the prostate. The superior fascia of the urogenital diaphragm invests the prostate and the commencement of the membranous portion of the urethra.

The base of the prostate is directed upward and is attached to the inferior surface of the urinary bladder. The greater part of this surface is directly continuous with the bladder wall. It is penetrated by the urethra nearer its anterior than its posterior border. A malignant growth in the base is most likely to involve the urinary bladder. The apex is directed downward, and is in contact with the superior fascia of the urogenital diaphragm.

The posterior surface is flattened from side to side and is slightly convex from above downward. It is separated from the rectum by its sheath and by some loose connective tissue, and is situated about 4 cm from the anus. Near its upper border there is a depression through which the two ejaculatory ducts enter the prostate. This depression divides the posterior surface into a larger lower part and a smaller upper part. The smaller upper part constitutes the middle lobe of the prostate and intervenes between the ejaculatory ducts and the urethra. It varies greatly in size, and in some cases is devoid of glandular tissue. The larger lower portion sometimes presents a shallow median depression, which imperfectly separates it into right and left lateral lobes. These lateral lobes form the main mass of the gland and are directly continuous with each other behind the urethra. In front of the urethra they are connected by a band called the isthmus, which consists of the same tissues as the capsule and is devoid of glandular substance.

The anterior surface measures about 2.5 cm from above downward but is narrow and convex from side to side. It is situated about 2 cm behind the pubic symphysis, from which it is separated by a plexus of veins and some loose fat. It is connected to the pubic bone on either side by the puboprostatic ligaments. The urethra emerges from this surface a little above and in front of the apex of the gland.

The lateral surfaces are prominent, and are covered by the anterior portions of the levatores ani, which are, however, separated from the gland by a plexus of veins.

pelvis

The prostate is perforated by the urethra and the ejaculatory ducts. The urethra usually lies along the junction of its anterior and middle thirds. The ejaculatory ducts pass obliquely downward and forward through the posterior part of the prostate and open into the prostatic portion of the urethra.

5.23

Answer: B   Base of the bladder and rectum

The seminal vesicles are two lobulated membranous pouches situated between the fundus of the bladder and the rectum. The act as reservoirs for the semen and also secrete a fluid that is added to the seminal fluid. Each sac is somewhat pyramidal in form, the broad end being directed backward, upward and laterally. They are usually about 7.5 cm in length, but vary in size, not only in different individuals, but also in the same individual on the two sides. The anterior surface is in contact with the fundus of the bladder, extending from near the termination of the ureter to the base of the prostate. The posterior surface lies on the rectum, from which it is separated by the rectovesical fascia. The upper extremities of the two vesicles diverge from each other, are related to the vasa deferentia and the terminations of the ureters, and are partly covered by peritoneum. The lower extremities are pointed and converge toward the base of the prostate, where each joins with the corresponding ductus deferens to form the ejaculatory duct. The ampulla of the ductus deferens runs along the medial margin of each vesicle.

Each vesicle consists of a single tube, coiled on itself, which gives off several irregular caecal diverticula. These separate coils and the diverticula are connected by fibrous tissue. When uncoiled, the tube is about the diameter of a quill, and varies in length from 10 cm to 15 cm. It ends posteriorly in a blind sac, while its anterior end becomes constricted into a narrow straight duct, which joins with the corresponding ductus deferens to form the ejaculatory duct.

pelvis

5.24

Answer: B   Middle rectal

The arteries supplying the seminal vesicles are derived from the middle and inferior vesical and middle rectal arteries. Of the options provided, ligation of middle rectal artery is most likely to affect the blood supply to seminal vesicles.

5.25

Answer: C   Ejaculatory duct

The ductus deferens is joined at an acute angle by the duct of the seminal vesicle to form the ejaculatory duct, which traverses the prostate behind its middle lobe and opens into the prostatic portion of the urethra, close to the orifice of the prostatic utricle.

The ductus deferens is a cylindrical structure that presents a hard and cord-like sensation to the fingers. Its walls are dense and its lumen is extremely small. At the fundus of the bladder it becomes enlarged and tortuous and this portion is called the ampulla. A long narrow tube, the inferior aberrant (the vas aberrans of Haller) is occasionally found connected with the lower part of the canal of the epididymis, or with the commencement of the ductus deferens. Its length varies from 3.5 cm to 35 cm, and it can become dilated toward its extremity; more commonly it retains the same diameter throughout. Its structure is similar to that of the ductus deferens. Occasionally it is found unconnected with the epididymis. A second tube, the superior aberrant ductule, is found in the head of the epididymis and this is connected to the rete testis. The small collection of convoluted tubules that is situated in front of the lower part of the cord, above the head of the epididymis, is known as the paradidymis. These tubes are lined with columnar ciliated epithelium, and probably represent the remains of a part of the Wolffian body.

pelvis

5.26

Answer: E   Superficial inguinal

The lymphatics from the anus pass forward and end with those of the skin of the perineum and scrotum in the superficial inguinal lymph nodes.

5.27

Answer: A   Internal iliac

The lymphatics from the anal canal accompany the middle and inferior rectal arteries and end in the internal iliac lymph nodes.

5.28

Answer: B   Fundus of the bladder

The anterior surface of the vagina is related to the fundus of the bladder and the urethra. A growth in the anterior wall is therefore most likely to involve the fundus of the urinary bladder and/or the urethra. The posterior surface is separated from the rectum by the rectouterine pouch in its upper quarter and by the rectovesical fascia in its middle two quarters, while the lower quarter is separated from the anal canal by the perineal body. Its sides are enclosed between the levatores ani muscles. As the terminal portions of the ureters pass forward and medially to reach the fundus of the bladder, they run close to the lateral fornices of the vagina, and as they enter the bladder they are slightly anterior to the anterior fornix.

5.29

Answer: B   Inferior epigastric

The surgeon must have ligated the inferior epigastric artery, as the rest of the options are all branches of the internal iliac artery. The inferior epigastric artery arises from the external iliac, immediately above the inguinal ligament. It curves forward in the subperitoneal tissue and then ascends obliquely along the medial margin of the abdominal inguinal ring. Continuing its course upward, it pierces the transversalis fascia and, passing in front of the linea semicircularis, ascends between the rectus abdominis and the posterior lamella of its sheath. It finally divides into numerous branches which anastomose above the umbilicus, with the superior epigastric branch of the internal mammary and with the lower intercostal arteries. As the inferior epigastric artery passes obliquely upward from its origin it lies along the lower and medial margins of the deep inguinal ring and behind the commencement of the spermatic cord. The ductus deferens, as it leaves the spermatic cord in the man and the round ligament of the uterus in the woman, winds around the lateral and posterior aspects of the artery.

The branches of the inferior epigastric artery are:

- The cremasteric artery, which accompanies the spermatic cord and supplies the cremaster and other coverings of the cord, anastomosing with the internal spermatic artery (in the woman it is very small and accompanies the round ligament)

- A pubic branch, which runs along the inguinal ligament and then descends along the medial margin of the femoral ring to the back of the pubis and there anastomoses with the pubic branch of the obturator artery

- Muscular branches, some of which are distributed to the abdominal muscles and peritoneum, anastomosing with the iliac circumflex and lumbar arteries

- Branches that perforate the tendon of the external oblique and supply the skin, anastomosing with branches of the superficial epigastric.

5.30

Answer: A   Haemorrhoidal plexus

The haemorrhoidal plexus (rectal venous plexus) surrounds the rectum. It communicates anteriorly with the vesical plexus in the male and the uterovaginal plexus in the female. It consists of two parts, an internal part in the submucosa, and an external part outside

pelvis

the muscular coat of the rectum. The internal plexus presents a series of dilated pouches which are arranged in a circle around the rectum, immediately above the anal orifice, and which are connected by transverse branches. The lower part of the external plexus is drained by the inferior haemorrhoidal (rectal) veins into the internal pudendal vein; the middle part is drained by the middle haemorrhoidal (rectal) vein, which joins the internal iliac vein; and the upper part is drained by the superior haemorrhoidal (rectal) vein, which forms the commencement of the inferior mesenteric vein, a tributary of the portal vein. The haemorrhoidal plexus is a site of free communication between the portal and systemic venous systems.

The prostatic veins form a well-marked prostatic plexus which lies partly in the fascial sheath of the prostate and partly between the sheath and the prostatic capsule. It communicates with the pudendal and vesical plexuses.

The uterine plexuses lie along the sides and superior angles of the uterus between the two layers of the broad ligament. They communicate with the ovarian and vaginal plexuses. They are drained by a pair of uterine veins on either side. The uterine veins arise from the lower part of the plexuses, opposite the external orifice of the uterus, and open into the corresponding internal iliac vein.

The vaginal plexuses are placed at the sides of the vagina. They communicate with the uterine, vesical, and haemorrhoidal plexuses, and are drained by the vaginal veins, one on either side, into the internal iliac veins.

The vesical plexus surrounds the lower part of the bladder and the base of the prostate and communicates with the pudendal and prostatic plexuses. It is drained by means of several vesical veins into the internal iliac veins.

SECTION 6:
HEAD AND NECK – ANSWERS

6.1

Answer: D   Superficial temporal

The external carotid artery is one of the two terminal branches of the common carotid artery. It supplies the external aspect of the head, the face, and the greater part of the neck. The external carotid artery begins opposite the upper border of the thyroid cartilage and, taking a slightly curved course, passes upward and forward, before inclining backward to the space behind the neck of the mandible. It is here that it divides into the superficial temporal and internal maxillary arteries. The branches of the external carotid artery may be divided into four sets of branches:

- Anterior branches:
    - superior thyroid artery
    - lingual artery
    - facial artery

- Posterior branches:
    - occipital artery
    - posterior auricular artery

- Ascending branch:
    - ascending pharyngeal artery

- Terminal branches:
    - superficial temporal artery
    - internal maxillary artery.

6.2

Answer: C   It is crossed by the branches of the facial nerve from behind forward

The facial artery arises in the carotid triangle a little above the lingual artery and, covered by the ramus of the mandible, passes obliquely up beneath the digastric and stylohyoid muscles. It arches over the stylohyoid muscle to enter a groove on the posterior surface of the submandibular gland. It then curves upward over the body of the mandible at the anteroinferior angle of the masseter muscle and passes forward and upward across the cheek to the angle of the mouth. It then ascends along the side of the nose and ends at the medial angle of the eye as the angular artery. The facial artery is remarkably tortuous, both in the neck and on the face. In the neck the tortuosity enables it to accommodate itself to the movements of the pharynx in swallowing. In the face this tortuosity allows it to accommodate movements of the mandible, lips and cheeks. It is crossed by the branches of the facial nerve from behind forward. The branches of the artery can be divided into two sets – branches given off in the neck (the cervical branches) and branches given off in the face (the facial branches):

- Cervical branches:
    - ascending palatine artery
    - tonsillar artery
    - glandular branches to the submaxillary gland
    - submental artery
    - muscular branches

- Facial branches:
    - inferior labial artery
    - superior labial artery
    - lateral nasal branch
    - angular artery
    - muscular branches.

head and neck

6.3

Answer: D   Posterior cricoarytenoid

The posterior cricoarytenoid is innervated by the inferior laryngeal nerve, which is a continuation of the recurrent laryngeal nerve. The posterior cricoarytenoid is the only muscle that abducts the vocal folds. If this muscle is denervated, the vocal folds may be paralysed in an adducted position, which would prevent air from entering the trachea. Arytenoid, lateral cricoarytenoid and thyroarytenoid all adduct the vocal folds. Cricothyroid is the only laryngeal muscle innervated by the external branch of the superior laryngeal. It tenses the vocal ligaments by tipping the thyroid cartilage forward relative to the cricoid cartilage.

6.4

Answer: A   Are formed by the superior free edge of the conus elasticus

The vocal folds are concerned with the production of sound and enclose two strong bands, the vocal ligaments. Each ligament consists of a band of yellow elastic tissue formed by the superior free edge of the conus elasticus, attached in front to the angle of the thyroid cartilage and behind to the vocal process of the arytenoid. Its lower border is continuous with the thin lateral part of the conus elasticus. Its upper border forms the lower boundary of the ventricle of the larynx. Laterally, the vocalis muscle lies parallel with it. It is covered medially by mucous membrane, which is extremely thin and closely adherent to its surface.

6.5

Answer: B   Sternocleidomastoid

The sternocleidomastoid passes obliquely across the side of the neck. It is thick and narrow at its central part, but broader and thinner at either end. It arises from the sternum and clavicle by two heads. The medial or sternal head is a rounded fasciculus, tendinous in front, fleshy behind, which arises from the upper part of the anterior surface of the manubrium sterni and is directed upward, lateralward and backward. The lateral or clavicular head, composed of fleshy and aponeurotic fibres, arises from the superior border and anterior surface of the medial third of the clavicle; it is directed almost vertically upward. The two heads are separated from one another at their origins by a triangular interval, but gradually blend, below the middle of the neck, into a thick, rounded muscle which is inserted by a strong tendon into the lateral surface of the mastoid process, from its apex to its superior border, and by a thin aponeurosis into the lateral half of the superior nuchal line of the occipital bone. This muscle divides the quadrilateral area of the side of the neck into two triangles, an anterior and a posterior. The sternocleidomastoid is supplied by the accessory nerve and branches from the anterior divisions of the second and third cervical nerves. When only one sternocleidomastoid acts, it draws the head toward the shoulder of the same side, assisted by the splenius and the obliquus capitis inferior of the opposite side. At the same time, it rotates the head so as to carry the face toward the opposite side. Acting together from their sternoclavicular attachments, the muscles will flex the cervical part of the vertebral column. If the head was fixed, the two muscles assist in elevating the thorax in forced inspiration.

6.6

Answer: A   Anterior scalene

The phrenic nerve contains motor and sensory fibres in the proportion of about two to one. It arises chiefly from the fourth cervical nerve, but receives a branch from the third and another from the fifth (the fibres from the fifth occasionally come through the nerve to the subclavius). It descends to the root of the neck, running obliquely across the front of the scalenus anterior and beneath the sternocleidomastoid, the inferior belly of the omohyoid and the transverse cervical and transverse scapular vessels. It next passes in front of the first part of the subclavian artery, between it and the subclavian vein and, as it enters the thorax, crosses the internal mammary artery near its origin. Within the thorax, it descends nearly vertically in front of the root of the lung and then between the pericardium and the mediastinal pleura, to the diaphragm, where it divides into branches which pierce that muscle and are distributed to its under surface. In the thorax, it is accompanied by the pericardiacophrenic branch of the internal mammary artery.

The two phrenic nerves differ in their length and also in their relations at the upper part of the thorax. The right nerve is situated more deeply and is shorter and more vertical in direction than the left; it lies lateral to the right innominate vein and superior vena cava. The left nerve is rather longer than the right, as a result of the inclination of the heart to the left side and of the diaphragm being lower on this than on the right side. At the root of the neck, it is crossed by the thoracic duct. In the superior mediastinal cavity it lies between the left common carotid and left subclavian arteries and crosses superficial to the vagus on the left side of the arch of the aorta.

Each nerve supplies filaments to the pericardium and pleura and at the root of the neck is joined by a filament from the sympathetic and, occasionally, by one from the ansa hypoglossi. Branches have been described as passing to the peritoneum. From the right nerve, one or two filaments pass to join in a small phrenic ganglion with phrenic branches of the coeliac plexus. Branches from this ganglion are distributed to the falciform and coronary ligaments of the liver, the suprarenal gland, inferior vena cava and right atrium. From the left nerve, filaments pass to join the phrenic branches of the coeliac plexus, but without any ganglionic enlargement; and a twig is distributed to the left suprarenal gland.

6.7

Answer: E   Common carotid artery, internal jugular vein, vagus nerve

The carotid sheath is an anatomical term for the fibrous connective tissue that surrounds the internal carotid artery and related structures in the neck. The carotid sheath extends from the base of the skull down to the root of the neck. The three major structures contained in the carotid sheath are the internal carotid artery (the common carotid artery below the carotid bifurcation), the internal jugular vein, and the vagus nerve. The carotid artery lies medial to the internal jugular vein, and the vagus nerve is situated posteriorly between the two vessels. In the upper part, the carotid sheath also contains the glossopharyngeal nerve, the accessory nerve, and the

head and neck

hypoglossal nerve, which pierce the fascia of the carotid sheath. The three major fascial layers in the neck, namely the investing fascia, the pretracheal fascia and the prevertebral fascia, contribute to the carotid sheath. The cervical part of the sympathetic trunk is embedded in prevertebral fascia immediately posterior to the sheath.

6.8

Answer: A Inferior border of the mandible, anterior of border of the sternocleidomostoid muscle, anterior midline of the neck

The side of the neck presents a somewhat quadrilateral outline. It is limited superiorly by the lower border of the body of the mandible and an imaginary line extending from the angle of the mandible to the mastoid process, inferiorly by the upper border of the clavicle, anteriorly by the midline of the neck, and posteriorly by the anterior margin of trapezius. This space is subdivided into two large triangles by the sternocleidomastoid muscle, which passes obliquely across the neck from the sternum and clavicle below to the mastoid process and occipital bone above. The triangular space anterior to the sternocleidomastoid is called the anterior triangle and the space posterior to it is called the posterior triangle.

The anterior triangle is bounded anteriorly by the midline of the neck and posteriorly by the anterior margin of the sternocleidomastoid. Its base, directed upward, is formed by the lower border of the body of the mandible and a line extending from the angle of the mandible to the mastoid process. Its apex is below at the sternum. This space is subdivided into four smaller triangles by the digastric superiorly and the superior belly of the omohyoid inferiorly. These smaller triangles are the inferior carotid, the superior carotid, the submaxillary, and the suprahyoid.

6.9

Answer: C   Thyroid/parathyroids, larynx/trachea, pharynx/ oesophagus

The correct order of visceral structures in the neck from superficial to deep is thyroid/parathyroids, larynx/trachea, pharynx/oesophagus.

6.10

Answer: D   The two bellies of the digastric muscle arise from two separate pharyngeal arches

The muscles attached to the hyoid bone are divided into suprahyoid and infrahyoid muscles. The suprahyoid muscles are:

- Digastric
- Mylohyoid
- Stylohyoid
- Geniohyoid.

The infrahyoid muscles are:

- Sternohyoid
- Thyrohyoid
- Sternothyroid
- Omohyoid.

The digastric muscle consists of two fleshy bellies united by an intermediate rounded tendon. It lies below the body of the mandible, and extends, in a curved form, from the mastoid process to the symphysis menti. The anterior belly takes origin from a depression on the inner side of the lower border of the mandible, close to the symphysis, and passes downward and backward. The posterior belly, longer than the anterior, takes origin from the mastoid notch of the temporal bone and passes downward and forward. The two bellies end in an intermediate tendon which perforates the stylohyoid muscle, and is held in connection with the side of the body and the greater cornu of the hyoid bone by a fibrous loop, which is sometimes lined by a mucous sheath. A broad aponeurotic layer, the suprahyoid aponeurosis, is given

head and neck

off from the tendon of the digastric on either side, to be attached to the body and greater cornu of the hyoid bone. The digastric divides the anterior triangle of the neck into three smaller triangles:

- The submandibular triangle, bounded superiorly by the lower border of the body of the mandible and a line drawn from its angle to the sternocleidomastoid, inferiorly by the posterior belly of the digastric and the stylohyoid, and anteriorly by the anterior belly of the digastric

- The carotid triangle, bounded superiorly by the posterior belly of the digastric and stylohyoid, posteriorly by the sternocleidomastoid, inferiorly by the omohyoid

- The suprahyoid or submental triangle, bounded laterally by the anterior belly of the digastric, medially by the midline of the neck from the hyoid bone to the symphysis menti, and inferiorly by the body of the hyoid bone.

The anterior belly of the digastric is supplied by the mylohyoid branch of the inferior alveolar nerve and the posterior belly of the digastric is supplied by the facial nerve. Developmentally, the anterior belly of the digastric is a derivative of first pharyngeal arch and the posterior belly is a derivative of the second pharyngeal arch.

6.11

Answer: A   Superior pharyngeal constrictor muscle

The pterygomandibular raphé (pterygomandibular ligament) is a tendinous band of the buccopharyngeal fascia, attached by one extremity to the hamulus of the medial pterygoid plate and by the other to the posterior end of the mylohyoid line of the mandible. Its medial surface is covered by the mucous membrane of the mouth. Its lateral surface is separated from the ramus of the mandible by adipose tissue. Its posterior border gives attachment to the superior pharyngeal constrictor; its anterior border, to part of the buccinator.

head and neck

6.12

Answer: B Posterior borber of the sternocleidomastoid muscle, the clavicle and anterior border of the trapezius muscle

The posterior triangle is bounded in front by the sternocleidomastoid; behind, by the anterior margin of the trapezius; its base is formed by the middle third of the clavicle; its apex, by the occipital bone. The space is crossed, about 2.5 cm above the clavicle, by the inferior belly of the omohyoid, which divides it into two triangles, an upper or occipital and a lower or subclavian.

6.13

Answer: A The thyrocervical trunk typically gives rises to the inferior thyroid artery, transverse cervical artery and suprascapular artery

The thyrocervical trunk is a short thick trunk which arises from the front of the first portion of the subclavian artery, close to the medial border of scalenus anterior, and divides almost immediately into three branches, the inferior thyroid, transverse scapular and transverse cervical arteries.

6.14

Answer: B Abduct the vocal process of the arteroid cartilages

Each posterior cricoarytenoid muscle arises from the broad depression on the corresponding half of the posterior surface of the lamina of the cricoid cartilage. Its fibres run upward and lateralward and converge to be inserted into the back of the muscular process of the arytenoid cartilage. The uppermost fibres are nearly horizontal, the middle oblique and the lowest almost vertical. These separate the vocal folds and consequently open the glottis by rotating the arytenoid cartilages outward around a vertical axis passing through the cricoarytenoid joints (abduction), so that their vocal processes and the vocal folds attached to them become widely separated. The nerve supply comes from recurrent laryngeal nerve.

head and neck

6.15

Answer: C   Facial vein

The anterior facial vein begins at the side of the root of the nose, and is a direct continuation of the angular vein. It lies behind the facial artery and follows a less tortuous course. It runs obliquely downward and backward, under the zygomaticus and the zygomatic head of the quadratus labii superioris. It descends along the anterior border and then on the superficial surface of the masseter. It crosses over the body of the mandible, and passes obliquely backward, deep to the platysma and cervical fascia and superficial to the submandibular gland, the digastric and stylohyoid. It unites with the posterior facial vein to form the common facial vein, which crosses the external carotid artery and enters the internal jugular vein at a variable point below the hyoid bone. From near its termination a communicating branch often runs down the anterior border of the sternocleidomastoid to join the lower part of the anterior jugular vein. The facial vein has no valves, and its walls are not as flaccid as most superficial veins. The anterior facial vein receives a branch of considerable size, the deep facial vein, from the pterygoid venous plexus. It is also joined by the superior and inferior palpebral, the superior and inferior labial, the buccinator and the masseteric veins. Below the mandible it receives the submental, palatine and submaxillary veins and, generally, the vena comitans of the hypoglossal nerve. The connection between the pterygoid venous plexus and the facial vein is the usual route of spread of infection to the cavernous sinus from the face.

6.16

Answer: E   Vertebral

The vertebral artery is the first branch of the subclavian and arises from the upper and back part of the first portion of the vessel. It is surrounded by a plexus of nerve fibres derived from the inferior cervical ganglion of the sympathetic trunk and ascends through the foramina in the transverse processes of the upper six cervical vertebrae; it then winds behind the superior articular process of the atlas and, entering the skull through the foramen magnum, unites at the lower border of the pons with the vessel of the opposite side to form the basilar artery.

head and neck

The vertebral artery may be divided into four parts. The first part runs upward and backward between the longus colli and the scalenus anterior. In front of it are the internal jugular and vertebral veins and it is also crossed by the inferior thyroid artery; the left vertebral is also crossed by the thoracic duct. Behind it are the transverse process of the seventh cervical vertebra, the sympathetic trunk and its inferior cervical ganglion. The second part runs upward through the foramina in the transverse processes of the upper six cervical vertebrae and is surrounded by branches from the inferior cervical sympathetic ganglion and by a plexus of veins which unite to form the vertebral vein at the lower part of the neck. It is situated in front of the trunks of the cervical nerves and pursues an almost vertical course as far as the transverse process of the atlas, above which it runs upward and lateralward to the foramen in the transverse process of the atlas. The third part issues from this foramen on the medial side of the rectus capitis lateralis and curves backward behind the superior articular process of the atlas, the anterior ramus of the first cervical nerve being on its medial side. It then lies in the groove on the upper surface of the posterior arch of the atlas and enters the vertebral canal by passing beneath the posterior atlanto-occipital membrane. This part of the artery is covered by the semispinalis capitis and is contained in the suboccipital triangle – a triangular space bounded by the rectus capitis posterior major, the superior oblique and the inferior oblique. The first cervical or suboccipital nerve lies between the artery and the posterior arch of the atlas. The fourth part pierces the dura mater and inclines medialward to the front of the medulla oblongata. It is placed between the hypoglossal nerve and the anterior root of the first cervical nerve and beneath the first digitation of the ligamentum denticulatum. At the lower border of the pons it unites with the vessel of the opposite side to form the basilar artery.

The branches of the vertebral artery can be divided into two sets, those given off in the neck and those within the cranium:

- Cervical branches:
    - spinal
    - muscular

- Cranial branches:
  - meningeal
  - posterior spinal
  - anterior spinal
  - posterior inferior cerebellar
  - medullary.

6.17

Answer: B   Anterior branches of the middle meningeal artery

The pterion is the point where the great wing of the sphenoid joins the sphenoidal angle of the parietal bone; it is situated 35 mm behind and 12 mm above the level of the frontozygomatic suture. It marks the junction between three bones, the sphenoid bone, the parietal bone and the temporal bone. Clinically, the pterion is relevant because the anterior branches of the middle meningeal artery run beneath it, on the inner side of the skull, which is quite thin at this point. A blow to the pterion (as in boxing) may rupture the artery, causing an extradural haematoma. The pterion receives its name from the Greek root *pteron*, meaning 'wing'. In Greek mythology, Hermes, messenger of the gods, was enabled to fly by winged sandals and wings on his head, which were attached at the pterion.

6.18

Answer: C   Sphenoid

The sphenoid bone is situated at the base of the skull, anterior to the temporals and basilar part of the occipital. It somewhat resembles a bat with its wings extended. It is divided into a median portion or body, two great wings and two small wings, extending outward from the sides of the body, and two pterygoid processes that project from it inferiorly. The optic foramen is situated in the body; the foramen rotundum, foramen ovale and foramen spinosum are located in the great wing; and the superior orbital fissure is located in the lesser wing of the sphenoid.

6.19

Answer: E   Can be injured by erroneous placement of a tympanic membrane shunt

The chorda tympani is a nerve that branches from the facial nerve (cranial nerve VII) inside the facial canal, just before the facial nerve exits the skull via the stylomastoid foramen. The chorda tympani carry two types of nerve fibres from their origin with the facial nerve to the lingual nerve that carries them to their destinations:

- Special sensory fibres providing taste sensation from the anterior two-thirds of the tongue

- Presynaptic parasympathetic fibres to the submandibular ganglion, providing secretomotor innervation to two salivary glands, the submandibular gland and the sublingual gland.

Rather than leave the skull with the facial nerve, the chorda tympani travels through the middle ear, where it runs from posterior to anterior across the tympanic membrane. It is here that it can be injured by erroneous placement of a tympanic membrane shunt. The nerve continues through the petrotympanic fissure, after which it emerges from the skull into the infratemporal fossa. It soon combines with the larger lingual nerve, a branch of the mandibular nerve (cranial nerve V3). The fibres of the chorda tympani travel with the lingual nerve to the submandibular ganglion. Here the preganglionic parasympathetic fibres of the chorda tympani synapse with postganglionic fibres which go on to innervate the submandibular and sublingual salivary glands. Special sensory (taste) fibres also extend from the chorda tympani to the anterior two-thirds of the tongue via the lingual nerve.

6.20

Answer: D   Compression at the internal acoustic meatus

The parasympathetic nerve supply originates from the lacrimal nucleus of the facial nerve in the pons and travels via the pterygopalatine ganglion and maxillary nerve to innervate the gland. Compression of the facial nerve at the internal acoustic meatus can

head and neck

damage the parasympathetic innervation to the lacrimal gland, resulting in dry eye.

6.21

Answer: B   Frontal

The supratrochlear nerve, the smaller of the two branches of the frontal nerve, passes above the pulley of the superior oblique and gives off a descending filament to join the infratrochlear branch of the nasociliary nerve. It then escapes from the orbit between the pulley of the superior oblique and the supraorbital foramen, curves up onto the forehead close to the bone, ascends beneath the corrugator and frontalis and dividing into branches which pierce these muscles, it supplies the skin of the lower part of the forehead close to the midline and sends filaments to the conjunctiva and skin of the upper eyelid.

6.22

Answer: C   They are in the same subcutaneous plane as the platysma muscle

The facial muscles are subcutaneous (just under the skin, in the same plane as the platysma) muscles that control facial expression. They generally originate on bone and insert on the skin of the face. The facial muscles are innervated by cranial nerve VII, also known as the facial nerve. The facial muscles are derived from the second pharyngeal arch.

6.23

Answer: A   Protrude the mandible

The lateral pterygoid is a short, thick muscle, somewhat conical in shape, which extends almost horizontally between the infratemporal fossa and the condyle of the mandible. It has two heads of origin. The upper head arises from the lower part of the lateral surface of the great wing of the sphenoid and from the infratemporal crest, while the lower head takes origin from the lateral surface of the lateral pterygoid plate. Its fibres pass horizontally backward and laterally to be inserted into the pterygoid fovea, which is a depression on the anterior aspect of the neck of the condyle of the mandible, and into the front margin of the articular disc of the temporomandibular joint. The lateral pterygoids, in common with other muscles of mastication, are supplied by the mandibular nerve. The lateral pterygoid assists in opening the mouth, but its main action is to draw forward the condyle and articular disc so that the mandible is protruded and the inferior incisors projected in front of the upper. The lateral pterygoid is assisted in this action by the medial pterygoid. If the medial and lateral pterygoid muscles of one side act, the corresponding side of the mandible is drawn forward while the opposite condyle remains comparatively fixed, facilitating side-to-side movements such those occurring during the trituration of food.

6.24

Answer: B   In the mandible

Below the second premolar tooth, on either side, midway between the upper and lower borders of the body of the mandible, is the mental foramen, for the passage of the mental vessels and nerve.

6.25

Answer: C   Preganglionic fibres synapse in the pterygopalatine ganglion

The parasympathetic innervation to the nose comes from the pterygopalatine ganglion, with the preganglionic fibres synpasing in the ganglion. The pterygopalatine ganglion (or sphenopalatine ganglion) is a parasympathetic ganglion found in the pterygopalatine fossa. The pterygopalatine ganglion (the ganglion of Meckel) is the largest of the parasympathetic ganglia that are associated with the branches of the trigeminal nerve. It is deeply placed in the pterygopalatine fossa, close to the sphenopalatine foramen. It is triangular or heart-shaped, reddish-grey in colour, and is situated just below the maxillary nerve as it crosses the fossa. The pterygopalatine ganglion supplies the lacrimal gland, paranasal sinuses, glands of the mucosa of the nasal cavity and pharynx, the gums, and the mucous

head and neck

membrane and glands of the hard palate. It communicates anteriorly with the nasopalatine nerve.

The pterygopalatine ganglion receives a sensory, a motor, and a sympathetic root. Its sensory root is derived from two sphenopalatine branches of the maxillary nerve: although the majority of their fibres pass directly into the palatine nerves, some enter the ganglion, forming its sensory root. Its motor root is derived from the nervus intermedius (a part of the facial nerve) through the greater petrosal nerve. In the pterygopalatine ganglion, the parasympathetic fibres form synapses with neurones whose postganglionic axons, vasodilator and secretory fibres, are distributed with the deep branches of the trigeminal nerve to the mucous membrane of the nose, soft palate, tonsils, uvula, roof of the mouth, upper lip and gums, and to the upper part of the pharynx. It also distributes postganglionic parasympathetic fibres to the lacrimal gland through the zygomatic nerve, a branch of the maxillary nerve (from the trigeminal nerve), which then connects with the lacrimal nerve (a branch of the ophthalmic nerve, also part of the trigeminal nerve) to arrive at the lacrimal gland. The ganglion also consists of sympathetic efferent (postganglionic) fibres from the superior cervical ganglion. These fibres, from the superior cervical ganglion, travel through the carotid plexus and then through the deep petrosal nerve. The deep petrosal nerve joins with the greater petrosal nerve to form the nerve of the pterygoid canal, which enters the ganglion.

6.26

Answer: B   Middle meatus

The middle meatus is inferolateral to the middle concha, and is continued anteriorly into a shallow depression, situated above the vestibule and called the atrium of the middle meatus. The lateral wall of the middle meatus is fully displayed by raising or removing the middle concha. There is a rounded elevation, the bulla ethmoidalis, on the lateral wall of the middle meatus, and anteroinferior to this is a curved cleft, the hiatus semilunaris. The bulla ethmoidalis is produced by the bulging of the middle ethmoidal cells, which open on or immediately above it, and the size of the bulla varies with that of the cells it contains. The hiatus semilunaris is bounded inferiorly by the sharp concave margin of the uncinate process of the ethmoid bone, and leads into a curved channel, the infundibulum, bounded superiorly by the bulla ethmoidalis and inferiorly by the lateral surface of the uncinate process of the ethmoid. The anterior ethmoidal cells open into the front part of the infundibulum: in slightly over 50% of people this is directly continuous with the frontonasal duct or passage leading from the frontal air sinus. #When the anterior end of the uncinate process fuses with the front part of the bulla, however, this continuity is interrupted and the frontonasal duct then opens directly into the anterior end of the middle meatus. In order to gain access to the frontal sinus via the nasal cavity, therefore, one would enter through the middle meatus. Below the bulla ethmoidalis, and partly hidden by the inferior end of the uncinate process, is the opening from the maxillary sinus (the ostium maxillare). In a frontal section this opening is seen to be located near the roof of the sinus. An accessory opening from the sinus is often found below the posterior end of the middle nasal concha.

6.27

Answer: B　　Are located in the anterior cranial fossa

The olfactory foramina are located in the anterior cranial fossa. These foramina are in the cribriform plate of the ethmoid bone for the passage of olfactory nerves.

6.28

Answer: C　　Is formed between two layers of meningeal dura

The inferior sagittal sinus is enclosed in the posterior half or two-thirds of the free margin of the falx cerebri. It is cylindrical in shape. It increases in size as it passes backward and ends in the straight sinus. It receives several veins from the falx cerebri and occasionally receives a few veins from the medial surfaces of the hemispheres.

head and neck

6.29

Answer: D   Would be affected by severance of the oculomotor
nerve (cranial nerve III)

The ciliary ganglion is a small parasympathetic ganglion. It is reddish-
grey in colour and about the size of a pinhead. It is situated in the
posterior part of the orbit, in some loose fat between the optic
nerve and the lateral rectus muscle, lying generally on the lateral
side of the ophthalmic artery.

It has three roots and these enter its posterior border. One, the
long or sensory root, is derived from the nasociliary nerve and joins
its posterosuperior angle. The second, the short or motor root, is
a thick nerve (occasionally divided into two parts) that is derived
from the branch of the oculomotor nerve to the inferior oblique,
and is connected to the posteroinferior angle of the ganglion.
The ciliary ganglion would therefore be affected by severance
of the oculomotor nerve. The motor root is thought to contain
sympathetic efferent fibres (preganglionic fibres) from the nucleus
of the third nerve in the midbrain to the ciliary ganglion, where they
form synapses with neurones whose fibres (postganglionic) pass to
the ciliary muscle and to the sphincter muscle of the pupil. The third
root, the sympathetic root, is a slender filament from the cavernous
plexus of the sympathetic; it is frequently blended with the long
root. The ciliary ganglion receives a communicating branch from the
sphenopalatine ganglion.

Its branches are the short ciliary nerves. These are delicate filaments,
from six to ten in number, which arise from the forepart of the
ganglion in two bundles, connected with its superior and inferior
angles; the lower bundle is the larger. They run forward with the
ciliary arteries in a wavy course, one set above and the other set
below the optic nerve, and are accompanied by the long ciliary
nerves from the nasociliary nerve. They pierce the sclera at the
posterior aspect of the bulb of the eye, pass forward in delicate
grooves on the inner surface of the sclera, and are distributed to the
ciliary muscle, iris and cornea. A small branch penetrates the optic
nerve with the central artery of retina.

6.30

Answer: A   Infraorbital nerve

The inferior palpebral branches are terminal twigs from the infraorbital branch of the maxillary nerve which ascend behind the orbicularis oculi. They supply the skin and conjunctiva of the lower eyelid, joining at the lateral angle of the orbit with the facial and zygomaticofacial nerves.

6.31

Answer: B   A branch of a nerve that exits through the stylomastoid foramen

The orbicularis oculi arises from the nasal part of the frontal bone, from the frontal process of the maxilla anterior to the lacrimal groove, and from the anterior surface and borders of the medial palpebral ligament. From this origin, the fibres are directed lateralward, forming a broad and thin layer, which occupies the eyelids or palpebrae, surrounds the circumference of the orbit, and spreads over the temple and downward on the cheek. The palpebral portion of the muscle is thin and pale. It arises from the bifurcation of the medial palpebral ligament, forms a series of concentric curves, and is inserted into the lateral palpebral raphé. The orbital portion is thicker and reddish in colour. Its fibres form a complete ellipse without interruption at the lateral palpebral commissure. The upper fibres of this portion blend with the frontalis and corrugator muscles. The lacrimal part (tensor tarsi) is a small, thin muscle, about 6 mm in breadth and 12 mm in length, situated behind the medial palpebral ligament and lacrimal sac. It arises from the posterior crest and the adjacent part of the orbital surface of the lacrimal bone and, passing behind the lacrimal sac, divides into two slips (upper and lower) which are inserted into the superior and inferior tarsi medial to the puncta lacrimalia; occasionally it is very indistinct. It is supplied by zygomatic branch of the facial nerve (cranial nerve VII), which exits through the stylomastoid foramen.

The muscle acts to close the eye and is the only muscle capable of doing this. Loss of function for any reason results in an inability to close the eye, necessitating treatment with eye drops at the very

head and neck

least, or even removal of the eye in extreme cases. The orbicularis oculi is the sphincter muscle of the eyelids. The palpebral portion acts involuntarily, closing the lids gently, as in sleep or in blinking; the orbital portion is subject to conscious control. When the entire muscle is brought into action, the skin of the forehead, temple and cheek is drawn toward the medial angle of the orbit and the eyelids are firmly closed, as in photophobia. When the skin is pulled in this way it is thrown into folds, particular into folds radiating from the lateral angle of the eyelids – these folds become permanent in old age, forming what are known as 'crow's feet'. The levator palpebrae superioris is the direct antagonist of this muscle. It raises the upper eyelid and exposes the front of the bulb of the eye. Each time the eyelids are closed through the action of the orbicularis, the medial palpebral ligament is tightened and the wall of the lacrimal sac is drawn laterally and forward, so that a vacuum is formed in it and the tears are sucked along the lacrimal canals into it. The lacrimal part of the orbicularis oculi draws the eyelids and the ends of the lacrimal canals medially and compresses them against the surface of the globe of the eye, thus placing them in the most favourable position for receiving the tears; it also compresses the lacrimal sac.

6.32

Answer: A   Decrease blood flow to some parts of the nasal septum

The facial artery arises in the carotid triangle a little above the lingual artery and, sheltered by the ramus of the mandible, passes obliquely up beneath the digastric and stylohyoid, over which it arches to enter a groove on the posterior surface of the submaxillary gland. It then curves upward over the body of the mandible at the antero-inferior angle of the masseter, passes forward and upward across the cheek to the angle of the mouth, then ascends along the side of the nose and ends at the medial commissure of the eye, under the name of the angular artery. This vessel, both in the neck and on the face, is remarkably tortuous: in the former situation, to accommodate itself to the movements of the pharynx in deglutition and, in the latter, to the movements of the mandible, lips and cheeks. Through the septal branch of the superior labial artery it supplies the nasal septum. As the superior labial artery is derived from the facial artery above the inferior border of the mandible blood supply to the nasal septum may therefore be affected on the side where the facial artery is ligated at the inferior border of mandible (see also *Answer* to **6.2**).

6.33

Answer: A   Laterally, to the right

The left lateral pterygoid muscle acting alone will shift the mandible laterally and to the right (see also *Answer* to **6.23**).

6.34

Answer: D   A muscle that both opens the auditory tube and tenses the palate is innervated by cranial nerve V

The tensor veli palatini (tensor palati) is a broad, thin, ribbon-like muscle in the head that tenses the soft palate. The tensor veli palatini is found lateral to the levator veli palatini muscle. It arises by a flat lamella from the scaphoid fossa at the base of the medial pterygoid plate, from the spina angularis of the sphenoid and from the lateral wall of the cartilage of the auditory tube. Descending vertically between the medial pterygoid plate and the medial pterygoid muscle, it ends in a tendon which winds around the pterygoid hamulus, being retained in this situation by some of the fibres of origin of the medial pterygoid muscle. Between the tendon and the hamulus is a small bursa. The tendon then passes medialward and is inserted into the palatine aponeurosis and into the surface behind the transverse ridge on the horizontal part of the palatine bone. The tensor veli palatini is innervated by the mandibular nerve, a branch of the trigeminal nerve (cranial nerve V). It is associated both with mastication and with the function (opening) of the auditory tube through its function of tensing the palate.

6.35

Answer: B   Trigeminal nerve

The tensor tympani muscle originates from the cartilaginous wall of the Eustachian tube (also called the auditory tube) and the bony

head and neck

wall surrounding the tube. The muscle inserts onto the handle of the malleus. When tensed, the action of the muscle is to pull the malleus medially, tensing the tympanic membrane, damping vibration in the ear ossicles and thereby reducing the amplitude of sounds. Innervation of the muscle is from branches of the mandibular division of the trigeminal nerve (cranial nerve V3), by way of the otic ganglion.

6.36

Answer: C   The iris

The iris has received its name from its various colours in different individuals. It is a thin, circular, contractile disc, suspended in the aqueous humour between the cornea and lens and perforated a little to the nasal side of its centre by a circular aperture, the pupil. At its periphery it is continuous with the ciliary body and is also connected to the posterior elastic lamina of the cornea by means of the pectinate ligament. Its surfaces are flattened and look forward and backward, the anterior toward the cornea, the posterior toward the ciliary processes and lens. The iris divides the space between the lens and the cornea into an anterior and a posterior chamber. The anterior chamber of the eye is bounded in front by the posterior surface of the cornea; behind by the front of the iris and the central part of the lens. The posterior chamber is a narrow chink behind the peripheral part of the iris and in front of the suspensory ligament of the lens and the ciliary processes. In the adult, the two chambers communicate through the pupil, but in the fetus up to the seventh month they are separated by the membrana pupillaris.

6.37

Answer: C   Abducent

The lateral rectus muscle is a muscle in the orbit. It is one of six extraocular muscles that control the movements of the eyeball and the only muscle innervated by the abducent nerve, cranial nerve VI. The Latin name for the sixth cranial nerve is nervus abducens: 'abducens' is more common in recent literature, while 'abducent' predominates in the older literature. The abducens nucleus is located in the pons, on the floor of the fourth ventricle, at the level

head and neck

of the facial colliculus. Axons from the facial nerve loop around the abducens nucleus, creating a slight bulge (the facial colliculus) that is visible on the dorsal surface of the floor of the fourth ventricle. The abducens nucleus is close to the midline, like the other motor nuclei that control eye movements (the oculomotor and trochlear nuclei). Motor axons leaving the abducens nucleus run ventrally and caudally through the pons. They pass lateral to the corticospinal tract (which runs longitudinally through the pons at this level) before exiting the brainstem at the pontomedullary junction.

The abducens nerve leaves the brainstem at the junction of the pons and the medulla, medial to the facial nerve. In order to reach the eye, it runs superiorly and then bends anteriorly. The nerve enters the subarachnoid space when it emerges from the brainstem. It runs upward between the pons and the clivus, and then pierces the dura mater to run between the dura and the skull. At the tip of the petrous temporal bone it makes a sharp turn forward to enter the cavernous sinus. In the cavernous sinus it runs alongside the internal carotid artery. It then enters the orbit through the superior orbital fissure and innervates the lateral rectus muscle of the eye.

The long course of the abducens nerve between the brainstem and the eye makes it vulnerable to injury at several levels. For example, fractures of the petrous temporal bone can selectively damage the nerve, as can aneurysms of the intracavernous carotid artery. Mass lesions that push the brainstem downward can damage the nerve by stretching it between the point where it emerges from the pons and the point where it hooks over the petrous temporal bone.

6.38

Answer: B   Tensor veli palatini

The tensor veli palatini (tensor palati) is a broad, thin, ribbon-like muscle in the head that tenses the soft palate. The tensor veli palatini is found lateral to the levator veli palatini muscle. It arises by a flat lamella from the scaphoid fossa at the base of the medial pterygoid plate, from the spina angularis of the sphenoid and from the lateral wall of the cartilage of the auditory tube. Descending vertically between the medial pterygoid plate and the medial pterygoid muscle, it ends in a tendon which winds around the pterygoid hamulus, being retained in this situation by some of the fibres of origin of the medial pterygoid muscle. Between the tendon and the hamulus is a small bursa. The tendon then passes medialward and is inserted into the palatine aponeurosis and into the surface behind the transverse ridge on the horizontal part of the palatine bone.

6.39

Answer: A   Visceral space

The thyroid gland is a highly vascular organ, situated at the front and sides of the neck in the visceral space. It consists of right and left lobes connected across the midline by a narrow portion, the isthmus. Its weight is somewhat variable, but is usually about 30 grams. It is slightly heavier in the woman, in whom it becomes enlarged during menstruation and pregnancy.

6.40

Answer: D   The recurrent laryngeal nerves run along its posterior surface

The arteries supplying the thyroid gland are the superior and inferior thyroids and sometimes an additional branch (thyroidea ima) from the innominate artery or the arch of the aorta, which ascends on the front of the trachea. The arteries are remarkable for their large size and frequent anastomoses. The veins form a plexus on the surface of the gland and on the front of the trachea. The superior, middle and inferior thyroid veins arise from this plexus; the superior and middle veins end in the internal jugular vein, the inferior in the innominate vein. The capillary blood vessels form a dense plexus in the connective tissue around the vesicles, between the epithelium of the vesicles and the endothelium of the lymphatics, which surround a greater or smaller part of the circumference of the vesicle. The lymphatic vessels run in the interlobular connective tissue, not uncommonly surrounding the arteries that they accompany, and communicate with a network in the capsule of the gland; they may contain colloid material. They end in the thoracic and right lymphatic trunks. The nerves are derived from the middle and inferior cervical ganglia of the sympathetic trunk.

The recurrent laryngeal nerve is best known for its importance in thyroid surgery, as it runs immediately posterior to this gland. If it is damaged during surgery, the patient will have a hoarse voice. Nerve damage can be assessed by laryngoscopy, during which a stroboscopic light confirms the absence of movement in the affected side of the vocal cords. Similar problems can also be caused by invasion of the nerve by a tumour or after trauma to the neck. If the damage is unilateral, the patient may present with voice changes, including hoarseness. Bilateral nerve damage can result in breathing difficulties and aphonia, the inability to speak. Galen is said to have first described the clinical syndrome of recurrent laryngeal nerve paralysis.

6.41

Answer: A   Skin, investing fascia, pretracheal fascia, thyroid gland, parathyroid glands

The lobes of the thyroid gland are conical in shape. Each lobe has an apex that is directed upward and laterally as far as the junction of the middle and lower thirds of the thyroid cartilage and a base that faces inferiorly and is on a level with the fifth or sixth tracheal ring. Each lobe measures about 5 cm in length, about 3 cm at its widest, and about 2 cm in thickness. The lateral or superficial surface is convex, and covered by the skin, the superficial and deep fasciae, the sternocleidomastoid, the superior belly of the omohyoid, and the sternohyoid and sternothyroid; and is covered beneath the sternothyroid by the pretracheal layer of the deep fascia that forms a capsule for the gland. The deep or medial surface is moulded over the underlying structures – the thyroid and cricoid cartilages, the trachea, the inferior pharyngeal constrictor and the posterior part of the cricothyroid, the oesophagus (particularly on the left side of the neck), the superior and inferior thyroid arteries, and the recurrent nerves. The anterior border is thin and inclines obliquely from above downward, toward the midline of the neck, while the posterior border is thick and overlaps the common carotid artery and, as a rule, the parathyroids.

The isthmus connects the lower thirds of the lobes. It is about 1.25 cm in breadth, and the same in depth, and usually covers the second and third rings of the trachea. Its situation and size can vary, however. It is covered by the skin and fascia in the midline of the neck, and

head and neck

by the sternothyroid on either side of the midline. Across its upper border runs an anastomotic branch uniting the two superior thyroid arteries; at its lower border are the inferior thyroid veins. Sometimes the isthmus is missing altogether.

A third lobe, conical in shape, called the pyramidal lobe, frequently arises from the upper part of the isthmus or from the adjacent portion of either lobe (but most commonly the left) and ascends as far as the hyoid bone. It is occasionally quite detached, or can be divided into two or more parts.

A fibrous or muscular band is sometimes found attached superiorly to the body of the hyoid bone, and inferiorly to the isthmus of the gland, or its pyramidal lobe. When it is muscular it is known as the levator glandulae thyroideae.

6.42

Answer: E   Transverse cervical

The transverse cervical nerve arises from the second and third cervical nerves, turns around the posterior border of the sternocleidomastoid about its middle and, passing obliquely forward beneath the external jugular vein to the anterior border of the muscle, it perforates the deep cervical fascia and divides beneath the platysma into ascending and descending branches, which are distributed to the anterolateral parts of the neck (anterior triangle).

6.43

Answer: B   Ansa cervicalis

The ansa cervicalis (or ansa hypoglossi in older literature) is a loop of nerves that are part of the cervical plexus. Branches from the ansa cervicalis innervate the sternohyoid, sternothyroid and the inferior belly of the omohyoid. Two roots make up the ansa cervicalis. The superior root of the ansa cervicalis is formed by a branch of spinal nerve C1. These nerve fibres travel in the hypoglossal nerve before leaving to form the superior root. The superior root goes around the occipital artery and then descends embedded in the carotid sheath. It sends a branch off to the superior belly of the omohyoid muscle and is then joined by the inferior root. The inferior root is formed by fibres from spinal nerves C2 and C3.

6.44

Answer: B Foramen rotundum and foramen ovale

The patient's neurological examination suggest injury to the maxillary and mandibular nerves. At the base of the skull in the middle cranial fossa, behind the medial end of the superior orbital fissure is the foramen rotundum, for the passage of the maxillary nerve. Behind and lateral to the foramen rotundum is the foramen ovale, which transmits the mandibular nerve, the accessory meningeal artery and the lesser superficial petrosal nerve.

6.45

Answer: D Middle meningeal artery

The middle meningeal artery is the largest of the arteries that supply the dura mater. It is typically the first branch of the first part (the retromandibular part) of the maxillary artery, which is one of the two terminal branches of the external carotid artery. It ascends between the sphenomandibular ligament and the lateral pterygoid, and between the two roots of the auriculotemporal nerve to the foramen spinosum of the sphenoid bone, through which it enters the cranium. It then runs forward in a groove on the great wing of the sphenoid bone and divides into two branches, anterior and posterior. The larger anterior branch crosses the great wing of the sphenoid to reach the groove, or canal, in the sphenoidal angle of the parietal bone, where it divides into branches which spread out between the dura mater and the internal surface of the cranium. Some of these branches pass upward as far as the vertex and others pass backward to the occipital region. The posterior branch curves backward on the squamous temporal bone and, reaching the parietal bone some distance in front of its mastoid angle, divides into branches which supply the posterior part of the dura mater and cranium. The branches of the middle meningeal artery are distributed partly to the dura mater, but chiefly to the bones. They anastomose with the arteries of the opposite side, and with the anterior and posterior meningeal arteries.

head and neck

The middle meningeal artery gives off the following branches on entering the cranium:

- Numerous small vessels that supply the semilunar ganglion and the dura mater

- A superficial petrosal branch, which enters the hiatus of the facial canal, supplies the facial nerve and anastomoses with the stylomastoid branch of the posterior auricular artery

- A superior tympanic artery, which runs in the canal for the tensor tympani and supplies this muscle and the lining membrane of the canal

- Orbital branches, which pass through the superior orbital fissure or through separate canals in the great wing of the sphenoid to anastomose with the lacrimal or other branches of the ophthalmic artery

- Temporal branches, which pass through foramina in the great wing of the sphenoid and anastomose in the temporal fossa with the deep temporal arteries.

An injured middle meningeal artery causes an epidural haematoma. A head injury (for example following a road traffic accident or sports injury) is required to rupture the artery. Emergency treatment requires decompression of the haematoma, usually by craniotomy. Subdural bleeding is usually venous in nature rather than arterial.

6.46

Answer: E   Is the only source of nutrients for the lens of the eye

The aqueous humour is a thick watery substance that is located in the eye. The anterior segment is the front third of the eye that includes the structures in front of the vitreous humour: the cornea, iris, ciliary body and lens. Within the anterior segment are two fluid-filled spaces divided by the iris plane:

- The anterior chamber, between the posterior surface of the cornea (the corneal endothelium) and the iris

- The posterior chamber, between the iris and the front of the vitreous.

Aqueous humour fills these spaces within the anterior segment to provide nutrients to the lens and corneal endothelium and its pressure maintains the convex shape of the cornea. In health, the aqueous humour does not mix with the firm, gel-like vitreous humour because of the lens and its suspensory ligaments between the two. The aqueous humour is secreted into the posterior chamber by the ciliary body, specifically the ciliary processes, and flows through the narrow cleft between the front of the lens and the back of the iris, to escape through the pupil into the anterior chamber and then to drain out of the eye via the trabecular meshwork into the aqueous veins and eventually into the veins of the orbit.

The aqueous humour:

- Maintains the intraocular pressure and inflates the globe of the eye

- Provides nutrition for the avascular ocular tissues: posterior cornea, trabecular meshwork, lens and anterior vitreous

- Carries away waste products from metabolism of these avascular ocular tissues

- May serve to transport ascorbate in the anterior segment to act as an antioxidant agent

- Has a role in the immune response, to defend against pathogens, as indicated by presence of immunoglobulins.

The composition of aqueous humour includes:

- Water: 98.8%

- Ions: HCO_3^-, buffers metabolic acids; Cl^-, preserves electric neutrality; Na^+; K^+; Ca^{2+}; PO_4^{3-}

- Proteins: albumin, β-globulins, very low density due to filtration

- Ascorbate: antioxidative, protects against ultraviolet rays

head and neck

- Glucose
- Lactate: produced by metabolism of anaerobic structures of the eye
- Amino acids: transported by ciliary epithelial cells.

6.47

Answer: B   Superior cervical ganglion

The cervical portion of the sympathetic trunk consists of three ganglia, named according to their positions as the superior, middle and inferior ganglia, and connected by intervening cords. This portion receives no white rami communicantes from the cervical spinal nerves. Its spinal fibres are derived from the white rami of the upper thoracic nerves, and enter the corresponding thoracic ganglia of the sympathetic trunk, through which they ascend into the neck.

The superior cervical ganglion, the largest of the three, is located opposite the second and third cervical vertebrae. It is reddish-grey in colour and usually fusiform in shape. It is thought to be formed by the coalescence of four ganglia, corresponding to the upper four cervical nerves. It is related anteriorly to the sheath of the internal carotid artery and the internal jugular vein and posteriorly to the longus capitis muscle. It contains neurones that supply sympathetic innervation to the face (including the dilator pupillae muscle of the iris).

6.48

Answer: A   Optic canal

The ophthalmic artery arises from the internal carotid, just as that vessel is emerging from the cavernous sinus, on the medial side of the anterior clinoid process and enters the orbital cavity through the optic foramen (canal), below and lateral to the optic nerve. It then passes over the nerve to reach the medial wall of the orbit and thence horizontally forward, beneath the lower border of the superior oblique and divides it into two terminal branches, the frontal and dorsal nasal. As the artery crosses the optic nerve it is accompanied by the nasociliary nerve and is separated from the frontal nerve by the rectus superior and levator palpebrae superioris.

6.49

Answer: A   External carotid artery

The external carotid artery begins opposite the upper border of the thyroid cartilage and, taking a slightly curved course, passes upward and forward and then inclines backward to the space behind the neck of the mandible, where it divides into the superficial temporal and internal maxillary arteries. It rapidly diminishes in size in its course up the neck, owing to the number and large size of the branches given off from it. In the child, it is somewhat smaller than the internal carotid; but in the adult, the two vessels are of nearly equal size. At its origin, this artery is more superficial and placed nearer the midline than the internal carotid and is contained within the carotid triangle.

The external carotid artery is covered by the skin, superficial fascia, platysma, deep fascia and anterior margin of the sternocleidomastoid. It is crossed by the hypoglossal nerve, by the lingual, ranine, common facial and superior thyroid veins; and by the digastric and stylohyoid; higher up it passes deeply into the substance of the parotid gland, where it lies deep to the facial nerve and the junction of the temporal and internal maxillary veins. It is here that it is in danger during surgery on the parotid gland. Medial to it are the hyoid bone, the wall of the pharynx, the superior laryngeal nerve and a portion of the parotid gland. Lateral to it, in the lower part of its course, is the internal carotid artery. Posterior to it, near its origin, is the superior laryngeal nerve; and higher up, it is separated from the internal carotid by the styloglossus and stylopharyngeus, the glossopharyngeal nerve, the pharyngeal branch of the vagus and part of the parotid gland. Its branches include:

- Superior thyroid artery
- Ascending pharyngeal artery
- Lingual artery
- Facial artery

head and neck

- Occipital artery

- Posterior auricular artery

- Maxillary artery (a terminal branch)

- Superficial temporal artery (a terminal branch).

6.50

Answer: D   The lateral rectus muscle of the right eye and cranial nerve III on the left side

The inferior oblique and the recti superior, inferior and medialis are supplied by the oculomotor nerve. The superior oblique is supplied by the trochlear nerve and the lateral rectus is supplied by the abducent nerve. The four recti are attached to the bulb of the eye in such a manner that, acting singly, they will turn its corneal surface either upward, downward, medialward, or lateralward, as expressed by their names. The movement produced by the rectus superior or rectus inferior is not such a simple one, for inasmuch as each passes obliquely lateralward and forward to the bulb of the eye, the elevation or depression of the cornea is accompanied by a certain deviation medialward, with a slight amount of rotation. These latter movements are corrected by the obliques, the inferior oblique correcting the medial deviation caused by the rectus superior and the superior oblique the deviation caused by the rectus inferior. Contraction of the rectus lateralis or rectus medialis, on the other hand, produce a purely horizontal movement. If any two neighbouring recti of one eye act together they carry the globe of the eye in the diagonal of these directions, viz. upward and medialward, upward and lateralward, downward and medialward, or downward and lateralward. Sometimes the corresponding recti of the two eyes act in unison and at other times the opposite recti act together. So, in turning the eyes to the right, the rectus lateralis of the right eye will act in unison with the rectus medialis of the left eye; but if both eyes are directed to an object in the midline at a short distance, the two recti mediales will act in unison. The movement of circumduction, as in looking around a room, is performed by the successive actions of the four recti. The obliques rotate the eyeball on its anteroposterior axis, the superior directing the cornea downward and lateralward and the inferior directing it upward and lateralward. These movements are required for the correct viewing of an object when the head is moved laterally, as from shoulder to shoulder, in order that the picture falls in all respects on the same part of the retina of either eye. So from this description it is clear that inability of a patient to gaze directly to the right with both eyes simultaneously will result from deficits in the lateral rectus muscle of the right eye and cranial nerve III on the left side (supplying the medial rectus of the left eye).

6.51

Answer: B   Is supplied by the ophthalmic nerve

The cornea is one of the most sensitive tissues of the body. It is densely innervated with sensory nerve fibres via the ophthalmic division of the trigeminal nerve by way of 70–80 long ciliary nerves and short ciliary nerves. The nerves enter the cornea via three levels, scleral, episcleral and conjunctival. Most of the bundles give rise by subdivision to a network in the stroma, from which fibres supply the different regions. The three networks are mid-stromal, subepithelial/Bowman's layer and epithelium. The receptive fields of each nerve ending are very large and may overlap.

6.52

Answer: C   External carotid

The lingual artery arises from the external carotid between the superior thyroid and external maxillary. It first runs obliquely upward and medialward to the greater cornu of the hyoid bone, it then curves downward and forward, forming a loop which is crossed by the hypoglossal nerve, and, passing beneath the digastric and stylohyoid, it runs horizontally forward, beneath the hyoglossus and, finally, ascending almost perpendicularly to the tongue, turns forward on its lower surface as far as the tip, under the name of the profunda linguae (deep lingual artery).

head and neck

6.53

Answer: D   The sublingual gland

The branches of the lingual artery:

- The hyoid branch runs along the upper border of the hyoid bone, supplying the muscles attached to it and anastomosing with its fellow of the opposite side.

- The dorsal lingual artery consists usually of two or three small branches which arise beneath the hyoglossus. They ascend to the back part of the dorsum of the tongue and supply the mucous membrane in this situation, the glossopalatine arch, the tonsil, soft palate and epiglottis, anastomosing with the vessels of the opposite side.

- The sublingual artery arises at the anterior margin of the hyoglossus and runs forward between the genioglossus and mylohyoid to the sublingual gland. It supplies the gland and gives branches to the mylohyoid and neighbouring muscles and to the mucous membrane of the mouth and gums. One branch runs behind the alveolar process of the mandible in the substance of the gum to anastomose with a similar artery from the other side; another pierces the mylohyoid and anastomoses with the submental branch of the external maxillary artery.

- The profunda linguae (deep lingual artery) is the terminal portion of the lingual artery. It pursues a tortuous course and runs along the undersurface of the tongue, below the longitudinalis inferior and above the mucous membrane; it lies on the lateral side of the genioglossus, accompanied by the lingual nerve. At the tip of the tongue, it is said to anastomose with the artery of the opposite side. In the mouth, these vessels are placed one on either side of the frenulum linguae.

6.54

Answer: C   Supplies blood to the lateral nasal wall and nasal septum

The sphenopalatine artery, a branch of the third part of the internal maxillary artery, passes through the sphenopalatine foramen into the cavity of the nose, at the back part of the superior meatus. Here it gives off its posterior lateral nasal branches, which spread forward over the conchae and meatuses, anastomose with the ethmoidal arteries and the nasal branches of the descending palatine and assist in supplying the frontal, maxillary, ethmoidal and sphenoidal sinuses. Crossing the undersurface of the sphenoid, the sphenopalatine artery ends on the nasal septum as the posterior septal branches; these anastomose with the ethmoidal arteries and the septal branch of the superior labial. One branch descends in a groove on the vomer to the incisive canal and anastomoses with the descending palatine artery.

6.55

Answer: D   Near the midline in the anterior aspect of the floor of the mouth

The submandibular duct (Wharton's duct) is about 5 cm long and its wall is much thinner than that of the parotid duct. It begins from numerous branches from the deep surface of the gland and runs forward between the mylohyoid and the hyoglossus and genioglossus, then between the sublingual gland and the genioglossus and opens by a narrow orifice on the summit of a small papilla, at the side of the frenulum linguae, near the midline in the anterior aspect of the floor of the mouth. On the hyoglossus it lies between the lingual and hypoglossal nerves, but at the anterior border of the muscle it is crossed laterally by the lingual nerve. The terminal branches of the lingual nerve ascend on its medial side.

head and neck

6.56

Answer: C   The hamulus of the medial pterygoid plate

The medial pterygoid plate of the sphenoid curves lateralward at its lower extremity into a hook-like process, the pterygoid hamulus, around which the tendon of the tensor veli palatini glides.

6.57

Answer: E   It acts on the tongue

The fauces (the Latin plural word for 'throat'; the singular 'faux' is rarely used) is the back part of the mouth, which leads into the pharynx. The fauces are the two pillars of mucous membrane. The anterior pillar is known as the palatoglossal arch and the posterior pillar is known as the palatopharyngeal arch. Between these two arches is the palatine tonsil. The palatoglossal arch (glossopalatine arch or anterior pillar of fauces) on either side runs downward, laterally and forward to the side of the base of the tongue, and is formed by the projection of the palatoglossus muscle (glossopalatinus) with its covering mucous membrane. The palatoglossus arises from the anterior surface of the soft palate, where it is continuous with the muscle of the opposite side. It passes downward, forward and laterally, anterior to the palatine tonsil, to be inserted into the side of the tongue. Some of the fibres of palatoglossus spread over the dorsum of the tongue and others pass deeply into the substance of the tongue to intermingle with the transversus linguae. The palatoglossus is the only muscle of the tongue that is not innervated by the hypoglossal nerve – it is innervated by the vagus nerve via the pharyngeal plexus.

6.58

Answer: C   It is crossed by the hypoglossal nerve

The lingual artery arises from the external carotid between the superior thyroid and external maxillary. It first runs obliquely upward and medialward to the greater cornu of the hyoid bone. It then curves downward and forward, forming a loop which is crossed by the hypoglossal nerve and, passing beneath the digastric and stylohyoid, it runs horizontally forward, beneath the hyoglossus and, finally, ascending almost perpendicularly to the tongue, then turns forward on its lower surface as far as the tip, under the name of the profunda linguae (deep lingual artery) (see also *Answer* to **6.53**).

6.59

Answer: E   General sensation to the anterior two-thirds of the tongue

The lingual nerve, a branch of the mandibular division of trigeminal nerve, supplies the mucous membrane of the anterior two-thirds of the tongue. It lies at first beneath the pterygoideus externus, medial to and in front of the inferior alveolar nerve, and is occasionally joined to this nerve by a branch, which may cross the internal maxillary artery. The chorda tympani also join it at an acute angle in this situation. The nerve then passes between the medial pterygoid and the ramus of the mandible and crosses obliquely to the side of the tongue, over the superior pharyngeal constrictor and styloglossus and then between the hyoglossus and deep part of the submandibular gland. It finally runs across the duct of the submandibular gland and along the tongue to its tip, lying immediately beneath the mucous membrane. Its branches of communication are with the facial (through the chorda tympani), the inferior alveolar and hypoglossal nerves and the submandibular ganglion. The branches to the submandibular ganglion are two or three in number; those connected with the hypoglossal nerve form a plexus at the anterior margin of the hyoglossus. Its branches of distribution supply the sublingual gland, the mucous membrane of the mouth, the gums and the mucous membrane of the anterior two-thirds of the tongue; the terminal filaments communicate, at the tip of the tongue, with the hypoglossal nerve.

6.60

Answer: B   Glossopharyngeal

The tympanic membrane separates the tympanic cavity from the bottom of the external acoustic meatus. It is a thin, semitransparent membrane, nearly oval in form, somewhat broader above than

head and neck

below and directed very obliquely downward and inward so as to form an angle of about 55° with the floor of the meatus. Its longest diameter is downward and forward and measures from 9 to 10 mm; its shortest diameter measures from 8 to 9 mm. The greater part of its circumference is thickened and forms a fibrocartilaginous ring, which is fixed in the tympanic sulcus at the inner end of the meatus. This sulcus is deficient superiorly at the notch of Rivinus and from the ends of this notch two bands, the anterior and posterior malleolar folds, are prolonged to the lateral process of the malleus. The small, triangular part of the membrane situated above these folds is lax and thin and is called the pars flaccida; in it a small orifice is sometimes seen. The manubrium of the malleus is firmly attached to the medial surface of the membrane as far as its centre, which it draws toward the tympanic cavity; the lateral surface of the membrane is therefore concave and the most depressed part of this concavity is called the umbo.

The arteries of the tympanic membrane are derived from the deep auricular branch of the internal maxillary, which ramifies beneath the cutaneous stratum; and from the stylomastoid branch of the posterior auricular and tympanic branch of the internal maxillary, which are distributed on the mucous surface. The superficial veins open into the external jugular. Those on the deep surface drain partly into the transverse sinus and the veins of the dura mater and partly into a plexus on the auditory tube. The membrane receives its chief nerve supply from the auriculotemporal branch of the mandibular; the auricular branch of the vagus and the tympanic branch of the glossopharyngeal also supply it.

6.61

Answer: B Hyoglossus

The lingual artery lies beneath the hyoglossus in the floor of the mouth. The hyoglossus, thin and quadrilateral, arises from the side of the body and from the whole length of the greater cornu of the hyoid bone and passes almost vertically upward to enter the side of the tongue, between the styloglossus and longitudinalis inferior. The fibres arising from the body of the hyoid bone overlap those from the greater cornu. It is supplied by the hypoglossal nerve. The hyoglossi depress the tongue and draw down its sides.

6.62

Answer: A   Valves do not exist in the veins of the face, scalp or diploic bone and they communicate directly with the dural venous sinuses

Valves do not exist in the veins of the face, scalp or diploic bone and they communicate directly with the dural venous sinuses. As a result, infection can be transmitted from the face or the scalp to the dural venous sinuses, with grave consequences.

6.63

Answer: A   Right lateral pterygoid muscle

The right lateral pterygoid muscle acting alone will shift the mandible laterally, to the left. So inability to move the mandible to the left would indicate paralysis of the right lateral pterygoid muscle (see also *Answer* to **6.23**).

6.64

Answer: E   Pharynx, pharyngotympanic tube, middle ear

The pharyngotympanic tube (the auditory or Eustachian tube) is the channel through which the tympanic cavity communicates with the nasal part of the pharynx. Hence infection from pharynx can be transferred to the middle ear. It is about 36 mm long and is directed downward, forward, and medially, forming an angle of about 45° with the sagittal plane and from 30° to 40° with the horizontal plane. It is formed partly of bone and partly of cartilage and fibrous tissue. The bony portion is about 12 mm in length. It begins in the carotid wall of the tympanic cavity, inferior to the processus cochleariformis, and, gradually narrowing, ends at the angle of the junction of the squamous and petrous portions of the temporal bone. Its extremity has a jagged margin which provides attachment to the cartilaginous portion. The cartilaginous portion is about 24 mm in length. It is formed from a triangular plate of elastic fibrocartilage, the apex of which is attached to the margin of the medial end of the bony portion of the tube, while its base lies directly under the mucous membrane of the nasal part of the

head and neck

pharynx, where it forms an elevation, the torus tubarius or cushion, behind the pharyngeal orifice of the tube. The upper edge of the cartilage is curled on itself, being bent laterally so as to present on transverse section the appearance of a hook; a groove or furrow is thus produced which is open below and laterally, and this part of the canal is completed by a fibrous membrane. The cartilage lies in a groove between the petrous part of the temporal bone and the great wing of the sphenoid. This groove ends opposite the middle of the medial pterygoid plate. The cartilaginous and bony portions of the tube are not in the same plane. The cartilaginous portion inclines downward a little more than the bony portion. The diameter of the tube is not uniform throughout, being greatest at the pharyngeal orifice, least at the junction of the bony and cartilaginous portions, and increasing again toward the tympanic cavity. The narrowest part of the tube is called the isthmus. The mucous membrane of the tube is continuous anteriorly with that of the nasal part of the pharynx and posteriorly with that of the tympanic cavity. It is covered with ciliated epithelium and is thin in the bony portion, while in the cartilaginous portion it contains many mucous glands and, near the pharyngeal orifice, a considerable amount of adenoid tissue, which Gerlach called the tube tonsil. The tube is opened during deglutition by the salpingopharyngeus and dilator tubae muscles. The latter arises from the hook of the cartilage and from the membranous part of the tube and blends below with the tensor veli palatini.

6.65

Answer: D   Meningeal and periosteal layers of the dura mater

The sinuses of the dura mater are venous channels which drain the blood from the brain. They are devoid of valves and are situated between the two layers of the dura mater (meningeal and periosteal) and lined by endothelium continuous with that lining the veins. They may be divided into two groups: a posterosuperior, at the upper and back part of the skull; and an anteroinferior, at the base of the skull.

The posterosuperior group comprises the:

- Superior sagittal sinus
- Inferior sagittal sinus

- Straight sinus
- Two transverse sinuses
- Occipital sinus.

The anteroinferior group of sinuses comprises the:

- Two cavernous sinuses
- Two intercavernous sinuses
- Two superior petrosal sinuses
- Two inferior petrosal sinuses
- Basilar plexus.

6.66

Answer: B   Is in direct contact with the tympanic membrane

The tympanic cavity contains a chain of three mobile ossicles, the malleus, incus and stapes. The malleus is attached to the tympanic membrane and the stapes to the circumference of the fenestra vestibule; the incus is located between them and connected to both by delicate articulations.

The malleus, so named because of its fancied resemblance to a hammer, consists of a head, a neck and three processes (the manubrium and the anterior and lateral processes). The head is the large upper extremity of the bone. It is oval in shape, and articulates posteriorly with the incus, being free along the rest of its extent. The facet for articulation with the incus is constricted near the middle, and consists of a larger upper part and a smaller lower part, which form nearly a right angle with each other. Opposite the constriction, the lower margin of the facet projects in the form of a process, the cogtooth or spur of the malleus. The neck is the narrow contracted part just beneath the head. Below the neck is a prominence to which the various processes are attached. The manubrium is connected by its lateral margin to the tympanic membrane. It is directed downward, medially and backward. It decreases in size toward its free end, which is curved slightly forward, and is flattened transversely. On its medial side, near its upper end, is a slight projection, into which the tendon of the tensor tympani is inserted. The anterior process is a delicate spicule, which arises from the eminence below the neck and is directed forward to the petrotympanic fissure, to which it is connected by ligamentous fibres. In the fetus this is the longest process of the malleus and is in direct continuity with the cartilage of Meckel. The lateral process is a slight conical projection which arises from the root of the manubrium. It is directed laterally, and is attached to the upper part of the tympanic membrane and, by means of the anterior and posterior malleolar folds, to the extremities of the notch of Rivinus.

6.67

Answer: C   Contracts when it receives postganglionic parasympathetic fibres that originate in the ciliary ganglion

The circular muscle fibres of the iris form the sphincter pupillae. They are arranged in a narrow band about 1 mm in width which surrounds the margin of the pupil toward the posterior surface of the iris; those near the free margin are closely aggregated; those near the periphery of the band are somewhat separated and form incomplete circles. The postsynaptic parasympathetic fibres that innervate the sphincter pupillae arise in the ciliary ganglion. The sphincter pupillae contracts in response to parasympathetic stimulation.

6.68

Answer: B   Maxillary artery

The middle meningeal artery is the largest of the arteries that supply the dura mater. It is typically the first branch of the first part (retromandibular part) of the maxillary artery; one of the two terminal branches of the external carotid artery (see also *Answer* to **6.45**).

6.69

Answer: E   Cricothyroid muscle

The cricothyroid, triangular in form, arises from the front and lateral part of the cricoid cartilage; its fibres diverge and are arranged in two groups. The lower fibres constitute a pars obliqua and slant backward and lateralward to the anterior border of the inferior cornu. The anterior fibres, forming pars recta, run upward, backward and lateralward to the posterior part of the lower border of the lamina of the thyroid cartilage. The external laryngeal branch of the superior laryngeal nerve supplies the cricothyroid. The cricothyroids produce tension and elongation of the vocal folds by drawing up the arch of the cricoid cartilage and tilting back the upper border of its lamina. The distance between the vocal processes and the angle of the thyroid is so increased and the folds are consequently elongated.

6.70

Answer: B   Inferior meatus

The nasolacrimal duct is a membranous canal, about 18 mm in length, which extends from the lower part of the lacrimal sac to the inferior meatus of the nose, where it ends by a somewhat expanded orifice, provided with an imperfect valve, the plica lacrimalis (Hasner's fold), formed by a fold of the mucous membrane. It is contained in an osseous canal, formed by the maxilla, the lacrimal bone and the inferior nasal concha. It is narrower in the middle than at either end and is directed downward, backward and a little lateralward. The mucous lining of the lacrimal sac and nasolacrimal duct is covered with columnar epithelium, which in places is ciliated.

6.71

Answer: B   Cranial nerve X

The palatoglossus and levator veli palatini are both innervated via the pharyngeal plexus by the vagus nerve (cranial nerve X).

head and neck

6.72

Answer: D   Postganglionic sympathetic and preganglionic parasympathetic

The pterygoid canal (also called the Vidian canal) is a passage in the skull leading from just anterior to the foramen lacerum in the middle cranial fossa to the pterygopalatine fossa. It runs through the medial pterygoid plate of the sphenoid bone to the back wall of the pterygopalatine fossa. It transmits the nerve of the pterygoid canal. The nerve of the pterygoid canal (Vidian nerve), formed by the junction of the great petrosal nerve and the deep petrosal nerve in the cartilaginous substance which fills the foramen lacerum, passes forward through the pterygoid canal with the corresponding artery and is joined by a small ascending sphenoidal branch from the otic ganglion. Finally, it enters the pterygopalatine fossa and joins the posterior angle of the sphenopalatine ganglion. The greater petrosal nerve carries preganglionic parasympathetic fibres and the deep petrosal nerve carries postsynaptic sympathetic fibres.

6.73

Answer: D   Middle meningeal artery

An injured middle meningeal artery is the cause of an epidural haematoma. A head injury (due to a road traffic accident or sports injury for example) is required to rupture the artery. Emergency treatment requires decompression of the haematoma, usually by craniotomy (see also *Answer* to **6.45**).

6.74

Answer: A   Supplied by the ophthalmic nerve

The sensory innervation to the lacrimal gland is from the lacrimal nerve, the smallest of the three branches of the ophthalmic branch of the trigeminal nerve. The parasympathetic nerve supply originates from the lacrimal nucleus of the facial nerve in the pons and travels via the pterygopalatine ganglion and maxillary nerve to innervate the gland. The sympathetic postganglionic fibres originate from the superior cervical ganglion and travel through the same route as the parasympathetic fibres from the pterygopalatine ganglion.

6.75

Answer: A   C1, C2

The rectus capitis anterior is a short, flat muscle, situated immediately behind the upper part of the longus capitis. It arises from the anterior surface of the lateral mass of the atlas and from the root of its transverse process and, passing obliquely upward and medialward, is inserted into the inferior surface of the basilar part of the occipital bone immediately in front of the foramen magnum. It is supplied from the loop between the first and second cervical nerves. Rectus capitis anterior and longus coli are the direct antagonists of the muscles at the back of the neck, serving to restore the head to its natural position after it has been drawn backward. These muscles also flex the head and, because of their obliquity, rotate it, so as to turn the face to one or other side.

6.76

Answer: A   Cricothyroid

The recurrent laryngeal nerve supplies all the muscles of the larynx except the cricothyroid. The ipsilateral cricothyroid will therefore be spared if the recurrent laryngeal nerve is severed on the same side.

6.77

Answer: A   Pterygopalatine fossa

The descending palatine artery, a branch of the third part of the internal maxillary artery, arises within the pterygopalatine fossa, descends through the pterygopalatine canal with the anterior palatine branch of the sphenopalatine ganglion and, emerging from the greater palatine foramen, runs forward in a groove on the medial side of the alveolar border of the hard palate to the incisive canal; the terminal branch of the artery passes upward through

head and neck

this canal to anastomose with the sphenopalatine artery. Branches are distributed to the gums, the palatine glands and the mucous membrane of the roof of the mouth. While in the pterygopalatine canal it gives off twigs which descend in the lesser palatine canals to supply the soft palate and palatine tonsil, anastomosing with the ascending palatine artery.

6.78

Answer: C   It is innervated by the glossopharyngeal nerve

Behind the angle of bifurcation of the common carotid artery is a reddish-brown oval body, known as the glomus caroticum (carotid body). It is similar in structure to the glomus coccygeum (coccygeal body) which is situated on the middle sacral artery. It measures changes in the composition of arterial blood flowing past it, including the partial pressures of oxygen and carbon dioxide, and is also sensitive to changes in pH and temperature. The chemoreceptors responsible for sensing changes in blood gasses are called glomus cells. While the central chemoreceptors in the brainstem are highly sensitive to CO_2, the carotid body is a peripheral chemoreceptor that provides afferent input to the respiratory centre that is highly O_2 dependent. Below an oxygen partial pressure of 60 mmHg, the carotid body cells release dopamine and trigger excitatory postsynaptic potentials in synapsed neurones leading to the respiratory centre. This event is mediated by a unique potassium channel that is responsive to the partial pressure of O_2. The peripheral chemoreceptor's input is secondary to CO_2-sensitive cells in the central chemoreceptors in healthy patients, but is the primary driver of ventilation in individuals who suffer from chronic hypercapnia (as in emphysema). It gives feedback to the medulla oblongata via the afferent branches of the glossopharyngeal nerve (cranial nerve IX). The medulla, in turn, regulates breathing and blood pressure.

6.79

Answer: D   Digastric

The digastric muscle consists of two fleshy bellies united by an intermediate rounded tendon. It lies below the body of the mandible and extends, in a curved form, from the mastoid process to the symphysis menti. The posterior belly, longer than the anterior, arises from the mastoid notch of the temporal bone and passes downward and forward. The anterior belly arises from a depression on the inner side of the lower border of the mandible, close to the symphysis and passes downward and backward. The two bellies end in an intermediate tendon, which perforates the stylohyoid muscle and is held in connection with the side of the body and the greater cornu of the hyoid bone by a fibrous loop, which is sometimes lined by a mucous sheath. A broad aponeurotic layer is given off from the tendon of the digastric on either side, to be attached to the body and greater cornu of the hyoid bone; this is known as the suprahyoid aponeurosis. The anterior belly of digastric is innervated by the mandibular division of the trigeminal nerve via the mylohyoid nerve; the posterior belly is innervated by the facial nerve. When the digastric muscle contracts, it acts to elevate the hyoid bone. If the hyoid is being held in place (by the infrahyoid muscles), it will tend to depress the mandible (open the mouth).

The digastric divides the anterior triangle of the neck into three smaller triangles:

- The submaxillary triangle, bounded above by the lower border of the body of the mandible and a line drawn from its angle to the sternocleidomastoid, below by the posterior belly of the digastric and the stylohyoid, in front by the anterior belly of the digastric

- The carotid triangle, bounded above by the posterior belly of the digastric and stylohyoid, behind by the sternocleidomastoid, below by the omohyoid

- The suprahyoid or submental triangle, bounded laterally by the anterior belly of the digastric, medially by the midline of the neck from the hyoid bone to the symphysis menti and inferiorly by the body of the hyoid bone.

head and neck

6.80

Answer: D   Inferior alveolar nerve

The inferior alveolar nerve is the largest branch of the mandibular nerve. It descends with the inferior alveolar artery, at first under the lateral pterygoid, and then between the sphenomandibular ligament and the ramus of the mandible to the mandibular foramen. It then passes forward in the mandibular canal, under the teeth, as far as the mental foramen, where it divides into two terminal branches, incisive and mental.

The branches of the inferior alveolar nerve are the mylohyoid, dental, incisive and mental. The mylohyoid nerve is derived from the inferior alveolar nerve just before it enters the mandibular foramen. It descends in a groove on the deep surface of the ramus of the mandible and, reaching the undersurface of the mylohyoid, supplies this muscle and the anterior belly of the digastric. The dental branches supply the molar and premolar teeth. They correspond in number to the roots of those teeth. Each nerve enters the orifice at the point of the root and supplies the pulp of the tooth. The incisive branch continues onward within the bone and supplies the canine and incisor teeth. The mental nerve emerges at the mental foramen, and divides beneath the depressor anguli oris into three branches. One of these branches descends to the skin of the chin and two ascend to the skin and mucous membrane of the lower lip. These branches communicate freely with the facial nerve.

6.81

Answer: A   Adduction

In considering the actions of the muscles of the larynx, they may be conveniently divided into two groups:

- Those that open and close the glottis
- Those that regulate the degree of tension of the vocal folds.

The posterior cricoarytenoids separate the vocal folds and, consequently open the glottis by rotating the arytenoid cartilages outward around a vertical axis passing through the cricoarytenoid joints, so that their vocal processes and the vocal folds attached to them become widely separated (abduction). The lateral cricoarytenoids close the glottis by rotating the arytenoid cartilages inward, so as to approximate their vocal processes (adduction). The arytenoid muscle approximates the arytenoid cartilages and so closes the opening of the glottis, especially at its back part (adduction). The cricothyroid muscles produce tension and elongation of the vocal folds by drawing up the arch of the cricoid cartilage and tilting back the upper border of its lamina. The distance between the vocal processes and the angle of the thyroid is so increased and the folds are consequently elongated.

The thyroarytenoid muscle, consisting of two parts with different attachments and different directions, are rather complicated as regards their action. Their main use is to draw the arytenoid cartilages forward toward the thyroid and so shorten and relax the vocal folds. However, owing to the connection of the deeper portion with the vocal fold, this part, if acting separately, is supposed to modify its elasticity and tension, while the lateral portion rotates the arytenoid cartilage inward and so narrows the rima glottidis by bringing the two vocal folds together.

6.82

Answer: C Contracts when it receives parasympathetic innervation from cranial nerve III

The ciliary muscle is a greyish, semi-transparent smooth muscle. It forms a circular band, about 3 mm broad, on the outer surface of the forepart of the choroid. It is thickest in front and consists of two sets of fibres, meridional and circular. The meridional fibres, much the more numerous, arise from the posterior margin of the scleral spur. They run backward and are attached to the ciliary processes and orbiculus ciliaris; one bundle is inserted into the sclera. The circular fibres are internal to the meridional ones and in a meridional section appear as a triangular zone behind the filtration angle and close to the circumference of the iris. They are well developed in hypermetropic eyes, but are rudimentary or absent in myopic eyes. The ciliary muscle is the chief agent in accommodation (adjusting the eye to the vision of near objects). When it contracts in response to parasympathetic stimulation supplied by postsynaptic fibres

head and neck

from ciliary ganglion (presynaptic fibres arising from oculomotor nerve), it draws the ciliary processes forward, and relaxes the suspensory ligament of the lens, thus allowing the lens to become more convex.

6.83

Answer: C   Is separated from the posterior chamber by the iris

The anterior segment is the front third of the eye that includes the structures in front of the vitreous humour: the cornea, iris, ciliary body and lens. Within the anterior segment are two fluid-filled spaces divided by the iris plane:

- The anterior chamber, between the posterior surface of the cornea (ie the corneal endothelium) and the iris

- The posterior chamber, between the iris and the front face of the vitreous.

Aqueous humour fills these spaces within the anterior segment to provide nutrients to the lens and corneal endothelium and its pressure maintains the convex shape of the cornea.

6.84

Answer: C   Superficial temporal artery

The superficial temporal artery, the smaller of the two terminal branches of the external carotid, appears, from its direction, to be the continuation of that vessel. It begins in the substance of the parotid gland, behind the neck of the mandible, and crosses over the posterior root of the zygomatic process of the temporal bone; about 5 cm above this process it divides into two branches, a frontal and a parietal. As it crosses the zygomatic process, it is covered by the auricularis anterior muscle and by a dense fascia. It is crossed by the temporal and zygomatic branches of the facial nerve and one or two veins and is accompanied by the auriculotemporal nerve, which lies immediately behind it. Besides some twigs to the parotid gland, to the temporomandibular joint and to the masseter muscle, its branches are:

- Transverse facial artery

- Middle temporal artery

- Anterior auricular artery

- Frontal artery

- Parietal artery.

6.85

Answer: B   Superior thyroid artery

The external laryngeal nerve is the smaller, external branch (ramus externus) of the superior laryngeal nerve. It descends on the larynx, beneath the sternothyroid muscle, to supply the cricothyroid muscle. It gives branches to the pharyngeal plexus and the superior portion of the inferior pharyngeal constrictor and communicates with the superior cardiac nerve behind the common carotid artery. The external branch is susceptible to damage during thyroidectomy, as it lies immediately deep to the superior thyroid artery.

6.86

Answer: B   Buccinator muscle

The parotid duct (Stensen's duct) is about 7 cm long. It begins by numerous branches from the anterior part of the gland, crosses the masseter and at the anterior border of this muscle turns inward nearly at a right angle, passes through the corpus adiposum of the cheek and pierces the buccinator. It then runs for a short distance obliquely forward between the buccinator and the mucous membrane of the mouth and opens on the oral surface of the cheek by a small orifice, opposite the second upper molar tooth. While crossing the masseter, it receives the duct of the accessory portion; in this position it lies between the branches of the facial nerve; the accessory part of the gland and the transverse facial artery are above it.

6.87

Answer: A   Recurrent laryngeal nerve

The nerves of the larynx are derived from the internal and external branches of the superior laryngeal nerve, from the recurrent nerve and from the sympathetic. The internal laryngeal branch is almost entirely sensory, but some motor filaments are said to be carried by it to the arytenoid. It enters the larynx by piercing the posterior part of the hyothyroid membrane above the superior laryngeal vessels and divides into a branch that is distributed to both surfaces of the epiglottis, a second to the aryepiglottic fold and a third, the largest, which supplies the mucous membrane over the back of the larynx and communicates with the recurrent nerve. The external laryngeal branch supplies the cricothyroid. The recurrent nerve passes upward beneath the lower border of the inferior pharyngeal constrictor immediately behind the cricothyroid joint. It supplies all the muscles of the larynx except the cricothyroid and perhaps a part of the arytenoid muscle and sensory innervation to the laryngeal mucosa inferior to the true vocal folds. The sensory branches of the laryngeal nerves form subepithelial plexuses, from which fibres pass to end between the cells covering the mucous membrane.

6.88

Answer: C   On either side of the larynx, within the laryngopharynx

On either side of the laryngeal orifice, within the laryngopharynx, is a recess called the piriform recess (sinus piriformis), which is bounded medially by the aryepiglottic fold, laterally by the thyroid cartilage and hyothyroid membrane.

6.89

Answer: D   Styloid process of the temporal bone

The styloid process is slender, pointed and of varying length; it projects downward and forward from the undersurface of the temporal bone. Its proximal part (tympanohyal) is ensheathed by the vaginal process of the tympanic portion, while its distal part (stylohyal)

gives attachment to the stylohyoid and stylomandibular ligaments and to the styloglossus, stylohyoid and stylopharyngeus muscles. The stylohyoid ligament extends from the apex of the process to the lesser cornu of the hyoid bone and in some instances is partially, and in others completely, ossified. As the styloid process is covered by the various muscles, it is not easily palpable in live subjects.

6.90

Answer: E   Epitympanic recess

The tympanic cavity consists of two parts: the tympanic cavity proper, opposite the tympanic membrane and the attic or epitympanic recess, above the level of the membrane. The latter contains the upper half of the malleus and the greater part of the incus. Including the attic, the vertical and anteroposterior diameters of the cavity are both about 15 mm. The transverse diameter measures about 6 mm above and 4 mm below; opposite the centre of the tympanic membrane it is only about 2 mm. The tympanic cavity is bounded laterally by the tympanic membrane; medially, by the lateral wall of the internal ear. It communicates behind with the tympanic antrum and through it with the mastoid air cells and in front with the auditory tube. The tympanic antrum and mastoid air cells are lined by a prolongation of the mucous membrane of the tympanic cavity and infection from the tympanic antrum and mastoid air cells can therefore be transmitted to the middle ear through the attic or epitympanic recess.

6.91

Answer: B   Inferior rectus muscle

The inferior rectus muscle is an extraocular muscle that depresses, adducts, and rotates the eye laterally. As with most of the muscles of the orbit (exceptions are the lateral rectus and superior oblique), it is innervated by the oculomotor nerve (cranial nerve III).

head and neck

6.92

Answer: C   Central artery of the retina

The central artery of the retina is the first and one of the smallest branches of the ophthalmic artery. It runs for a short distance within the dural sheath of the optic nerve, but about 1.25 cm behind the eyeball it pierces the nerve obliquely and runs forward in the centre of its substance to the retina. The artery immediately bifurcates into an upper and a lower branch and each of these again divides into a medial or nasal and a lateral or temporal branch, which at first run between the hyaloid membrane and the nervous layer, but soon enter the latter and pass forward, dividing dichotomously. From these branches a minute capillary plexus is given off which does not extend beyond the inner nuclear layer. The macula receives two small branches (superior and inferior macular arteries) from the temporal branches and small twigs directly from the central artery. These do not, however, reach as far as the fovea centralis, which has no blood vessels. The branches of the central artery of retina do not anastomose with each other – in other words, they are terminal arteries.

6.93

Answer: A   Hypoglossal nerve (cranial nerve XII)

The occipital artery arises from the posterior part of the external carotid, opposite the external maxillary, near the lower margin of the posterior belly of the digastric, and ends in the posterior part of the scalp. At its origin it is covered by the posterior belly of the digastric and the stylohyoid, and the hypoglossal nerve winds around it from behind forward; higher up, it crosses the internal carotid artery, the internal jugular vein and the vagus and accessory nerves. It next ascends to the interval between the transverse process of the atlas and the mastoid process of the temporal bone and passes horizontally backward, grooving the surface of the latter bone, being covered by the sternocleidomastoid, splenius capitis, longissimus capitis and digastric and resting on the rectus capitis lateralis, the superior oblique and semispinalis capitis. It then changes its course and runs vertically upward, pierces the fascia connecting the cranial attachment of the trapezius with the sternocleidomastoid and ascends in a tortuous course in the superficial fascia of the scalp, where it divides into

head and neck

numerous branches, which reach as high as the vertex of the skull and anastomose with the posterior auricular and superficial temporal arteries. Its terminal portion is accompanied by the greater occipital nerve. The branches of the occipital artery are:

- Muscular
- Sternocleidomastoid
- Auricular
- Meningeal
- Descending.

6.94

Answer: D   Maxillary vein

The pterygoid venous plexus is of considerable size and is situated between the temporalis and lateral pterygoid and partly between the lateral and medial pterygoids. It receives tributaries corresponding to the branches of the internal maxillary artery, so it receives the sphenopalatine, the middle meningeal, the deep temporal, the pterygoid, masseteric, buccinator, alveolar and some palatine veins and a branch which communicates with the ophthalmic vein through the inferior orbital fissure. This plexus communicates freely with the anterior facial vein; it also communicates with the cavernous sinus, by branches through the foramen of Vesalius, foramen ovale and foramen lacerum. The (internal) maxillary vein is a short trunk which accompanies the first part of the (internal) maxillary artery. It is formed by a confluence of the veins of the pterygoid plexus and passes backward between the sphenomandibular ligament and the neck of the mandible and unites with the temporal vein to form the posterior facial vein. It carries blood away from the infratemporal fossa.

head and neck

6.95

Answer: C   Middle meatus

The maxillary sinus is a large pyramidal cavity within the body of the maxilla: its apex, directed lateralward, is formed by the zygomatic process; its base, directed medialward, by the lateral wall of the nose. Its walls are everywhere exceedingly thin and correspond to the nasal orbital, anterior and infratemporal surfaces of the body of the bone. Its nasal wall, or base, presents, in the disarticulated bone, a large, irregular aperture, communicating with the nasal cavity. In the articulated skull this aperture is much reduced in size by the following bones: the uncinate process of the ethmoid above, the ethmoidal process of the inferior nasal concha below, the vertical part of the palatine behind and a small part of the lacrimal above and in front. The sinus communicates with the middle meatus of the nose, generally by two small apertures left between the above-mentioned bones. In the fresh state, usually only one small opening exists, near the upper part of the cavity; the other is closed by mucous membrane. On the posterior wall are the alveolar canals, transmitting the posterior superior alveolar vessels and nerves to the molar teeth. The floor is formed by the alveolar process of the maxilla and, if the sinus is of an average size, is on a level with the floor of the nose; if the sinus is large it reaches below this level. Projecting into the floor of the antrum are several conical processes, corresponding to the roots of the first and second molar teeth; in some cases the floor is perforated by the fangs of the teeth. The infraorbital canal usually projects into the cavity as a well-marked ridge extending from the roof to the anterior wall; additional ridges are sometimes seen in the posterior wall of the cavity and are caused by the alveolar canals. The size of the cavity varies in different skulls and even on the two sides of the same skull.

6.96

Answer: C   Lateral pterygoid plate of the sphenoid bone

The infratemporal fossa is an irregularly shaped cavity, situated below and medial to the zygomatic arch. It is bounded, in front, by the infratemporal surface of the maxilla and the ridge which descends from its zygomatic process; behind, by the articular tubercle of the temporal and the spinal angularis of the sphenoid; above, by the great wing of the sphenoid below the infratemporal crest and by the undersurface of the temporal squama; below, by the alveolar border of the maxilla; and medially by the lateral pterygoid plate of sphenoid bone. It contains the lower part of the temporalis, the medial and lateral pterygoid muscles, the internal maxillary vessels and the mandibular and maxillary nerves. The foramen ovale and foramen spinosum open on its roof and the alveolar canals on its anterior wall. At its upper and medial part are two fissures, which together form a T-shaped fissure, the horizontal limb being called the inferior orbital fissure and the vertical one the pterygomaxillary fissure.

6.97

Answer: D   Beside the lingual frenulum through the sublingual caruncle

The submandibular duct (Wharton's duct) opens by a narrow orifice on the summit of a small papilla, at the side of the frenulum linguae (see also *Answer* to **6.55**).

6.98

Answer: C   Facial nerve

The stapedius is the smallest striated muscle in the human body. At just over one millimeter in length, its purpose is to stabilise the smallest bone in the body, the stapes. It prevents excess movement by the stapes, helping to control the conduction of sound waves from the external environment to the inner ear. Paralysis of the stapedius allows wider oscillation of the stapes, resulting in heightened reaction of the auditory ossicles to sound vibration. Loud noises become deafening. The stapedius is innervated by a branch of cranial nerve VII, the facial nerve.

head and neck

6.99

Answer: A   Facial expression

The facial nerve is the seventh of twelve paired cranial nerves. It emerges from the brainstem between the pons and the medulla. It controls the muscles of facial expression and supplies taste fibres to the anterior two-thirds of the tongue. It also supplies preganglionic parasympathetic fibres to several head and neck ganglia. Its branches and distribution is as follows:

Inside the facial canal (proximal to the stylomastoid foramen):

- Greater petrosal nerve – provides parasympathetic innervation to the lacrimal gland, as well as special taste sensory fibres to the palate via the nerve of pterygoid canal

- Nerve to stapedius – provides motor innervation for the stapedius muscle in the middle ear

- Chord tympani – provides parasympathetic innervation to the submandibular and sublingual glands and special sensory taste fibres for the anterior two-thirds of the tongue

Outside the skull (distal to the stylomastoid foramen):

- Posterior auricular nerve – controls the movements of some of the scalp muscles around the ear

- Five major facial branches (in the parotid gland), from top to bottom:

    - temporal branch
    - zygomatic branch
    - buccal branch
    - marginal mandibular branch
    - cervical branch.

Helpful mnemonics for remembering these major branches are the phrases, 'To Zanzibar by motor car', 'Two zebras bit my cat', or 'Tell Ziggy Bob Marley called'. From the description given above it is obvious that injury to the facial nerve distal to the stylomastoid foramen will affect facial expression.

head and neck

6.100

Answer: A   Middle pharyngeal constrictor

The hyoid bone is shaped like a horseshoe and is attached to the tips of the styloid processes of the temporal bones by the stylohyoid ligaments. It consists of five segments - a body, two greater cornua, and two lesser cornua. The body or central part is quadrilateral in shape. Its anterior surface is convex and is directed forward and upward. It is crossed in its upper half by a well-marked transverse ridge with a slight downward convexity, and in many cases a vertical median ridge divides it into two lateral halves. The anterior surface gives insertion to the geniohyoid in the greater part of its extent, both above and below the transverse ridge; a portion of the origin of the hyoglossus notches the lateral margin of the geniohyoid attachment. The mylohyoid, sternohyoid and omohyoid are inserted below the transverse ridge. The posterior surface is smooth, concave, directed backward and downward, and is separated from the epiglottis by the hyothyroid membrane and some loose areolar tissue; a bursa intervenes between it and the hyothyroid membrane. The superior border is rounded and gives attachment to the hyothyroid membrane and some aponeurotic fibres of the genioglossus. The inferior border provides insertion medially to the sternohyoid and laterally to the omohyoid and occasionally to a portion of the thyrohyoid. It also gives attachment to the levator glandulae thyroideae when this muscle is present. In early life the lateral borders are connected to the greater cornua by synchondroses. The synchondroses are usually replaced by bony union after middle life.

The greater cornua project backward from the lateral borders of the body. They are flattened from above downward and diminish in size from the front backward. Each cornu ends in a tubercle which provides attachment to the lateral hyothyroid ligament. The upper surface is rough close to its lateral border, for muscular attachments. The largest of these attachments are the origins of the hyoglossus and middle pharyngeal constrictor, which extend along the whole length of the cornu. The digastric and stylohyoid have small insertions in front of the origins of the hyoglossus and middle pharyngeal constrictor, near the junction of the body with the cornu. The hyothyroid membrane is attached to the medial border, while the anterior half of the lateral border gives insertion to the thyrohyoid.

head and neck

The lesser cornua are two small, conical eminences, attached by their bases to the angles of junction between the body and greater cornua. They are connected to the body of the bone by fibrous tissue, and occasionally to the greater cornua by distinct diarthrodial joints, which usually persist throughout life, but occasionally become ankylosed. The lesser cornua are situated in the line of the transverse ridge on the body and appear to be morphological continuations of it. The apex of each cornu gives attachment to the stylohyoid ligament while the chondroglossus arises from the medial side of the base.

6.101

Answer: B   The ophthalmic nerve as a single structure does not reach the interior of the globe

The ophthalmic nerve, or first division of the trigeminal, is a sensory nerve. It supplies branches to the cornea, ciliary body and iris; to the lacrimal gland and conjunctiva; to part of the mucous membrane of the nasal cavity; and to the skin of the eyelids, eyebrow, forehead and nose. It is the smallest of the three divisions of the trigeminal and arises from the upper part of the semilunar ganglion as a short, flattened band, about 2.5 cm long, which passes forward along the lateral wall of the cavernous sinus, below the oculomotor and trochlear nerves. Just before entering the orbit, through the superior orbital fissure, it divides into three branches, lacrimal, frontal and nasociliary. The ophthalmic nerve is joined by filaments from the cavernous plexus of the sympathetic and communicates with the oculomotor, trochlear and abducent nerves; it gives off a recurrent filament which passes between the layers of the tentorium.

6.102

Answer: B   Inferior belly of the omohyoid

The posterior triangle is bounded in front by the sternocleido-mastoid; behind, by the anterior margin of the trapezius; its base is formed by the middle third of the clavicle; its apex, by the occipital bone. The space is crossed, about 2.5 cm above the clavicle, by the inferior belly of the omohyoid, which divides it into two triangles, an upper or occipital and a lower or subclavian. It contains the accessory nerve, which crosses the triangle from the upper third of sternocleidomastoid to the lower two-thirds of trapezius. It is particularly vulnerable to damage during lymph node biopsy, when damage results in an inability to shrug the shoulders or raise the arm above the head (brushing hair).

6.103

Answer: B   C4

The common carotid arteries differ in length and in their mode of origin. The right begins at the bifurcation of the innominate artery behind the sternoclavicular joint and is confined to the neck. The left springs from the highest part of the arch of the aorta to the left of and on a plane posterior to the innominate artery and therefore consists of a thoracic and a cervical portion. The thoracic portion of the left common carotid artery ascends from the arch of the aorta through the superior mediastinum to the level of the left sternoclavicular joint, where it is continuous with the cervical portion. The cervical portions of the common carotids resemble each other closely. Each vessel passes obliquely upward, from behind the sternoclavicular articulation, to the level of the upper border of the thyroid cartilage (C4 cervical vertebra), where it divides into the external and internal carotid arteries.

6.104

Answer: C   Investing fascia

The deep cervical fascia (fascia colli) lies under cover of the platysma and invests the neck. It also forms sheaths for the carotid vessels and for the structures situated in front of the vertebral column. The investing portion of the fascia is attached behind to the ligamentum nuchae and to the spinous process of the seventh cervical vertebra. It forms a thin covering for trapezius and at the anterior border of this muscle is continued forward as a rather loose areolar layer, covering the posterior triangle of the neck. At the level of the posterior border of the sternocleidomastoid it begins to assume the appearance of a fascial membrane. Along the posterior edge of the sternocleidomastoid it divides to enclose the muscle and at the

head and neck

anterior margin again forms a single layer, which covers the anterior triangle of the neck and reaches forward to the midline. Here it is continuous with the corresponding part from the opposite side of the neck. In the midline of the neck it is attached to the symphysis menti and the body of the hyoid bone. Superiorly the fascia is attached to the superior nuchal line of the occipital, to the mastoid process of the temporal, and to the whole length of the inferior border of the body of the mandible. Opposite the angle of the mandible the fascia is very strong and binds the anterior edge of the sternocleidomastoid firmly to that bone. Between the mandible and the mastoid process it encloses the parotid gland – the layer that covers the gland extends upward under as the parotideomasseteric fascia and is fixed to the zygomatic arch. From the part which passes under the parotid gland a strong band extends upward to the styloid process, forming the stylomandibular ligament.

Two other bands, the sphenomandibular and the pterygospinous ligaments, are also identifiable. The sphenomandibular ligament is a flat, thin band which is attached above to the angular spine of the sphenoid bone and, becoming broader as it descends, is fixed to the lingula of the mandibular foramen. Its lateral surface is related superiorly to the lateral pterygoid and inferiorly it is separated from the neck of the condyle by the internal maxillary vessels. Further inferiorly, the inferior alveolar vessels and nerve and a lobule of the parotid gland lie between it and the ramus of the mandible. Its medial surface is related to the medial pterygoid. The pterygospinous ligament stretches from the upper part of the posterior border of the lateral pterygoid plate to the spinous process of the sphenoid. It occasionally ossifies and a foramen is then formed between its upper border and the base of the skull, which transmits the branches of the mandibular nerve to the muscles of mastication.

6.105

Answer: C   Sternocleidomastoid

The superior carotid, or carotid triangle, is bounded posteriorly by the sternocleidomastoid, inferiorly by the superior belly of the omohyoid, and superiorly by the stylohyoid and the posterior belly of the digastric. It is covered by the skin, superficial fascia, and platysma and deep fascia containing the branches of the facial and cutaneous cervical nerves. Its floor is formed by parts of the thyrohyoid, hyoglossus, and the middle and inferior pharyngeal constrictors. This space when dissected is seen to contain the upper part of the common carotid artery, which bifurcates opposite the upper border of the thyroid cartilage into the external and internal carotid arteries. These vessels are overlapped by the anterior margin of the sternocleidomastoid. The external and internal carotids lie side by side, the external being the more anterior of the two. The following branches of the external carotid are also contained in this space:

- The superior thyroid artery, running forward and downward

- The lingual artery, directly forward

- The external maxillary artery, running forward and upward

- The occipital artery, running backward

- The ascending pharyngeal artery, running directly upward on the medial side of the internal carotid.

The veins in this triangle include:

- The internal jugular vein, which lies on the lateral side of the common and internal carotid arteries

- Veins corresponding to the above-mentioned branches of the external carotid, namely the superior thyroid, lingual, common facial, ascending pharyngeal, and (sometimes) occipital, all of which end in the internal jugular vein.

The nerves in this space are as follows. In front of the sheath of the common carotid is the ramus descendens hypoglossi. The hypoglossal nerve crosses both the internal and external carotids above, curving around the origin of the occipital artery. Within the sheath, between the artery and vein, and behind both, is the vagus nerve. The sympathetic trunk lies behind the sheath. On the lateral side of the vessels the accessory nerve runs for a short distance before it pierces the sternocleidomastoid. On the medial side of the external carotid, just below the hyoid bone, lies the internal branch of the superior laryngeal nerve. Further inferiorly lies the external

head and neck

branch of the superior laryngeal nerve. The upper portion of the larynx and the lower portion of the pharynx are also found in the anterior part of this space.

6.106

Answer: A Ciliary muscle

The sympathetic efferent fibres of the oculomotor nerve probably arise from cells in the anterior part of the oculomotor nucleus, which is located in the tegmentum of the midbrain. These preganglionic fibres run with the third nerve into the orbit and pass to the ciliary ganglion where they terminate by forming synapses with sympathetic motor neurones whose axons, postganglionic fibres, proceed as the short ciliary nerves to the eyeball. Here they supply motor fibres to the ciliary muscle and the sphincter pupillae muscle. Therefore, injury to these fibres will affect the function of these involuntary muscles associated with accommodation reflex.

6.107

Answer: B Connective tissue

The scalp is the anatomical area bounded by the face anteriorly and the neck to the sides and posteriorly. It is usually described as having five layers, which can be remembered with the help of the mnemonic, 'scalp':

- **S** The **s**kin on the head from which head hair grows. It is richly supplied with blood vessels and can be subject to such conditions as dandruff and cutis verticis gyrata.

- **C** **C**onnective tissue, a thin layer of fat and fibrous tissue, lies beneath the skin. It is continuous behind with the superficial fascia at the back of the neck and laterally is continued over the temporal fascia. It contains the superficial vessels and nerves and a great deal of granular fat between its layers.

- **A** The **a**poneurosis (or galea aponeurotica) is the next layer. It is a tough layer of dense fibrous tissue which runs from the frontalis muscle anteriorly to the occipitalis posteriorly.

- **L** The **l**oose areolar connective-tissue layer provides an easy plane of separation between the upper three layers and the pericranium. In the barbaric practice of scalping, the scalp is torn off through this layer. It also provides a plane of access in craniofacial surgery and neurosurgery. This layer is sometimes referred to as the 'danger zone' because of the ease with which infectious agents can spread through it to emissary veins, which then drain into the cranium. The loose areolar tissue in this layer is made up of random collagen type I bundles and collagen type III, and is highly vascular and cellular. It is also rich in glycosaminoglycans and is formed of more matrix than fibres.

- **P** The **p**ericranium is the periosteum of the skull bones and provides nutrition to the bone and the capacity for repair. It can be lifted from the bone to allow removal of bone windows (craniotomy).

6.108

Answer: D   From the brachiocephalic trunk

The thyroidea ima artery, when present, arises from the brachiocephalic trunk (innominate artery) and ascends in front of the trachea to the lower part of the thyroid gland, which it supplies. It varies greatly in size and appears to compensate for deficiency or absence of one of the other thyroid vessels. It occasionally arises from the aorta, the right common carotid, the subclavian or the internal mammary.

6.109

Answer: C   Foramen magnum

The foramen magnum is a large oval aperture in the occipital bone, with its long diameter anteroposterior. It is wider behind than in

head and neck

front, where it is encroached upon by the condyles. It transmits the medulla oblongata and its membranes, the accessory nerves, the vertebral arteries, the anterior and posterior spinal arteries and the membrana tectoria and alar ligaments.

6.110

Answer: D   Internal acoustic meatus

The internal acoustic meatus is a large orifice near the centre of the posterior surface of the petrous part of the temporal bone, the size of which varies considerably. Its margins are smooth and rounded and it leads into a short canal, about 1 cm in length, which runs lateralward. It transmits the facial and acoustic (vestibulocochlear) nerves and the internal auditory branch of the basilar artery.

6.111

Answer: A   Jugular foramen

The jugular foramen is situated between the lateral part of the occipital and the petrous part of the temporal. The anterior portion of this foramen transmits the inferior petrosal sinus. The posterior portion transmits the transverse sinus and some meningeal branches from the occipital and ascending pharyngeal arteries. The intermediate portion transmits the glossopharyngeal, vagus and accessory nerves.

6.112

Answer: D   Internal acoustic meatus

The internal acoustic meatus transmits the vestibulocochlear nerve (see also *Answer* to **6.110**).

head and neck

6.113

Answer: C   Foramen magnum

The foramen magnum transmits the dura mater (see also *Answer* to **6.109**).

6.114

Answer: E   Foramen ovale

In the middle cranial fossa, behind and lateral to the foramen rotundum, is the foramen ovale, which transmits the mandibular nerve, the accessory meningeal artery and the lesser superficial petrosal nerve.

6.115

Answer: B   Foramen ovale

The mandibular nerve exits the cranial cavity by way of the foramen ovale (see also *Answer* to **6.114**).

6.116

Answer: A   Oculomotor nerve

The signs in this patient are suggestive of damage to the oculomotor nerve as it supplies the levator palpebrae superioris and the sphincter pupillae. The levator palpebrae superioris (or levator muscle of the upper eyelid) is the muscle in the orbit that elevates the superior (upper) eyelid.

6.117

Answer: E   Glossopharyngeal nerve

The otic ganglion is a small, oval-shaped, flattened ganglion of a reddish-grey colour, situated immediately below the foramen ovale. It lies on the medial surface of the mandibular nerve, and surrounds the origin of the nerve to the medial pterygoid. It is related

head and neck

laterally to the trunk of the mandibular nerve at the point where the motor and sensory roots join; medially to the cartilaginous part of the auditory tube and the origin of the tensor veli palatini; and posteriorly to the middle meningeal artery. It is connected by two or three short filaments to the nerve to the medial pterygoid, from which it may obtain a motor, and possibly a sensory root. It communicates with the glossopharyngeal and facial nerves through the lesser superficial petrosal nerve continued from the tympanic plexus. It probably receives a root from the glossopharyngeal nerve and a motor root from the facial nerve through the lesser superficial petrosal nerve. Its sympathetic root consists of a filament from the plexus surrounding the middle meningeal artery. The fibres from the glossopharyngeal nerve which pass to the otic ganglion in the small superficial petrosal nerve are considered to be sympathetic efferent (preganglionic) fibres from the dorsal nucleus or the inferior salivatory nucleus of the medulla. Fibres (postganglionic) from the otic ganglion with which these form synapses are thought to pass with the auriculotemporal nerve to the parotid gland. A slender filament (sphenoidal) ascends from it to the nerve of the pterygoid canal, and a small branch connects it to the chorda tympani. Its branches of distribution are a filament to the tensor tympani and a branch to the tensor veli palatini. The branch to the tensor tympani passes backward, lateral to the auditory tube; the branch to the tensor veli palatini arises from the ganglion, near the origin of the nerve to the medial pterygoid, and is directed forward. The fibres of these nerves are, however, mainly derived from the nerve to the medial pterygoid.

6.118

Answer: A   Sphenoid

The sphenoid bone is situated at the base of the skull in front of the temporal and basilar part of the occipital. It somewhat resembles a bat with its wings extended and is divided into a median portion or body, two great and two small wings extending outward from the sides of the body and two pterygoid processes which project from it below. The foramen ovale is present in the great wing of the sphenoid.

head and neck

6.119

Answer: C   Edinger–Westphal nucleus

The neuronal pathway of accommodation involves the retina, the optic nerve, the chiasma and tract, the lateral geniculate body, the optic radiation, the visual area of the cortex, the superior longitudinal association tract, the frontal eye field, the third nerve nucleus (Edinger–Westphal nucleus), the third cranial nerve (the nerve to the inferior oblique containing preganglionic parasympathetic fibres that begin in the Edinger–Westphal nucleus), the ciliary ganglion, the short ciliary nerves and the ciliary and sphincter pupillae muscles.

6.120

Answer: D   Cavernous and transverse sinuses

The superior petrosal sinus is small and narrow and connects the cavernous with the transverse sinus. It runs lateralward and backward, from the posterior end of the cavernous sinus, over the trigeminal nerve and lies in the attached margin of the tentorium cerebelli and in the superior petrosal sulcus of the temporal bone; it joins the transverse sinus where the latter curves downward on the inner surface of the mastoid part of the temporal. It receives some cerebellar and inferior cerebral veins and veins from the tympanic cavity.

6.121

Answer: C   Inferior thyroid

The inferior thyroid artery, a branch of the thyrocervical trunk, passes upward, in front of the vertebral artery and longus colli. It then turns medialward behind the carotid sheath and its contents and also behind the sympathetic trunk, the middle cervical ganglion lying on the vessel. Reaching the lower border of the thyroid gland it divides into two branches, which supply the posteroinferior parts of the gland and anastomose with the superior thyroid and with the corresponding artery of the opposite side. The recurrent nerve passes upward, generally behind, but occasionally in front of the artery. The branches of the inferior thyroid are:

head and neck

415

- Inferior laryngeal
- Tracheal
- Ascending cervical
- Oesophageal
- Muscular.

6.122

Answer: B   Elevation of the upper eyelid

The frontal nerve is the largest branch of the ophthalmic nerve, and can be regarded on the basis of both size and direction, as the continuation of that nerve. It enters the orbit through the superior orbital fissure, and runs forward between the levator palpebrae superioris and the periosteum. The levator palpebrae superioris is thin, flat, and triangular in shape. It takes origin from the undersurface of the small wing of the sphenoid, anterosuperior to the optic foramen, from which it is separated by the origin of the rectus superior. At its origin it is narrow and tendinous, but soon becomes broad and fleshy, and ends anteriorly in a wide aponeurosis which splits into three layers. The superficial layer blends with the upper part of the orbital septum, and is prolonged forward above the superior tarsus to the palpebral part of the orbicularis oculi, and to the deep surface of the skin of the upper eyelid. The middle layer, largely made up of smooth muscular fibres, is inserted into the upper margin of the superior tarsus, while the deepest layer blends with an expansion from the sheath of the rectus superior and with it is attached to the superior fornix of the conjunctiva. The upper part of the sheath of the levator palpebrae becomes thickened in front and forms a transverse ligamentous band above the anterior part of the muscle which is attached to the sides of the orbital cavity. On the medial side it is mainly attached to the pulley of the superior oblique, but some fibres are attached to the bone behind the pulley and a slip passes forward and bridges over the supraorbital notch. On the lateral side it is fixed to the capsule of the lacrimal gland and to the frontal bone. In front of the transverse ligamentous band the sheath is continued over the aponeurosis of the levator palpebrae as a thin connective-tissue layer which is fixed to the upper orbital margin immediately behind the attachment of the orbital septum. When the levator palpebrae contracts, the lateral and medial parts of the ligamentous band are stretched and check the action of the muscle. The retraction of the upper eyelid is checked also by the orbital septum coming into contact with the transverse part of the ligamentous band. The levator palpebrae superioris is supplied by the oculomotor nerve. It elevates the upper eyelid and directly opposes the action of the orbicularis oculi.

6.123

Answer: D   C3, C4 and C5

The suprascapular artery passes over the phrenic nerve to enter the posterior triangle of the neck. The phrenic nerve contains motor and sensory fibres in the proportion of about two to one. It arises chiefly from the fourth cervical nerve, but receives a branch from the third and another from the fifth (the fibres from the fifth occasionally come through the nerve to the subclavius) (see also *Answer* to **6.6**).

6.124

Answer: B   Brachiocephalic vein

The veins of thyroid gland form a plexus on the surface of the gland and on the front of the trachea. The superior, middle and inferior thyroid veins arise from this plexus; the superior and middle end in the internal jugular, the inferior in the brachiocephalic vein (see also *Answer* to **6.40**).

6.125

Answer: D   Temporal

The internal carotid artery supplies the anterior part of the brain, the eye and its appendages, and the forehead and nose. In the adult it is the same size as the external carotid, but in the child it is larger than the external carotid. It is remarkable for the number of curvatures that it presents in different parts of its course. It occasionally has one or two curvatures near the base of the skull, while in its passage

head and neck

through the carotid canal in the petrous part of the temporal bone and along the side of the body of the sphenoid bone it describes a double curvature and resembles an italic letter 's'. The carotid canal is found on the inferior surface of the petrous part of the temporal bone. It ascends vertically at first and then bends and runs horizontally forward and medially. It transmits the internal carotid artery and the carotid plexus of nerves into the cranium.

SECTION 7:
BRAIN AND CRANIAL NERVES
– ANSWERS

7.1

Answer: B   Epidural

An epidural haemorrhage is a bleed into the space between the dura and the skull. These haemorrhages are usually caused by rupturing the middle meningeal artery, which supplies blood to the dura and the bones of the cranial vault. This haemorrhage results in compression of the dura mater and the brain; if it is not drained, it may result in the brain herniating through the tentorium and death. A subdural haemorrhage is characterised by a collection of blood beneath the dura, often caused by a head injury. An intracerebral haemorrhage is a haemorrhage within the cerebral hemispheres. A subaponeurotic haemorrhage could be a collection of blood under the aponeurosis of the scalp, but this is not really a brain haemorrhage and is not as clinically significant as the other choices. A subarachnoid haemorrhage is an acute condition where blood collects in the area between the pia mater and arachnoid mater. This is often secondary to a head injury or a ruptured aneurysm.

7.2

Answer: A   Cerebral aqueduct

The cerebral aqueduct is the part of the ventricular system that carries cerebrospinal fluid (CSF) from the third ventricle to the fourth ventricle. Therefore, this must be the part of the ventricular system that was blocked. The central canal is the space where CSF flows through the spinal cord. It is continuous with the fourth ventricle. The interventricular foramina are passages from the lateral ventricles that allow the CSF to leave to enter the third ventricle. The foramen of Luschka and foramen of Magendie are small foramina in the fourth ventricle that allow the CSF to leave the ventricular system and enter the subarachnoid space.

7.3

Answer: B   Abducens

Cranial nerves are nerves that emerge directly from the brain, in contrast to spinal nerves, which emerge from segments of the spinal cord. Conventionally, there are 12 recognised cranial nerves in humans. The nerves from the third onward arise from the brainstem. Except for the tenth and the eleventh nerves, they primarily serve the motor and sensory systems of the head and neck region. However, unlike peripheral nerves, that are separated to achieve segmental innervation, cranial nerves are divided to serve one or a few specific functions in wider anatomical territories. The table below summarises the 12 cranial nerves.

#	Name	Type of fibres	Nuclei	Function
I	Olfactory	Special sensory	Anterior olfactory nucleus	Sense of smell
II	Optic	Special sensory	Lateral geniculate nucleus	Transmits visual information to the brain
III	Oculomotor	Somatic motor, sympathetic efferent	Oculomotor nucleus, Edinger–Westphal nucleus	Controls most of the eye movements; controls accommodation and pupillary reflexes
IV	Trochlear	Somatic motor only	Trochlear nucleus	Rotates the eye away or down from the nose
V	Trigeminal	Somatic motor, somatic sensory	Principal sensory trigeminal nucleus, spinal trigeminal nucleus, mesencephalic trigeminal nucleus, trigeminal motor nucleus	Gives sensations to the face, controls movements of muscles of mastication
VI	Abducent (or abducens)	Somatic motor only	Abducens nucleus	Controls each eye's ability to move away from the midline

#	Name	Type of fibres	Nuclei	Function
VII	Facial	Somatic sensory, sympathetic afferent, taste, somatic motor and sympathetic efferent	Facial nucleus, solitary nucleus, superior salivary nucleus	Controls facial expression and taste to anterior two-thirds of the tongue, vasodilatory to salivary glands, conveys sensory impulses from the middle ear region
VIII	Vestibulocochlear (or auditory, vestibular)	Special sensory	Vestibular nuclei, cochlear nuclei	Senses sound, rotation and gravity (essential for balance and movement)
IX	Glossopharyngeal	Somatic sensory, sympathetic afferent, taste, somatic motor and sympathetic efferent	Nucleus ambiguus, inferior salivary nucleus, solitary nucleus	Controls various sensations including taste to the posterior third of the tongue, glands and muscles
X	Vagus	Somatic sensory, sympathetic afferent, somatic motor, sympathetic efferent, (taste fibres to hard palate)	Nucleus ambiguus, dorsal motor vagus nucleus, solitary nucleus	Supplies motor parasympathetic fibres to nearly all internal organs
XI	Accessory (or cranial accessory and spinal accessory)	Somatic motor only	Nucleus ambiguus, spinal accessory nucleus	Controls muscles of the neck and overlaps with functions of the vagus
XII	Hypoglossal	Somatic motor only	Hypoglossal nucleus	Controls most of the tongue muscles as well as others

brain

7.4

Answer: A   VII

Cranial nerve VII (facial nerve) exits through the stylomastoid foramen and therefore will be affected by a tumour in this location (see also *Answer* to **6.99**).

7.5

Answer: D   Result in general sensory deficit to the pharynx

The glossopharyngeal nerve is the ninth of the twelve cranial nerves. It exits the brainstem out from the sides of the upper medulla, just rostral (closer to the nose) to the vagus nerve. There are a number of functions of the glossopharyngeal nerve:

- It receives sensory fibres from the posterior third of the tongue, the tonsils, the pharynx, the middle ear and the carotid body.

- It supplies parasympathetic fibres to the parotid gland via the otic ganglion.

- It supplies motor fibres to stylopharyngeus muscle.

- It contributes to the pharyngeal plexus.

Lesions of the glossopharyngeal nerve will affect all or some of these functions.

7.6

Answer: B   Trigeminal

The trigeminal nerve, or fifth cranial nerve is responsible for sensation in the face. Its three branches, the ophthalmic, maxillary and mandibular branches, leave the skull through three separate foramina: the superior orbital fissure, the foramen rotundum and the foramen ovale: the mnemonic, 'standing room only' can be used to remember that V1 passes through the superior orbital fissure, V2 passes through the foramen rotundum, and V3 passes through the foramen ovale.

The sensory fibres of the ophthalmic nerve are distributed to the scalp and forehead, the upper eyelid, the conjunctiva and cornea of the eye, the nose (including the tip of the nose), the nasal mucosa, the frontal sinuses and parts of the meninges (the dura and blood vessels). The sensory fibres of the maxillary nerve are distributed to the lower eyelid and cheek, the nares and upper lip, the upper teeth and gums, the nasal mucosa, the palate and roof of the pharynx, the maxillary, ethmoid and sphenoid sinuses, and parts of the meninges. The sensory fibres of the mandibular nerve are distributed to the lower lip, the lower teeth and gums, the floor of the mouth, the anterior two-thirds of the tongue, the chin and jaw (except the angle of the jaw, which is supplied by C2–C3), parts of the external ear, and parts of the meninges. The mandibular nerve carries touch/position and pain/temperature sensation from the mouth. It does not carry taste sensation, but one of its branches, the lingual nerve, carries multiple types of nerve fibres that do not originate in the mandibular nerve. Taste fibres from the anterior two-thirds of the tongue are initially carried in the lingual nerve (which is anatomically a branch of V3) but then enter the chorda tympani, a branch of cranial nerve VII.

7.7

Answer: E   Cranial nerve V ganglion

The trigeminal nerve is the largest of the cranial nerves. Its name derives from the fact that it has three major branches: (i) the ophthalmic nerve (V1); (ii) the maxillary nerve (V2); and (iii) the mandibular nerve (V3). The ophthalmic and maxillary nerves are purely sensory. The mandibular nerve has both sensory and motor functions. The three branches converge on the trigeminal ganglion (also called the semilunar ganglion or Gasserian ganglion), which contains the cell bodies of incoming sensory nerve fibres. The trigeminal ganglion is analogous to the dorsal root ganglia of the spinal cord, which contain the cell bodies of incoming sensory fibres from the rest of the body. From the trigeminal ganglion, a single large sensory root enters the brainstem at the level of the pons. Immediately adjacent to the sensory root, a smaller motor root emerges from the pons at the same level. Motor fibres pass through the trigeminal ganglion on their way to peripheral muscles, but their

brain

cell bodies are located in the motor nucleus of the fifth nerve, deep within the pons. Motor fibres are distributed (together with sensory fibres) in branches of the mandibular nerve. The sensory function of the trigeminal nerve is to provide the tactile, proprioceptive and nociceptive afference of the face and mouth. The posterior scalp and the neck are innervated by C2–C3, not by the trigeminal nerve. The brain parenchyma itself does not have sensory receptors, but the meninges do. The areas of cutaneous distribution (dermatomes) of the three branches of the trigeminal nerve have sharp borders with relatively little overlap (unlike dermatomes in the rest of the body, which show considerable overlap). Injection of local anaesthetics such as lidocaine results in complete loss of sensation from well-defined areas of the face and mouth. For example, the teeth on one side of the jaw can be numbed by injecting the mandibular nerve.

7.8

Answer: B   X

The vagus nerve (cranial nerve X) supplies efferent parasympathetic fibres to all the organs except the suprarenal glands, from the neck down to the second segment of the transverse colon. The vagus also supplies a few skeletal muscles, namely:

- Levator veli palatini
- Salpingopharyngeus
- Palatoglossus (muscle in the palatoglossal arch)
- Palatopharyngeus
- Superior, middle and inferior pharyngeal constrictors
- Muscles of the larynx (speech).

This means that the vagus nerve is responsible for such varied tasks as heart rate, gastrointestinal peristalsis, sweating and quite a few muscle movements in the mouth, including speech (via the recurrent laryngeal) and keeping the larynx open for breathing. It also receives some sensation from the outer ear, via the auricular branch (also known as Alderman's nerve) and part of the meninges.

7.9

Answer: C　Internal carotid artery

The cerebral arterial circle of Willis is a roughly pentagon-shaped circle of arteries on the ventral surface of the brain. It is an important anastomosis between the four arteries at the base of the brain that supply the brain (two internal carotid and two vertebral arteries). It is formed in front by the anterior cerebral arteries, branches of the internal carotid, which are connected by the anterior communicating; and behind by the two posterior cerebral arteries, branches of the basilar artery, which are connected on either side with the internal carotid by the posterior communicating. The parts of the brain included within this arterial circle are the lamina terminalis, the optic chiasma, the infundibulum, the tuber cinereum, the mamillary bodies, and the posterior perforated substance. The three arteries which together supply each cerebral hemisphere arise from the arterial circle of Willis. From its anterior part arise the two anterior cerebrals, from its anterolateral parts arise the middle cerebrals, and from its posterior part arise the posterior cerebrals. Each of these principal arteries gives origin to two different systems of secondary vessels. One of these is the ganglionic system and this supplies the thalami and corpora striata. The other is the cortical system whose vessels ramify in the pia mater and supply the cortex and subjacent brain substance. These ganglionic and cortical systems do not communicate at any point of their peripheral distribution, resulting in the presence of a watershed area between the parts supplied by the two systems.

7.10

Answer: A　In (medially), then down

The trochlear nerve (the fourth cranial nerve, also called the fourth nerve or simply IV) is a motor nerve (a 'somatic efferent' nerve) that innervates a single muscle: the superior oblique muscle of the eye. An older name is the pathetic nerve, which refers to the dejected appearance (head bent forward) that is characteristic of patients with fourth nerve palsies. The trochlear nerve is unique among the cranial nerves in several respects. It is the smallest nerve in terms of the number of axons it contains. It has the greatest intracranial

brain

length. It is the only cranial nerve that decussates (crosses to the other side) before innervating its target. Finally, it is the only cranial nerve that exits from the dorsal aspect of the brainstem.

To understand the actions of the superior oblique muscle, it is useful to imagine the eyeball as a sphere that is constrained – like the trackball of a computer mouse – in such a way that only certain rotational movements are possible. Allowable movements for the superior oblique are: (i) rotation in a vertical plane – looking down and up (depression and elevation of the eyeball) and (ii) rotation in the plane of the face (intorsion and extorsion of the eyeball). The body of the superior oblique muscle is located behind the eyeball, but the tendon (which is redirected by the trochlea) approaches the eyeball from the front. The tendon attaches to the top (superior aspect) of the eyeball at an angle of 51° with respect to the primary position of the eye (looking straight forward). The force of the tendon's pull therefore has two components: a forward component that tends to pull the eyeball downward (depression) and a medial component that tends to rotate the top of the eyeball toward the nose (intorsion). The relative strength of these two forces depends on which way the eye is looking. When the eye is adducted (looking toward the nose), the force of depression increases. When the eye is abducted (looking away from the nose), the force of intorsion increases, while the force of depression decreases. When the eye is in the primary position (looking straight ahead), contraction of the superior oblique produces depression and intorsion in roughly equal amounts.

To summarise, the actions of the superior oblique muscle are: depression of the eyeball, especially when the eye is adducted; and intorsion of the eyeball, especially when the eye is abducted. The clinical consequences of weakness in the superior oblique (caused, for example, by fourth nerve palsies) are discussed below. This summary of the superior oblique muscle describes its most important functions. However, it is an oversimplification of the actual situation. For example, the tendon of the superior oblique inserts behind the equator of the eyeball in the frontal plane, so contraction of the muscle also tends to abduct the eyeball (turn it outward). In fact, each of the six extraocular muscles exerts rotational forces in all three planes (elevation–depression, adduction–abduction, intorsion–extorsion) to varying degrees, depending on which way the eye is looking. The relative forces change every time the eyeball moves – every time the direction of gaze changes. The central control of this process, which involves the continuous, precise adjustment of forces on twelve different tendons to point both eyes in exactly the same direction, is truly remarkable.

Injury to the trochlear nerve causes weakness of downward eye movement with consequent vertical diplopia (double vision). The affected eye drifts upward relative to the normal eye, due to the unopposed actions of the remaining extraocular muscles. The patient sees two visual fields (one from each eye), separated vertically. To compensate for this, patients learn to tilt the head forward (tuck the chin in) to bring the fields back together – to fuse the two images into a single visual field. This accounts for the 'dejected' appearance of patients with 'pathetic nerve' palsies.

As would be expected, the diplopia gets worse when the affected eye looks toward the nose – the contribution of the superior oblique muscle to downward gaze is greater in this position. Common activities requiring this type of convergent gaze are reading the newspaper and walking down stairs. Diplopia associated with these activities may be the initial symptom of a fourth nerve palsy. Trochlear nerve palsy also affects torsion (rotation of the eyeball in the plane of the face). Torsion is a normal response to tilting the head sideways. The eyes automatically rotate in an equal and opposite direction, so that the orientation of the environment remains unchanged – vertical things remain vertical. Weakness of intorsion results in torsional diplopia, in which two different visual fields, tilted with respect to each other, are seen at the same time. To compensate for this, patients with trochlear nerve palsies tilt their heads to the opposite side, to fuse the two images into a single visual field. The characteristic appearance of patients with fourth nerve palsies (head tilted to one side, chin tucked in) suggests the diagnosis, but other causes must be ruled out. For example, torticollis can produce a similar appearance.

brain

7.11

Answer: D Hyoglassus

The hypoglossal nerve is the twelfth cranial nerve (XII). The nerve arises from the hypoglossal nucleus and emerges from the medulla oblongata in the periolivary sulcus separating the olive and the pyramid. It then passes through the hypoglossal canal. On emerging from the hypoglossal canal, the nerve picks up a branch from the anterior ramus of C1. It spirals behind the vagus nerve and passes between the internal carotid artery and the internal jugular vein lying on the carotid sheath. After passing deep to the posterior belly of the digastric muscle, it passes to the tongue. It supplies motor fibres to all of the muscles of the tongue, except the palatoglossus, which is innervated by the vagus nerve (X). To test the function of the nerve, a person is asked to poke out their tongue. If there is a loss of function on one side (unilateral paralysis) the tongue will point towards the affected side. The strength of the tongue can be tested by getting the person to poke at the inside of their cheek and feeling how strongly they can push a finger pushed against their cheek – a more elegant way of testing than directly touching the tongue. The tongue can also be looked at for signs of lower motor neurone disease, such as fasciculation and atrophy.

7.12

Answer: C Fibres of the corpus callosum

The two lateral ventricles, containing cerebrospinal fluid, are irregular cavities situated in the lower and medial parts of the cerebral hemispheres, one on either side of the midline. They are separated from each other by the septum pellucidum which is a median vertical partition. The two lateral ventricles, lined by the ependyma, communicate with the third ventricle and indirectly with each other through the interventricular foramen. Each lateral ventricle consists of a central part or body and three extensions from it which are known as the cornua or horns.

The posterior cornu or horn is directed backward and medially and passes into the occipital lobe. Its roof is formed by the fibres of the corpus callosum passing to the temporal and occipital lobes, which are likely to be compressed by a tumour in the roof of the posterior horn of the lateral ventricle. On its medial wall is a longitudinal eminence, the calcar avis (hippocampus minor), which is an involution of the ventricular wall produced by the calcarine fissure. Above this the forceps posterior of the corpus callosum, sweeping around to enter the occipital lobe, causes another projection, the bulb of the posterior cornu. The calcar avis and the bulb of the posterior cornu are extremely variable in their degree of development, being poorly defined in some people and much more prominent in others.

7.13

Answer: C   Posterior part of the septum pellucidum

The central part or body of the lateral ventricle extends from the interventricular foramen to the splenium of the corpus callosum. It is an irregularly curved cavity, triangular on transverse section, with a roof, a floor and a medial wall. The roof is formed by the undersurface of the corpus callosum; the floor by the following parts, enumerated in their order of position, from before backward: the caudate nucleus of the corpus striatum, the stria terminalis and the terminal vein, the lateral portion of the upper surface of the thalamus, the choroid plexus and the lateral part of the fornix; the medial wall is the posterior part of the septum pellucidum, which separates it from the opposite ventricle. A tumour in the medial wall of the body of the lateral ventricle will involve the posterior part of the septum pellucidum.

7.14

Answer: B   Hippocampus

The inferior cornu of the lateral ventricle is the largest of the three cornua. It traverses the temporal lobe of the brain, forming in its course a curve around the posterior end of the thalamus. It passes at first backward, lateralward and downward and then curves forward to within 2.5 cm of the apex of the temporal lobe, its direction being fairly well indicated on the surface of the brain by that of the superior temporal sulcus. Its roof is formed chiefly by the inferior surface of the tapetum of the corpus callosum, but the tail of the caudate nucleus and the stria terminalis also extend forward in the roof of the inferior cornu to its extremity; the tail of the caudate nucleus joins the putamen. Its floor presents the following parts: the hippocampus, the fimbria hippocampi, the collateral eminence and the choroid plexus. All these structures are likely to be compressed by a tumour in this location. When the choroid plexus is removed, a cleft-like opening is left along the medial wall of the inferior cornu; this cleft constitutes the lower part of the choroidal fissure.

7.15

Answer: C   Posterior inferior cerebellar

Lateral medullary syndrome (also called Wallenberg's syndrome and posterior inferior cerebellar artery syndrome or PICA syndrome) is a disease in which the patient has difficulty with swallowing or speaking or both, owing to one or infarcts caused by interrupted blood supply to the lateral parts of the medulla oblongata. PICA syndrome presents with the following clinical features:

- Contralateral deficits in pain and temperature sensation from the body (dysfunction of the lateral spinothalamic tract)
- Ipsilateral loss of pain and temperature sensation from the face (dysfunction of the spinal trigeminal nucleus)
- Ipsilateral dysphagia, hoarseness, diminished gag reflex (dysfunction of the nucleus ambiguus, which affects the vagus and glossopharyngeal nerves)
- Vestibular dysfunction (vertigo, diplopia, nystagmus, vomiting)
- Ipsilateral Horner's syndrome (dysfunction of descending sympathetic fibres).

The patient may present with ataxia on the side of lesion, or might present with hiccoughs. There will be facial numbness on the side of the lesion whereas there will be contralateral body numbness.

7.16

Answer: E   Optic radiation

Hemianopia indicates a loss of half of the visual field. Homonymous hemianopia indicates that the same half of each visual field is lost, that is, all the vision on the left, or on the right, of the midline. Such a pattern of visual loss is caused by damage to the more distal part of the optic radiation, most commonly by a stroke.

7.17

Answer: B   Internal cerebral veins

The great cerebral vein (great vein of Galen), formed by the union of the two internal cerebral veins, is a short median trunk which curves backward and upward around the splenium of the corpus callosum and ends in the anterior extremity of the straight sinus. It is prone to congenital defects, such as vein of Galen aneurysmal malformation and vein of Galen aneurysmal dilatation.

7.18

Answer: E   Superior sagittal sinus

The superior cerebral veins, eight to twelve in number, drain the superior, lateral and medial surfaces of the cerebral hemispheres and are mainly lodged in the sulci between the gyri, but some run across the gyri. They open into the superior sagittal sinus. The anterior veins runs nearly at right angles to the sinus. The posterior and larger veins are directed obliquely forward and open into the sinus in a direction more or less opposed to the current of the blood contained within it.

7.19

Answer: C   Contralateral hemiplegia

The middle cerebral artery is one of the three major paired arteries that suppy blood to the brain. The middle cerebral artery arises from the internal carotid and continues into the lateral sulcus where it then branches and projects to many parts of the lateral cerebral cortex. It also supplies blood to the anterior temporal lobes and the insular cortices. The middle cerebral arteries rise from trifurcations of the internal carotid arteries and so are connected to the anterior cerebral arteries and the posterior communicating arteries, which connect to the posterior cerebral arteries. The middle cerebral arteries are not considered a part of the circle of Willis. Areas supplied by the middle cerebral artery include:

- The bulk of the lateral surface of the hemisphere. Exceptions are the superior inch of the frontal and parietal lobes and the inferior part of the temporal lobe and the occipital pole, which are supplied by the posterior cerebral artery.

- Part of the internal capsule and basal ganglia.

Occlusion of the middle cerebral artery may result in the following defects:

- Paralysis of the contralateral face, arm and leg

- Sensory loss in the contralateral face, arm and leg

- Aphasia (eg Broca's, Wernicke's, conduction and anomic types) when the dominant hemisphere (usually the left hemisphere for right-handed individuals) is affected

- Left-sided neglect with damage to the right hemisphere

- Homonymous hemianopia or quadrantanopia.

7.20

Answer: A   Abducent

The fourth ventricle, or cavity of the hindbrain, is situated in front of the cerebellum and behind the pons and upper half of the medulla oblongata. It is lined by ciliated epithelium and is continuous below with the central canal of the medulla oblongata. Superiorly it communicates with the cavity of the third ventricle through the cerebral aqueduct. It presents four angles, and possesses a roof or dorsal wall, a floor or ventral wall, and lateral boundaries.

The floor of the fourth ventricle is called the rhomboid fossa because of its shape. It is formed by the posterior surface of the pons and the posterior surface of the open part of the medulla oblongata. It is lined by a thin layer of neuroglia which constitutes the ependyma of the ventricle and supports a layer of ciliated epithelium. Deep to the floor is a thin layer of grey substance that is continuous with that of the spinal medulla. The floor of the fourth ventricle consists of three parts – superior, intermediate and inferior. The superior part is triangular in shape and limited laterally by the superior cerebellar peduncle. It has an apex directed upward that is continuous with the cerebral aqueduct. Its base is represented by an imaginary line at the level of the upper ends of the superior foveae. The intermediate part extends from this level to that of the horizontal portions of the teniae of the ventricle. It is narrow superiorly where it is limited laterally by the middle peduncle but widens inferiorly and is prolonged into the lateral recesses of the ventricle. The inferior part is triangular. It has a downwardly-directed apex called the calamus scriptorius that is continuous with the central canal of the closed part of the medulla oblongata. Among the prominent features of the floor of the fourth ventricle are the:

- Facial colliculus, formed by the internal part of the facial nerve as it loops around the abducens nucleus in the lower pons

- Sulcus limitans, which represents the border between the alar plate and the basal plate of the developing neural tube

- Obex, which represents the caudal tip of the fourth ventricle. The obex is also a marker for the level of the foramen magnum of the skull and is therefore a marker for the imaginary dividing line between the medulla and spinal cord

brain

SECTION 8:
BACK AND SPINAL CORD – ANSWERS

8.1

Answer: B   Iliac crest

The fourth lumbar vertebra (L4) is a relatively safe level for performing a lumbar puncture. Since the conus medullaris is at the inferior border of L1 or the superior border of L2, it should be safe to insert a needle either above or below L4. The anatomical landmark used to identify L4 is the top of the iliac crest. The line connecting the top of the two iliac crests, the supracrestal line, passes through the spinous process of the L4 vertebra. Therefore, by finding the tops of the iliac crests, you should be able to identify L4.

8.2

Answer: E   Internal vertebral venous plexus

The veins of the internal vertebral venous plexus are clinically significant because they are valveless and can serve as a route for metastases. Cancerous cells can travel freely in vertebral veins and lodge somewhere else in the body. The other veins all have valves that would direct the flow of blood and stop some of the metastatic spread.

8.3

Answer: A   Accessory

The accessory nerve innervates the trapezius muscle, which is the muscle responsible for elevating the acromion of the scapula, also known as the tip of the shoulder. If a patient has damaged her accessory nerve, she will be unable to elevate her acromion. The dorsal scapular nerve innervates three muscles: rhomboideus major, rhomboideus minor and the lower portion of levator scapulae. The rhomboids and trapezius retract the scapula toward the midline. Therefore, if the dorsal scapular nerve is injured and the rhomboids are paralysed, retraction of the scapula on the affected side will be weakened. The greater occipital nerve supplies cutaneous sensation to the posterior scalp. Damage to the greater occipital nerve would not result in any loss of muscular function. Spinal nerve C4 refers to the nerve formed by the dorsal and ventral roots of C4. This nerve does not innervate trapezius. Although branches from the ventral primary rami of C3 and C4 combine with the accessory nerve to form the subtrapezial plexus, C3 and C4 provide only proprioception and are not involved with the motion of the trapezius. Finally, the thoracodorsal nerve innervates latissimus dorsi. Latissimus dorsi is the muscle used to extend the arm or raise the trunk to the arms, as if climbing or doing chin-ups. If the thoracodorsal nerve was injured, a patient would be unable to complete these movements.

8.4

Answer: A   Accessory (cranial nerve XI)

If the accessory nerve is damaged and the trapezius is denervated, a person will no longer be able to raise the acromion of the shoulder. The dorsal scapular nerve innervates rhomboideus major, rhomboideus minor and levator scapulae. If the dorsal scapular nerve is damaged, the rhomboids will be denervated and retraction of the scapula will be weakened. An injury to the greater occipital nerve will result in a loss of sensation on the posterior scalp but no muscular deficit. The axillary nerve and suprascapular nerve will have been covered with the upper limb, but for completeness, note that the axillary nerve innervates the deltoid muscle. If this nerve is damaged, the deltoid may atrophy and the person will be unable to abduct the arm. If the suprascapular nerve is injured, lateral rotation of the humerus will be severely weakened.

8.5

Answer: B   Dorsal primary ramus of C7

Dorsal and ventral primary rami are the first branches off spinal nerves. Dorsal rami provide sensory innervation to the skin over the back and give motor innervation to the true back muscles; ventral rami supply sensory innervation to the skin over the limbs and the skin over the ventral side of the trunk. Ventral rami also give motor innervation to the skeletal muscles of the neck, trunk and extremities. Therefore, if the skin over the spine of your scapula began to itch, the sensation of that area would be transmitted by the dorsal primary ramus of C7. The accessory nerve, which innervates the trapezius, is not responsible for any sensory innervation. The dorsal and ventral roots of spinal nerves are not directly responsible for any sensory innervation to the skin. Dorsal and ventral rootlets emerge from the spinal cord to form the dorsal and ventral roots. The ventral roots contain efferent motor fibres to skeletal muscles, while the dorsal roots contain afferent sensory fibres. These roots combine to form the spinal nerve, which then gives off the primary rami.

8.6

Answer: A   Lumbar triangle

The lumbar triangle is the site of a lumbar hernia. It is a triangle defined by the border of the latissimus dorsi medially, the external abdominal oblique laterally and the iliac crest inferiorly. This is the exact site of the hernia that is described here, so that is the answer. The triangle of auscultation is a triangle located below the inferior angle of the scapula, bounded by the trapezius medially, rhomboideus major superiorly and the latissimus dorsi inferiorly. This is a place where you can place your stethoscope and auscultate the lungs. The inguinal triangle is bounded medially by rectus abdominis, inferiorally by the inguinal ligament and superolaterally by the inferior epigastric artery. It is the site of a direct inguinal hernia. The triangle of Calot is a triangle found near the gallbladder. It is bounded by the cystic artery, cystic duct and common hepatic duct. Finally, the greater sciatic foramen is a pelvic structure created by the sacrospinous ligament and the sacrotuberous ligament.

back and spine

8.7

Answer: C   Scapular retraction on the right would be weakened

The dorsal scapular nerve is a motor nerve off the C5 nerve root that innervates the rhomboids and levator scapulae. These muscles help to retract and elevate the scapula, so these movements would be weakened following that damage. The skin of the upper back on the right side is innervated by the dorsal primary rami of a spinal nerve. The point of the right shoulder, the acromion, is elevated by trapezius. Trapezius is innervated by the accessory nerve, so the point of the shoulder would droop if the accessory nerve was damaged. Latissimus dorsi, innervated by the thoracodorsal nerve, allows for extension and adduction of the arm.

8.8

Answer: D   Trapezius

The transverse cervical artery supplies blood to trapezius. Levator scapulaes and the rhomboids receive blood from the dorsal scapular artery. Latissimus dorsi receives blood from the thoracodorsal artery.

8.9

Answer: C   Greater occipital nerve

The greater occipital nerve is the dorsal primary ramus of spinal nerve C2 – it provides cutaneous innervation to the skin of the back of the head. The accessory nerve is cranial nerve XI – it innervates trapezius. The great auricular nerve, the lesser occipital nerve and ansa cervicalis are all structures from the cervical plexus, which is made of ventral primary rami.

8.10

Answer: C   The vertebrae in the upper three regions of the column are known as true vertebrae

The vertebral column is a flexible column composed of a series of bones called vertebrae. There are 33 vertebrae in total. These are grouped regionally into cervical, thoracic, lumbar, sacral and coccygeal vertebrae: there are seven cervical vertebrae, 12 thoracic vertebrae, five lumbar vertebrae, five sacral vertebrae and four coccygeal vertebrae. This number is sometimes increased by an additional vertebra in one region, or it can be diminished in one region, the deficiency often compensated for by an additional vertebra in another. The number of cervical vertebrae is, however, constant. The cervical, thoracic and lumbar vertebrae remain distinct throughout life and are known as true or movable vertebrae. In contrast, the sacral and coccygeal vertebrae are called false or fixed vertebrae because they are united with one another in the adult to form two bones – five forming the upper bone or sacrum, and four forming the terminal bone or coccyx. With the exception of the first and second cervical vertebrae, the remaining true or movable vertebrae present certain common characteristics which are best studied by examining one from the middle of the thoracic region.

8.11

Answer: B   The vertebral arch consists of a pair of pedicles and a pair of laminae

A typical vertebra consists of two essential parts – an anterior segment, the body and a posterior part, the vertebral or neural arch; these enclose a foramen, the vertebral foramen. The vertebral arch consists of a pair of pedicles and a pair of laminae and supports seven processes – four articular, two transverse and one spinous. When the vertebrae are articulated with each other the bodies form a strong pillar for the support of the head and trunk, and the vertebral foramina constitute a canal for the protection of the medulla spinalis (spinal cord), while between every pair of vertebrae are two apertures, the intervertebral foramina, one on either side, for the transmission of the spinal nerves and vessels.

8.12

Answer: D   Has a few small apertures for the passage of nutrient vessels on its anterior surface

The body is the largest part of a vertebra and is cylindrical in shape. Its upper and lower surfaces are flattened and rough and give attachment to the intervertebral fibrocartilages and each presents a rim around its circumference. In front, the body is convex from side to side and concave from above downward. Behind, it is flat from above downward and slightly concave from side to side. Its anterior surface presents a few small apertures for the passage of nutrient vessels; on the posterior surface is a single large, irregular aperture, or occasionally more than one, for the exit of the basivertebral veins from the body of the vertebra.

8.13

Answer: A   The spinous process serves for the attachment of muscles and ligaments

A typical thoracic vertebra has seven processes – four articular, two transverse and one spinous. The spinous process is directed backward and downward from the junction of the laminae and serves for the attachment of muscles and ligaments. The articular processes, two superior and two inferior, spring from the junctions of the pedicles and laminae. The superior project upward and their articular surfaces are directed more or less backward; the inferior project downward and their surfaces look more or less forward. The articular surfaces are coated with hyaline cartilage. The transverse processes, two in number, project one at either side from the point where the lamina joins the pedicle, between the superior and inferior articular processes. They serve for the attachment of muscles and ligaments.

8.14

Answer: D   Has a foramen transversarium for the passage of the vertebral artery

The most distinctive characteristic of this vertebra is the existence of a long and prominent spinous process, hence the name vertebra prominens. This process is thick, nearly horizontal in direction, not bifurcated, but terminating in a tubercle to which the lower end of the ligamentum nuchae is attached. The transverse processes are of considerable size, their posterior roots are large and prominent, while the anterior are small and faintly marked. The upper surface of each usually has a shallow sulcus for the eighth spinal nerve and its extremity seldom presents more than a trace of bifurcation. The foramen transversarium may be as large as that in the other cervical vertebrae, but is generally smaller on one or both sides; occasionally it is double, sometimes it is absent. On the left side, it occasionally gives passage to the vertebral artery; more frequently the vertebral vein traverses it on both sides; but the usual arrangement is for both artery and vein to pass in front of the transverse process and not through the foramen. Sometimes the anterior root of the transverse process attains a large size and exists as a separate bone, which is known as a cervical rib.

8.15

Answer: A   Axial

The grey matter of the spinal cord is arranged in three horns. The anterior is motor, the lateral is visceral efferent and afferent in function and the posterior is sensory in function. The anterior horn is divided into a ventral part, the head and a dorsal part, the base. The nuclei in the anterior horn innervate the skeletal muscles. The cells in the anterior horn are arranged in the following three main groups:

- Medial group: present throughout the entire extent of the spinal cord and innervates the axial muscles of the body

- Lateral group present only in the cervical and lumbar enlargements and supplies the musculature of the limbs. It is subdivided into three subgroups:

  - the anterolateral supplies the proximal muscles of the limbs (shoulder and arm/gluteal region and thigh)
  - the posterolateral supplies the intermediate muscles of the limbs (forearm/leg)
  - the post-posterolateral supplies the distal muscles of the limbs (hand/foot).

- Central group: present only in the upper cervical segments as the phrenic nerve nucleus and the nucleus of the spinal tract of the accessory nerve.

Hence, a disease process involving the medial group of nuclei in the anterior horn will affect the function of the axial muscles.

8.16

Answer: E   Substantia gelatinosa

There are four main afferent nuclei in the posterior grey column. These include:

- Nucleus dorsalis: also known as the thoracic nucleus, at the medial part of the base of the posterior horn, extending from C8 to L3 segments. It is a relay nuclear column for reflex or unconscious proprioceptive impulses to the cerebellum and its axons give rise to the posterior spinocerebellar tract.

- Nucleus proprius: lies subjacent to the substantia gelatinosa throughout the entire extent of cord. It is concerned with the sensory associative mechanism.

- Substantia gelatinosa: found at the tip of the posterior horn through the entire extent of spinal cord. It acts as a relay station for pain and temperature fibres and is concerned with the sensory associative mechanism. Its axons give rise to the lateral spinothalamic tract.

- Posteromarginal nucleus: a thin layer of neurones

back and spine

that caps the posterior horn. It receives some of the incoming dorsal root fibres.

The intermediolateral nucleus acts as both visceral efferent and afferent nuclear columns. So, the substantia gelatinosa will have to be involved by a disease process if the pain and temperature sensations are affected.

8.17

Answer: D   It invests the cauda equina

The spinal part of the arachnoid is a thin, delicate, tubular membrane loosely investing the spinal cord. Above, it is continuous with the cranial arachnoid; below, it widens out and invests the cauda equina and the nerves proceeding from it. It is separated from the dura mater by the subdural space, but here and there this space is traversed by isolated connective-tissue trabeculae, which are most numerous on the posterior surface of the spinal cord. The arachnoid surrounds the cranial and spinal nerves and encloses them in loose sheaths as far as their points of exit from the skull and vertebral canal. The arachnoid consists of bundles of white fibrous and elastic tissue intimately blended together. Its outer surface is covered with a layer of low cuboidal mesothelium. The inner surface and the trabeculae are likewise covered by a somewhat low type of cuboidal mesothelium, which in places is flattened to a pavement type. Vessels of considerable size, but few in number, and a rich plexus of nerves derived from the motor root of the trigeminal, the facial and the accessory nerves, are found in the arachnoid.

8.18

Answer: C   It separates the anterior from the posterior nerve roots

The ligamentum denticulatum is a narrow fibrous band of pia mater situated on either side of the spinal cord throughout its entire length and separating the anterior from the posterior nerve roots. Its medial border is continuous with the pia mater at the side of the spinal cord. Its lateral border presents a series of triangular tooth-like processes, the points of which are fixed at intervals to the dura mater. These processes are 21 in number, on either side, the first being attached to the dura mater, opposite the margin of the foramen magnum, between the vertebral artery and the hypoglossal nerve; and the last near the lower end of the medulla spinalis.

8.19

Answer: A   Cisterna basalis

At the base of the brain and around the brainstem the subarachnoid space forms intercommunicating pools, called cisterns, which reinforce the protective effect of cerebrospinal fluid on the vital centres situated in the medulla. The subarachnoid cisterns are as follows:

- The cerebellomedullary cistern (cisterna magna), which is triangular on sagittal section, and results from the arachnoid bridging over the interval between the medulla oblongata and the undersurfaces of the hemispheres of the cerebellum. It is continuous with the subarachnoid cavity of the spinal medulla at the level of the foramen magnum.

- The pontine cistern, a considerable space on the ventral aspect of the pons. It contains the basilar artery and is continuous behind with the subarachnoid cavity of the spinal medulla and with the cerebellomedullary cistern. It is continuous with the basal cistern in front of the pons.

- The interpeduncular cistern (basal cistern), a wide cavity where the arachnoid extends across between the two temporal lobes. It encloses the cerebral peduncles and the structures contained in the interpeduncular fossa. It contains the arterial circle of Willis.

- The cisterna chiasmatis, formed in front of the basal cistern as it extends forward across the optic chiasma. (The basal cistern then extends on to the upper surface of the corpus callosum, as the arachnoid

back and spine

stretches across from one cerebral hemisphere to the other, immediately beneath the free border of the falx cerebri, leaving a space in which the anterior cerebral arteries are contained.)

- The cisterna fossae cerebri lateralis, formed in front of either temporal lobe by the arachnoid bridging across the lateral fissure. This cavity contains the middle cerebral artery.

- The cistern of the great cerebral vein occupies the interval between the splenium of the corpus callosum and the superior surface of the cerebellum. It extends between the layers of the tela chorioidea of the third ventricle and contains the great cerebral vein.

8.20

Answer: D It communicates with the general ventricular cavity of the brain by three openings

The subarachnoid cavity (subarachnoid space) is the space between the arachnoid and pia mater. It is traversed by a network of arachnoid trabeculae which give it a sponge-like appearance. It contains the cerebrospinal fluid and the large vessels of the brain. Cranial nerves pass through this space. This cavity is small on the surface of the hemispheres of the brain. The pia mater and the arachnoid are in close contact on the summit of each gyrus but in the sulci between the gyri the pia mater dips into the sulci whereas the arachnoid bridges across these sulci, resulting in the formation of triangular spaces in which the subarachnoid trabecular tissue is found. At certain parts of the base of the brain, the arachnoid is separated from the pia mater by wide intervals, which communicate freely with each other and are known as subarachnoid cisterns. The subarachnoid tissue is less abundant in the cisterns.

The spinal part of the subarachnoid cavity is a very wide space, and is at its largest at the lower part of the vertebral canal, where the arachnoid encloses the nerves which form the cauda equina. Superiorly it is continuous with the cranial subarachnoid cavity and inferiorly it ends at the level of the lower border of the second sacral vertebra. It is partially divided by a longitudinal septum, the subarachnoid septum, which connects the arachnoid with the pia mater opposite the posterior median sulcus of the medulla spinalis and forms a partition, incomplete and cribriform above, but more perfect in the thoracic region. The spinal subarachnoid cavity is further subdivided by the ligamentum denticulatum. The subarachnoid cavity communicates with the general ventricular cavity of the brain by three openings: the midline foramen of Magendie, situated in the inferior part of the roof of the fourth ventricle; and the two lateral foramina of Luschka, which are located at the extremities of the lateral recesses of fourth ventricle, posterior to the upper roots of the glossopharyngeal nerves.

SECTION 9:
DEVELOPMENTAL ANATOMY
– ANSWERS

9.1

Answer: B   Chiasmata separate during anaphase I

Meiosis is the process that allows one diploid cell to divide in a special way to generate haploid cells in eukaryotes. The word "meiosis" comes from the Greek *meioun*, meaning "to make smaller," since it results in a reduction in chromosome number. Meiosis is essential for sexual reproduction. It therefore occurs in most eukaryotes, including single-celled organisms. Meiosis does not occur in archea or prokaryotes, which reproduce by asexual cell division processes.

Meiosis has two stages: meiosis I and meiosis II. Meiosis I consists of segregating the homologous chromosomes from each other, then dividing the tetraploid cell into two diploid cells each containing one of the segregates. Meiosis II consists of decoupling each chromosome's sister strands (chromatids), segregating the DNA into two sets of strands (each set containing one of each homolog), and dividing both diploid cells to produce four haploid cells. Meiosis I and II are both divided into prophase, metaphase, anaphase, and telophase subphases, similar in purpose to their analogous subphases in the mitotic cell cycle. Therefore, meiosis encompasses the interphase (G_1, S, G_2), meiosis I (prophase I, metaphase I, anaphase I, telophase I), and meiosis II (prophase II, metaphase II, anaphase II, telophase II). The chiasmata separate during anaphase I as a result chromosomes, each with two chromatids, move to separate poles.

development

9.2

Answer: A Are developed from the primitive germ cells which are embedded in the substance of the ovaries

The ova are developed from the primitive germ cells, which are embedded in the substance of the ovaries. Each primitive germ cell gives rise, by repeated divisions, to a number of smaller cells called oögonia, from which the ova or primary oöcytes are developed. Human ova are extremely small, measuring about 0.2 mm in diameter, and are enclosed within the egg follicles of the ovaries. By the enlargement and subsequent rupture of a follicle at the surface of the ovary, an ovum is liberated and conveyed by the uterine tube to the cavity of the uterus. Unless it is fertilised it undergoes no further development and is discharged from the uterus, but if fertilisation take place it is retained within the uterus and develops into a new being.

9.3

Answer: C Increased left atrial pressure

Since the oxygen in the fetus is in the placenta, the system must necessarily undergo a change to adjust to gaseous exchange in the lungs at the point of birth. At birth, the placental blood supply is removed and the pulmonary circuit changes from a high-resistance to a low-resistance circuit when it is exposed to oxygen by breathing. The systemic circulation now becomes the high-pressure circuit and there is now no longer a pressure gradient to drive blood flow across the ductus arteriosus from the pulmonary artery to the aorta. When exposed to oxygenated blood and prostaglandins released at birth, the ductus constricts and closes in the following 24–72 hours. This increases the amount of blood flowing through the lungs and results in an increase in left atrial pressure. This, in turn, pushes the atrial septum primum against the septum secundum, functionally closing the foramen ovale. The ductus venosus in the liver closes when placental flow stops. So, at birth the system changes from a pulmonary and systemic system in parallel to a double circulation in series.

9.4

Answer: A In early fetal life, the heart lies immediately below the mandibular arch and is relatively large

The chief peculiarities of the fetal heart are the direct communication between the atria through the foramen ovale and the large size of the valve of the inferior vena cava. The following peculiarities are also notable:

- In early fetal life the heart lies immediately below the mandibular arch and is relatively large. With the growth of the fetus it is gradually drawn within the thorax. Although the heart initially lies in the midline, toward the end of pregnancy it gradually becomes oblique in direction.

- For a time the atria are larger than the ventricles and the walls of the ventricles are of equal thickness. However, toward the end of fetal life the ventricles become larger than the atria and the wall of the left ventricle becomes thicker than the wall of the right ventricle.

- The cardiac size is large in comparison with the rest of the body, with the proportion at the second month being 1 to 50. At birth this proportion is 1 to 120, while in the adult the average proportion is about 1 to 160.

9.5

Answer: C Efferent ductules

Early in the fourth week, nephric tubules begin to develop within a pair of elongated swellings – the mesonephric ridges – from the upper thoracic to the third lumbar level. About 40 mesonephric tubules are produced, in craniocaudal succession. The cranial ones regress as the more caudal ones form, so there are never more than 30 pairs. By the fifth week, there is a massive regression of the cranial ones, leaving about 20 pairs in the first three lumbar levels. These mesonephric tubules will develop into excretory units (renal corpuscle plus tubule) that look like an abbreviated version of the adult (metanephric) kidney tubules. Their duct, the bilateral

development

mesonephric or Wolffian duct, arises on about day 24 as a pair of solid longitudinal rods. The rods grow caudally toward and fuse with the ventrolateral surface of the cloaca (about day 26). The region of fusion will become part of the posterior wall of the future bladder. As the rods fuse with the cloaca, they begin to canalise (develop a lumen) from their caudal toward their cranial end. The mesonephric tubules fuse with the mesonephric duct, which provides a passage to the cloaca. The mesonephric excretory units function from about weeks 6 to 10, producing a small amount of urine. After week 10, they stop functioning and regress. Note that in the man, a few modified mesonephric tubules and the mesonephric duct will persist. The former will become the ductuli efferentes (efferent ductules) of the testis and the latter will giver rise to the epididymis and vas deferens. In the woman, these structures will regress.

9.6

Answer: C   Lesser horn of the hyoid bone

Each branchial (pharyngeal) arch has a cartilaginous bar, a muscle component that differentiates from the cartilaginous tissue, an artery and a cranial nerve. There are six pharyngeal arches, but in humans the fifth arch only exists transiently during embryological growth and development. Since no human structures result from the fifth arch, the arches in humans are I, II, III, IV and VI. More is known about the fate of the first arch than the remaining four. The first three contribute to structures above the larynx, while the last three contribute to the larynx. The second or hyoid arch assists in forming the side and front of the neck. From its cartilage are developed the styloid process, stylohyoid ligament and lesser cornu of the hyoid bone. The muscular derivatives include the muscles of facial expression, stapedius, stylohyoid and the posterior belly of the digastric. These muscles are innervated by cranial nerve VII but migrate into the area of the first arch.

9.7

Answer: B   Coronary sinus

The derivatives of the embryonic sinus venosus include: the smooth part of the right atrium (sinus venarum), the 'valve' of the superior vena cava and the sinoatrial node from the right horn; the coronary sinus and the valve of coronary sinus from the left horn; the border of smooth part of right atrium (crista terminalis) from the right half of the valve of the sinus venosus and part of the atrial septum from the left half of the valve of the sinus venosus.

9.8

Answer: C   The heart begins to beat in the fourth week

The primordium of the heart forms in the cardiogenic plate located at the cranial end of the embryo. Angiogenic cell clusters, which lie in a horseshoe-shape configuration in the plate, coalesce to form two endocardial tubes. These tubes are then forced into the thoracic region due to cephalic and lateral foldings, where they fuse together forming a single endocardial tube during the third week. The heart begins to beat in the fourth week at about the same time that the septum primum appears and the bulboventricular loop is formed. From the fourth week onwards, septa begin to grow in the atria, ventricle and bulbus cordis to form right and left atria, right and left ventricles and the two great vessels – the pulmonary artery and the aorta. By the end of the eighth week, partitioning is completed and the fetal heart has formed.

9.9

Answer: A   Metanephric glomeruli are derived from a distal
              (caudal) dorsal region of the mesoderm

The kidney is derived from the middle embryonic layer or mesoderm. Mesodermic cells also give origin to the cardiovascular and musculoskeletal systems. The pronephros is a rudimentary kidney that develops first during vertebrate embryogenesis. It develops from the most anterior (cephalic) dorsal aspect of the mesoderm. The mesonephros evolves from the mid-dorsal region of

development

the mesoderm. It is functional during the first third of embryonic life and then becomes gradually atrophic. Metanephric glomeruli are derived from a distal (caudal) dorsal region of the mesoderm. The metanephric ureters, renal pelvis, renal calyces and renal tubules develop as outpouchings of mesonephric duct remnants. The branching renal tubules eventually reach the vascular glomerular capillary network and encapsulate glomerular tufts.

9.10

Answer: B   Adrenal medulla

Derivatives of ectoderm include the epidermis of the skin, nails, hair, sweat glands, mammary glands, sebaceous glands, the central nervous system, the peripheral nervous system, the retina and lens of eye, the pupillary muscle of the iris (this is the only muscle of ectodermal origin), the pineal body, the posterior pituitary, the adrenal medulla, melanocytes, Schwann cells and odontoblasts.

9.11

Answer: B   The heart tube is formed

During fourth week of intrauterine life:

- The embryo measures 4 mm in length and begins to curve into a 'C' shape.

- Somites, the divisions of the future vertebra, form.

- The heart bulges, develops further and begins to beat in a regular rhythm.

- Branchial arches, grooves that will form structures of the face and neck, form.

- The neural tube closes.

- The ears begin to form as otic pits.

- Arm buds and a tail are visible.

development

9.12

Answer: C   Epithelial part of the tympanic cavity

Derivatives of endoderm include the epithelium of the gastrointestinal tract and its associated glands as well as glandular cells of the liver and pancreas, epithelium of the urachus and urinary bladder, epithelium of respiratory passages (the pharynx, trachea, bronchi and alveoli), epithelial parts of the tonsils, thyroid, parathyroids, tympanic cavity and thymus and epithelial parts of the anterior pituitary.

9.13

Answer: D   Gives rise to the sphenomandibular ligament

The first pharyngeal arch or mandibular arch is involved with development of the face. It develops two processes, maxillary and mandibular, which form the upper and lower jaws respectively. Bones and muscles of this region are developed from mesoderm in the arch. Meckel's cartilage is the first arch cartilage. It ossifies to form the malleus and incus in the middle ear. The sphenomandibular ligament is derived from its perichondrium. The rest of the cartilage disappears after the mandible forms around it by intramembranous ossification. The muscles derived from the first arch include temporalis, masseter, medial and lateral pterygoids, anterior belly of the digastric, mylohyoid, tensor tympani and tensor palati. The trigeminal nerve is the motor supply of the mandibular arch.

9.14

Answer: B   Caecum

The midgut forms a primary intestinal loop and gives rise to the duodenum (distal half), jejunum, ileum, caecum, ascending colon and transverse colon (proximal two-thirds).

development

9.15

Answer: A   The ductus arteriosus receives blood from the pulmonary artery

The fetal blood is returned from the placenta to the fetus by the umbilical vein. This vein enters the abdomen at the umbilicus and passes upward along the free margin of the falciform ligament of the liver to the undersurface of the liver. Here it gives off two or three branches, one large branch to the left lobe, and others to the quadrate lobe and caudate lobe. At the porta hepatis (the transverse fissure of the liver) the umbilical vein divides into two branches. After being joined by the portal vein the larger branch enters the right lobe, while the smaller branch (the ductus venosus) continues upward and joins the inferior vena cava. The blood carried by the umbilical vein therefore passes to the inferior vena cava via three different routes:

- A considerable quantity of blood circulates through the liver with the portal venous blood before entering the inferior vena cava by the hepatic veins.

- Some blood enters the liver directly and is carried to the inferior cava by the hepatic veins.

- The remainder passes directly into the inferior vena cava through the ductus venosus.

In the inferior vena cava the blood carried by the ductus venosus and hepatic veins becomes mixed with that returning from the lower extremities and abdominal wall. It enters the right atrium and, guided by the valve of the inferior vena cava, passes through the foramen ovale into the left atrium, where it mixes with a small quantity of blood returned from the lungs by the pulmonary veins. From the left atrium it passes into the left ventricle. From the left ventricle the blood then passes into the aorta, by means of which it is distributed almost entirely to the head and upper extremities, a small quantity probably being carried into the descending aorta. From the head and upper extremities the blood is returned by the superior vena cava to the right atrium, where it mixes with a small portion of the blood from the inferior vena cava. From the right atrium it descends into the right ventricle, and thence passes into the pulmonary artery. Because the fetal lungs are inactive only a small quantity of the blood in the pulmonary artery is distributed to them via the right and left pulmonary arteries and returned by the pulmonary veins to the left atrium. The greater part of the pulmonary artery blood passes through the ductus arteriosus into the aorta, where it mixes with a small quantity of the blood transmitted by the left ventricle into the aorta. The blood then descends through the aorta and is in part distributed to the lower extremities and the viscera of the abdomen and pelvis, but most of the blood is conveyed to the placenta by the umbilical arteries.

9.16

Answer: B   The valve of the inferior vena cava serves to direct the blood from that vessel through the foramen ovale into the left atrium

The foramen ovale, situated at the lower part of the atrial septum, forms a free communication between the atria until the end of fetal life. The valve of the inferior vena cava serves to direct the blood from the inferior vena cava through the foramen ovale into the left atrium. The ductus arteriosus is a short tube, about 1.25 cm in length at birth, with a diameter similar to that of a goose quill. In early fetal life it forms the continuation of the pulmonary artery and opens into the aorta just distal to the origin of the left subclavian artery. It therefore transmits the greater part of the blood from the right ventricle into the aorta. Later in fetal life the ductus arteriosus is mainly connected to the left pulmonary artery when the branches of the pulmonary artery have become larger relative to it. The hypogastric arteries run along the sides of the bladder and then upward on the posterior aspect of the anterior abdominal wall to the umbilicus. They pass out of the abdomen through the umbilicus and are continued as the umbilical arteries in the umbilical cord to the placenta. They convey the fetal blood to the placenta.

development

9.17

Answer: C   The neurenteric canal is a transitory communication between the neural tube and the primitive digestive tube

The ectodermal wall of the neural tube forms the rudiment of the nervous system. After the coalescence of the neural folds over the anterior end of the primitive streak, the blastopore no longer opens on the surface but into the closed canal of the neural tube and so a transitory communication, the neurenteric canal, is established between the neural tube and the primitive digestive tube. The coalescence of the neural folds occurs first in the region of the hindbrain and from there extends forward and backward. The cephalic end of the neural groove exhibits several dilatations, which, when the tube is closed, assume the form of three vesicles; these constitute the three primary cerebral vesicles and correspond respectively to the future forebrain (prosencephalon), midbrain (mesencephalon) and hindbrain (rhombencephalon). The walls of the vesicles are developed into the nervous tissue and neuroglia of the brain and their cavities are modified to form its ventricles. The remainder of the tube forms the medulla spinalis or spinal cord; from its ectodermal wall the nervous and neuroglial elements of the medulla spinalis are developed, while the cavity persists as the central canal.

9.18

Answer: D   Gives rise to the anterior part of the tongue

The first branchial arch (mandibular arch) lies between the first branchial groove and the stomodeum. From it are developed the lower lip, the mandible, the muscles of mastication and the anterior part of the tongue. Its cartilaginous bar is formed by what are known as Meckel's cartilages (right and left); above this, the incus is developed. The dorsal end of each cartilage is connected with the ear capsule and is ossified to form the malleus. The ventral ends meet each other in the region of the symphysis menti and are usually regarded as undergoing ossification to form that portion of the mandible which contains the incisor teeth. The intervening part of the cartilage disappears; the portion immediately adjacent to the malleus is replaced by fibrous membrane, which constitutes the sphenomandibular ligament, while from the connective tissue covering the remainder of the cartilage the greater part of the mandible is ossified. From the dorsal ends of the mandibular arch a triangular process, the maxillary process, grows forward on either side and forms the cheek and lateral part of the upper lip.

9.19

Answer: E   The ventral portions of the cartilages of the fourth and fifth arches unite to form the thyroid cartilage

A total of six branchial or visceral arches are formed in the human embryo, on either side of the developing pharynx, but of these only the first four are visible externally. These arches are formed by thickening of the mesoderm. Each arch has a dorsal and a ventral end. The dorsal ends of these arches are attached to the sides of the head, while the ventral ends ultimately meet in the midline of the neck. Only the first two arches have distinct names. In each arch a cartilaginous bar develops, consisting of right and left halves. In addition, one of the primitive aortic arches is associated with each pharyngeal arch. The first arch is the mandibular arch. The second or hyoid arch assists in forming the side and front of the neck – the styloid process, stylohyoid ligament and lesser cornu of the hyoid bone develop from its cartilage. The stapes probably arises in the upper part of this arch. The cartilage of the third arch gives origin to the greater cornu of the hyoid bone. The ventral ends of the second and third arches unite with those of the opposite side and form a transverse band, from which the body of the hyoid bone and the posterior part of the tongue develop. The ventral portions of the cartilages of the fourth and fifth arches unite to form the thyroid cartilage. The cricoid and arytenoid cartilages and the cartilages of the trachea develop from the cartilages of the sixth arch.

development

9.20

Answer: D   Opens into the digestive tube by a long narrow tube, the vitelline duct

The yolk sac is situated on the ventral aspect of the embryo; it is lined by endoderm, outside which is a layer of mesoderm. It is filled with fluid, the vitelline fluid, which may possibly be utilized for the nourishment of the embryo during the earlier stages of its existence. Blood is conveyed to the wall of the sac by the primitive aorta and after circulating through a wide-meshed capillary plexus, is returned by the vitelline veins to the tubular heart of the embryo. This constitutes the vitelline circulation and, by means of it, nutritive material is absorbed from the yolk sac and conveyed to the embryo. At the end of the fourth week, the yolk sac presents the appearance of a small pear-shaped vesicle (umbilical vesicle) opening into the digestive tube by a long narrow tube, the vitelline duct. The vesicle can be seen in the afterbirth as a small, somewhat oval-shaped body whose diameter varies from 1 mm to 5 mm; it is situated between the amnion and the chorion and may lie on or at a varying distance from the placenta. As a rule, the duct undergoes complete obliteration during the seventh week, but in about 3% of cases its proximal part persists as a diverticulum from the small intestine, Meckel's diverticulum, which is situated about 1 m (3–4 ft) above the ileocolic junction and may be attached by a fibrous cord to the abdominal wall at the umbilicus. Sometimes a narrowing of the lumen of the ileum is seen opposite the site of attachment of the duct.

9.21

Answer: E   Is carried backward with the development of the hind-gut and then opens into the cloaca or terminal part of the hindgut

The allantois arises as a tubular diverticulum of the posterior part of the yolk sac. It is carried backward with the hindgut as a result of its development and opens into the cloaca or terminal part of the hindgut. It grows out into the body stalk, which is a mass of mesoderm that lies below and around the tail end of the embryo. The allantois is lined by endoderm and covered by mesoderm, which contains the allantoic or umbilical vessels. In reptiles, birds and many mammals the allantois becomes expanded into a vesicle which projects into the extra-embryonic coelom. In man and other primates the nature of the allantois is entirely different from that in birds and reptiles, existing merely as a narrow, tubular diverticulum of the hindgut. It never assumes the shape of a vesicle outside the embryo. With the formation of the amnion the embryo is, in most animals, entirely separated from the chorion, and is only reunited with it when the allantoic mesoderm spreads over and becomes applied to its inner surface. The human embryo, on the other hand, is never wholly separated from the chorion as its tail end is connected with the chorion right from start by means of a thick band of mesoderm called the body stalk.

9.22

Answer: A   Contains liquor amnii by about the fourth week of development

The amnion is a membranous sac that surrounds and protects the embryo. It is developed in reptiles, birds and mammals, which are therefore called 'Amniota' but not in amphibia and fish, which are consequently called 'Anamnia.' The amnion appears in the inner cell mass as a cavity. This cavity is roofed in by a single stratum of flattened, ectodermal cells, the amniotic ectoderm, and its floor consists of the prismatic ectoderm of the embryonic disc – the continuity between the roof and floor being established at the margin of the embryonic disc. By about the fourth or fifth week fluid (liquor amnii) begins to accumulate within it. The liquor amnii increases in quantity up to the sixth or seventh month of pregnancy, after which it diminishes somewhat; at the end of pregnancy it amounts to about 1 litre. It contains less than 2% solids, consisting of urea and other waste products, inorganic salts, a small amount of protein and frequently a trace of sugar.

9.23

Answer: E   Is filled with jelly of Wharton

The umbilical cord attaches the fetus to the placenta; its length at full term, as a rule, is about equal to the length of the fetus, ie about

development

50 cm, but it may be greatly diminished or increased. The rudiment of the umbilical cord is represented by the tissue which connects the rapidly growing embryo with the extra-embryonic area of the ovum. Included in this tissue are the body stalk and the vitelline duct – the former containing the allantoic diverticulum and the umbilical vessels, the latter forming the communication between the digestive tube and the yolk sac. The cord is covered by a layer of ectoderm, which is continuous with that of the amnion, and its various constituents are enveloped by embryonic gelatinous tissue, jelly of Wharton. The vitelline vessels and duct, together with the right umbilical vein, undergo atrophy and disappear, and so the cord, at birth, contains a pair of umbilical arteries and one (the left) umbilical vein.

9.24

Answer: A   Consists of the villi of the chorion laeve

The chorion consists of an outer layer, formed by the primitive ectoderm or trophoblast, and an inner layer formed by the somatic mesoderm. The amnion is in contact with the inner layer of the chorion. The trophoblast is made up of an internal layer of cubical or prismatic cells, the cytotrophoblast or layer of Langhans, and an external layer of richly nucleated protoplasm which is devoid of cell boundaries, the syncytiotrophoblast. It undergoes rapid proliferation and forms numerous processes, the chorionic villi, which invade and destroy the uterine decidua and at the same time absorb from it nutritive materials for the growth of the embryo. The chorionic villi are at first small and non-vascular and consist of trophoblast only. However they are vascularised when the mesoderm (carrying branches of the umbilical vessels) grows into them. They also increase in size and ramify. Blood is carried to the villi by the branches of the umbilical arteries and, after circulating through the capillaries of the villi, is returned to the embryo by the umbilical veins. Until about the end of the second month of pregnancy the villi cover the entire chorion, and are almost uniform in size but after this they develop unequally. The greater part of the chorion is in contact with the decidua capsularis and over this portion the villi and the vessels they contain atrophy, so that by the fourth month scarcely a trace of them is left – this part of the chorion therefore becomes smooth and is known as the chorion laeve. The

development

chorion laeve takes no part in the formation of the placenta and is therefore called the non-placental part of the chorion. On the other hand, the villi on that part of the chorion which is in contact with the decidua placentalis increase greatly in size and complexity, and this part is therefore called the chorion frondosum.

9.25

Answer: B   The cerebral hemispheres appear as hollow buds

During the fourth week the embryo is markedly curved on itself and when viewed in profile is almost circular in outline. The cerebral hemispheres appear as hollow buds and the elevations which form the rudiments of the auricula are visible. The limbs now appear as oval flattened projections (see also *Answer* to **9.11**).

9.26

Answer: E   The cloacal tubercle is evident

During the fifth week the embryo is less curved and the head is relatively large. Differentiation of the limbs into their segments occurs. The nose forms a short, flattened projection. The cloacal tubercle is evident.

9.27

Answer: A   The eyelids are present in the shape of folds above
and below the eye

During the second month of development the flexure of the head is gradually reduced and the neck is somewhat lengthened. The upper lip is completed and the nose is more prominent. The nostrils are directed forward and the palate is not completely developed. The eyelids are present in the shape of folds above and below the eye and the different parts of the auricula are distinguishable. By the end of the second month, the fetus measures from 28 to 30 mm in length.

development

9.28

Answer: C   The loop of gut that projected into the umbilical cord is withdrawn within the fetus

During the fourth month, the loop of gut that projected into the umbilical cord is withdrawn within the fetus. The hair begin to make their appearance. There is a general increase in size so that by the end of the fourth month the fetus measures from 12 to 13 cm in length, but if the legs were included it measures from 16 to 20 cm. It is during the fifth month that the first movements of the fetus are usually observed. The eruption of hair on the head commences and the vernix caseosa begins to be deposited. By the end of the fifth month the total length of the fetus, including the legs, is from 25 to 27 cm.

9.29

Answer: B   The testis descends with the vaginal sac of the peritoneum

During the seventh month, the pupillary membrane atrophies and the eyelids are open. The testis descends with the vaginal sac of the peritoneum. From vertex to heels, the total length at the end of the seventh month is from 35 to 36 cm. The weight is a little over 1.4 kg (3 lb). It is during the eighth month that the skin assumes a pink colour and is now entirely coated with vernix caseosa, and the lanugo begins to disappear. Subcutaneous fat has been developed to a considerable extent and the fetus presents a plump appearance. The total length, ie from head to heels, at the end of the eighth month is about 40 cm and the weight varies between 2 kg and 2.5 kg (4.5–5.5 lb).

9.30

Answer: B   The baby weighs from 3 kg to 3.5 kg (6.5–8 lb)

The lanugo has largely disappeared from the trunk. The umbilicus is almost in the middle of the body and the testes are in the scrotum. At full term, the fetus weighs 3 kg to 3.5 kg (6.5–8 lb) and measures from head to heels about 50 cm.

9.31

Answer: D   Stylohyoid muscle

The second or hyoid arch assists in forming the side and front of the neck. From its cartilage are developed the styloid process, stylohyoid ligament and lesser cornu of the hyoid bone. The muscular derivatives include the muscles of facial expression, stapedius, stylohyoid and the posterior belly of the digastric. These muscles are innervated by cranial nerve VII but migrate into the area of the first arch.

9.32

Answer: C   The fourth right aortic arch forms the right subclavian as far as the origin of its internal mammary branch

The first and second arches disappear early, but the dorsal end of the second gives origin to the stapedial artery, a vessel that atrophies in man but persists in some mammals. The third aortic arch constitutes the commencement of the internal carotid artery and is therefore called the carotid arch. The fourth right arch forms the right subclavian as far as the origin of its internal mammary branch; and the fourth left arch constitutes the arch of the aorta between the origin of the left carotid artery and the termination of the ductus arteriosus. The fifth arch disappears on both sides. The sixth right arch disappears; the sixth left arch gives off the pulmonary arteries and forms the ductus arteriosus. This duct remains open during the whole of fetal life, but is obliterated a few days after birth.

9.33

Answer: D   The mesenchyme of the pharyngeal arches forms connective tissue, and lymphatic and blood vessels of the tongue

The development of the tongue starts during the end of the fourth week of gestation with the appearance of a triangular elevation in the floor of the pharynx. This elevation is called the median tongue bud. The proliferation of mesenchymal cells in the ventromedial areas of the first pharyngeal arches causes the formation of two oval buds on either side of the distal part of the tongue. The oral part of the tongue forms when these distal tongue buds rapidly enlarge and fuse to overgrow the median tongue bud. Sensory innervation of this part is provided by the lingual branch of the mandibular division of the trigeminal nerve, which originates in the first pharyngeal arch. Behind the foramen caecum, two elevations called the copula and the hypobranchial eminence (also referred to as the tuberculum impar) form to create the pharyngeal part of the tongue. The copula is eventually overgrown by the hypobranchial eminence. The median and pharyngeal sections of the organ then become joined at the terminal sulcus. This posterior section of the tongue is innervated by the glossopharyngeal nerve, derived from the third pharyngeal arch. The growing tongue extends out into the oral cavity, covered by a layer of ectodermal epithelium. The root of the tongue, however, is covered with endodermal epithelium. These two tissues merge eventually so that their boundaries are undetectable. However, it is only the epithelial and mucosal tissues of the tongue which develop from the four pharyngeal swellings described above. The musculature of the tongue can be traced to another source. The majority of this muscle tissue descends from myoblasts which differentiate after migrating from the myotomes of the occipital cervical somites. The hypoglossal nerve, which is the motor nerve for the tongue musculature, accompanies these myoblasts. The mesenchyme of the pharyngeal arches forms connective tissue in the tongue region, lymphatic and blood vessels of the tongue, and probably some muscle tissue as well.

9.34

Answer: E   The ventral pancreatic bud forms part of the head and uncinate process of the pancreas

The pancreas is developed in two parts, a dorsal and a ventral. The dorsal part arises as a diverticulum from the dorsal aspect of the duodenum a short distance above the hepatic diverticulum. It grows upward and backward into the dorsal mesogastrium and forms a part of the head and uncinate process and the whole of the body and tail of the pancreas. The ventral part appears in the form of a diverticulum from the primitive bile duct and forms the remainder of the head and uncinate process of the pancreas. The duct of the dorsal part (the accessory pancreatic duct) therefore opens independently into the duodenum, while that of the ventral part (the pancreatic duct) opens with the common bile duct. About the sixth week, the two parts of the pancreas meet and fuse and a communication is established between their ducts. After fusion of the dorsal and ventral pancreatic buds the terminal part of the accessory duct (the part between the duodenum and the point of meeting of the two ducts) undergoes little or no enlargement, while the pancreatic duct increases in size and forms the main duct of the gland. The opening of the accessory duct into the duodenum is sometimes obliterated, and even when it remains patent it is probable that the whole of the pancreatic secretion is conveyed through the pancreatic duct. At first the pancreas is directed upward and backward between the two layers of the dorsal mesogastrium, which provide it with a complete peritoneal investment, and its surfaces face to the right and left. With the change in the position of the stomach, the dorsal mesogastrium is drawn downward and to the left, and the right side of the pancreas is directed backward and the left side forward. The right surface becomes applied to the posterior abdominal wall and the peritoneum which covered it undergoes absorption. This is why the gland appears to lie behind the peritoneal cavity in the adult. The pancreas is endodermal in origin.

9.35

Answer: C   The posterior lobe of the pituitary is neuroectodermal in origin

The pituitary gland in the adult consists of a large anterior, consisting of the pars anterior and the pars intermedia and a small posterior lobe: the former is derived from the ectoderm of the stomodeum, the latter from the floor of the forebrain. About the fourth week, there appears a pouch-like diverticulum of the ectodermal lining of the roof of the stomodeum. This diverticulum, the pouch of Rathke, is the rudiment of the anterior lobe of the hypophysis; it extends upward in front of the cephalic end of the notochord and the remnant of the buccopharyngeal membrane and comes into contact with the undersurface of the forebrain. It is then constricted off to form a closed vesicle, but remains for a time connected to the ectoderm of the stomodeum by a solid cord of cells. Masses of epithelial cells form on either side and in the front wall of the vesicle

development

and by the growth between these of a stroma from the mesoderm the development of the anterior lobe is completed. The upwardly directed hypophyseal involution becomes applied to the anterolateral aspect of a downwardly directed diverticulum from the base of the forebrain. This diverticulum constitutes the future infundibulum in the floor of the third ventricle while its inferior extremity becomes modified to form the posterior lobe of the hypophysis. In some of the lower animals, the posterior lobe contains nerve cells and nerve fibres, but in man and the higher vertebrates these are replaced by connective tissue.

9.36

Answer: D   The anterior part of the ventral mesogastrium forms the falciform and coronary ligaments

The liver arises as an endodermal diverticulum or hollow outgrowth from the ventral surface of the developing descending part of the duodenum. This diverticulum grows upward and forward into the septum transversum, a mass of mesoderm between the vitelline duct and the pericardial cavity, and there gives off two solid buds of cells which represent the right and the left lobes of the liver. The solid buds of cells grow into columns or cylinders, called the hepatic cylinders, which branch and anastomose to form a close meshwork. This network invades the vitelline and umbilical veins, and breaks these vessels up into a series of capillary-like vessels called sinusoids, which ramify in the meshes of the cellular network and ultimately form the venous capillaries of the liver. The mass of the liver is gradually formed as a result of the continued growth and ramification of the hepatic cylinders. The original diverticulum from the duodenum forms the common bile duct, and from this the cystic duct and gallbladder arise as a solid outgrowth, which later acquires a lumen. The opening of the common duct is at first in the ventral wall of the duodenum. However, as a result of rotation of the gut, the opening is carried to the left and then dorsally to the position it occupies in the adult. As the liver undergoes enlargement, both it and the ventral mesogastrium of the foregut are gradually differentiated from the septum transversum. The liver projects downward into the abdominal cavity from the undersurface of the septum transversum. The growth of the liver leads to division of the ventral mesogastrium into an anterior part that forms the falciform and coronary ligaments and a posterior part that forms the lesser omentum. At about the third month the liver almost fills the abdominal cavity and its lobes are nearly equal in size. From the third month onward, the relative development of the liver becomes less active, particularly the left lobe, which actually undergoes some degeneration and becomes smaller than the right lobe. However, up to the end of fetal life the liver remains relatively larger than it is in the adult.

9.37

Answer: E The thyroid gland is developed from a median diverticulum that appears on the summit of the tuberculum impar

The development of the thyroid gland starts during the fourth week in the pharyngeal floor, with the appearance of a midline solid endodermal cord of cells, the median thyroid diverticulum, between the tuberculum impar and the hypobranchial eminence. It grows downward and backward as a tubular duct, which bifurcates and subsequently subdivides into a series of cellular cords, from which the isthmus and lateral lobes of the thyroid gland are developed. The ultimo-branchial bodies from the fifth pharyngeal pouches are enveloped by the lateral lobes of the thyroid gland. They undergo atrophy, however, and do not form true thyroid tissue. The connection of the diverticulum with the pharynx is called the thyroglossal duct. The thyroglossal duct eventually degenerates. Its upper end is represented by the foramen caecum of the tongue and its lower end by the pyramidal lobe of the thyroid gland. The parenchyma of the gland is endodermal in origin, while the stroma is mesodermal in origin.

9.38

Answer: C Is accompanied by anticlockwise rotation of the herniated gut loop

Development of the human gut takes place during the first months of fetal life. In the normal embryo, physiological herniation of the gut through the umbilicus at 6 weeks is accompanied by a 270°

development

anticlockwise rotation of the developing intestine around the superior mesenteric artery. By 10–12 weeks, the intestine returns to the abdomen and assumes its normal adult anatomical position. Normal small-bowel mesentery has a broad attachment stretching diagonally from the duodenojejunal junction (in the left upper quadrant) to the caecum (in the right lower quadrant). The point of attachment at the duodenojejunal junction is referred to as the ligament of Treitz.

9.39

Answer: A An atrioventricular septal defect

The terms endocardial cushion defect, atrioventricular septal defect and common atrioventricular canal defect, are interchangeable in describing defects in the formation of the atrioventricular (AV) valves, the anterior portion of the atrial septum and the posterior portion of the ventricular septum. Endocardial cushions are masses of mesenchymal tissue that form components of the AV valves, atrial septum and ventricular septum. Defects range from incomplete (also called partial, such as ostium primum atrial septal defect with 'cleft mitral valve') to transitional (large ostium primum defect and small 'inlet' or posterior ventricular septal defect) to complete (large ostium primum atrial septal defect, large inlet ventricular septal defect, common AV valve).

9.40

Answer: B Gastric

This child has a Meckel's diverticulum. Meckel's diverticulum is present in about 2–4% of the population. Typically, it is a blindly ending pouch a few centimetres long on the antimesenteric border of the ileum within 100 cm of the ileocaecal junction. It is a remnant of an embryological structure called the vitelline duct, which once connected the yolk sac with the developing midgut. Usually the vitelline duct disappears completely. Meckel's diverticulum may produce no symptoms. However, sometimes it can become inflamed, or it might have ectopic gastric or pancreatic cells in its walls leading to ulceration. In some cases, a fibrous strand connects the diverticulum to the inner aspect of the umbilicus and a loop of small intestine can become twisted around this (volvulus) causing obstruction. The symptoms may closely mimic those of appendicitis. It is useful to remember the 'rule of twos' associated with Meckel's diverticulum: present in 2% of the population, occurs within 0.6 m (2 ft) of the ileocaecal valve, contains two types of ectopic mucosa (gastric and pancreatic) and is usually symptomatic by the age of 2 years.

development

INDEX

(The number in bold indicates the section and the number in italics indicates the question number)